BONE SURGERY IN SMALL ANIMALS

RESOLUTION OF THE MOST FREQUENT FRACTURES

Plaza Antonio Beltrán Martínez nº 1, planta 8 - letra I
(Centro empresarial El Trovador)
50002 Zaragoza - Spain

First printing: September 2015

This book was originally published in Spanish under the title:
Traumatología en pequeños animales. Resolución de las fracturas más frecuentes
© 2013 Grupo Asís Biomedia, SL
ISBN Spanish edition: 978-84-940402-4-5

Translation:
Anna Frandsen

ISBN: 978-84-16315-21-5
DL: Z 1387-2015

Design, layout and printing:
Servet editorial - Grupo Asís Biomedia, SL
www.grupoasis.com
info@grupoasis.com

Servet is the publishing house of Grupo Asís

Printed by Tipolinea SA, Zaragoza, Spain, July 2023

Bone surgery
in small animals

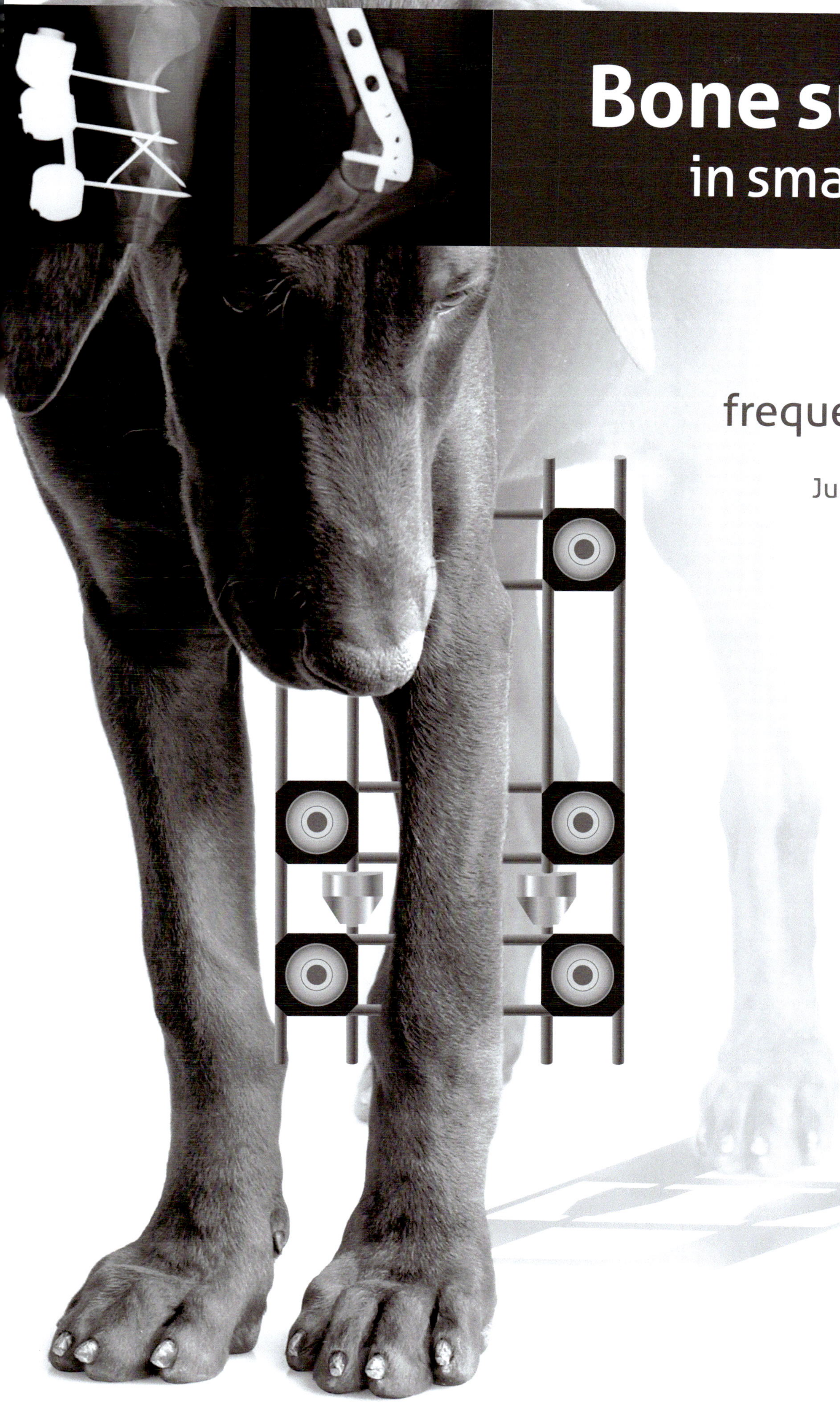

Resolution of the most frequent fractures

Juan Pablo Zaera Polo

SERVET

To Silvia,
for allowing me to bear her

ACKNOWLEDGEMENTS

To all people, veterinary surgeons or non-veterinary surgeons, that have contributed to my training, without the help of which, not surprisingly, I would never have come to perfect myself as a surgeon in the musculoskeletal area; and to many other people, without whom, this book would not have been possible.

To all that have helped me with the photography during the surgical interventions, without whom I would not have been able to obtain the graphic material found in this book: students and veterinary surgeons of the Veterinary Hospital of the School of Veterinary Sciences of the Universidad de Las Palmas de Gran Canaria (Spain) and the veterinary surgeons and intern veterinary surgeons of the Sierra de Madrid Veterinary Hospital (HVSM, Spain).

To Diagnoscan of HVSM for the cession of computerised tomography images and the great quality of their images in 3D reconstructions.

Special thanks to Silvia Piñol Brussotto (HVSM-Diagnoscan) and Oliver Rodríguez Lozano (FULP) for their collaboration in the diagnosis, assistance during surgery and follow-up of many of the cases presented.

To the following veterinary surgeons and their centres for the cession of the images for the chapter on infrequent fractures: to Ángel Rubio of the Veterinary Centre Indautxu (Bilbao, Spain), to Andrés Somaza of the Veterinary Clinic Somaza-Pérez (Ferrol, A Coruña, Spain) and to Javier Tabar of the Veterinary Hospital Raspeig (San Vicente, Alicante, Spain).

AUTHOR

JUAN PABLO ZAERA POLO

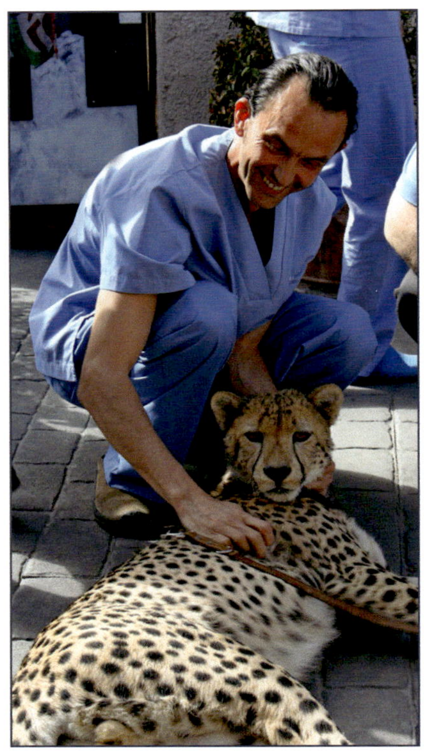

Degree in Veterinary Sciences at the Universidad Complutense de Madrid (UCM, Spain) in 1988. Intern of the *Deutscher Akademischer Austauschdienst* (German Academic Exchange Service, DAAD) in Hanover during the 1989-90 school year. In 1993, he received the title of Doctor from the Universidad Complutense de Madrid, where he worked as a lecturer. He has carried out various residencies in the Surgery Clinic of the University of Munich and in the Orthopaedics Department of the University of Michigan, United States.

Juan Pablo has collaborated in the publication of several books, monographs and articles, and has participated in various speeches at national and international conferences, courses and workshops.

He is a member of the Scientific Committee of the GEVO and AO-Vet.

Currently, he is a lecturer of Surgery at the School of Veterinary Sciences of the Universidad de Las Palmas de Gran Canaria (ULPGC, Spain) and Head of the Traumatology, Arthroscopy, Spine Surgery and Computerised Tomography (musculoskeletal) Department of the Veterinary Hospital Sierra de Madrid (HVSM, Spain).

PREFACE

Reaching the twenty-fifth anniversary of getting my degree and after twenty-four and a half years of training in bone surgery, orthopaedics and spine surgery, I decided to try to organise all the knowledge my teachers worked so hard to instil within me. I have attempted - and I hope I have been successful - to bring my personal experience to transmit some ideas that may be of help to veterinary surgeons that, like me, enjoy attempting to "repair" the musculoskeletal system of our dear fellow sufferers.

After an entire professional life alternating between university and non-university teaching and clinical activity - without which I think it would be completely impossible to enthuse students or help colleagues -, I decided to write this book. With this publication I have tried to transmit, in an eminently graphic manner, certain knowledge that may serve as a solid foundation for students who would like to initiate themselves in bone surgery as well as for those veterinary surgeons willing to improve in "the art of healing bones".

Given that it is impossible, due to limitations of space, to cover all of the fractures that can affect bones, a series of cases of uncommon fractures have been added at the end of the book in which the treatment applied and the reasons for choosing it have been reflected.

I hope that this book will be useful to my colleagues as well as to our patients.

Juan Pablo Zaera Polo

FOREWORD

This book is an excellent contribution to orthopaedic literature and osteosynthesis knowledge.

It has been clearly structured in two parts. In the first part, the characteristics of the bone tissue as well as the principal basic osteosynthesis techniques are described in a simple manner. The large amount of figures, carefully selected and designed, that accompany each osteosynthesis system, combined with the real, intraoperative images, perfectly illustrate the operating bases and the steps to be followed for the correct use and application of each technique. Along with the classical techniques, novel orthopaedic treatments are also included.

The study of the primary errors that can be committed with each system may also be of great use as well as how to avoid and correct them. The X-ray material, carefully selected, enables the reader to visually understand which fixation system or implant can or should be used in each case.

This first part of the book allows both veterinary students as well as professionals to increase their knowledge in veterinary bone surgery.

The second part of the book focuses on the in-depth study of the characteristics of each bone, placing emphasis on their anatomical and biomechanical peculiarities. From the very beginning, the possible treatments that can be applied in each case, along with the factors that should be taken into account for their proper selection, are tied together in a simple and educational manner. Each type of fracture is dealt with by assessing the characteristics of the bone and its location, taking into consideration other factors that may orient the surgeon towards the most suitable system for its treatment. The graphic material in this part also makes the information presented easy to understand.

In summary, thanks to its structure, the great amount of graphic material that it provides, the clearly comprehensible language and its eminently practical focus, this book will be of great use to both veterinary students and surgeons specialising in bone surgery. They will surely use this work to streamline their decision-making in orthopaedic cases encountered in their daily practice.

Professor Dr. R. Köstlin
Dipl. ECVS, PhD
Munich, Germany, July 9th 2013

TABLE OF CONTENTS

OVERVIEW

1 BONE TISSUE

2 BONE GROWTH AND HEALING

3 CLASSIFICATION OF FRACTURES

4 BONE STIMULATION

5 OSTEOSYNTHESIS SYSTEMS AND BIOMECHANICS

6 COMPLICATIONS IN THE BONE HEALING PROCESS

FRACTURES

7 HEAD FRACTURES

8 FORELIMB FRACTURES

10 CLINICAL CASES OF UNCOMMON FRACTURES

Bone tissue

1

OVERVIEW

Before beginning a more in-depth study of fractures and osteosynthesis systems used for their treatment, understanding the type of tissue involved is essential.

As a starting point, it must be taken into account that bone tissue is a living material, that is, it should not be considered as simply a "piece of wood", as it is commonly compared to. In fact, it is quite the contrary. "Specialists in bone surgery must no longer be considered carpenters, their work is that of a gardener that treats the roots of the bone with great care, where the subsistence of the surrounding soft tissues depends on them".

FUNCTION

Bone tissue carries out various functions in the organism:

a. Mechanical support: this is its primary function. Due to its hardness, bones provide support to the organism and act as a rigid frame. Also, they allow the extremities to move by transforming muscle contraction into joint movements.

b. Protection of vital structures: the resistance of this tissue is used by nature to protect the vital structures from external aggressions. The more important an organ is for survival, the more protection it receives. For example, the brain is completely surrounded by the cranium, and the heart and lungs are protected by the ribs. The haematopoietic tissue, essential to our survival, is found in the epiphysis and internal cavities of flat bones.

c. Storage of ions: although this is a secondary function, from an orthopaedic perspective, bones store and maintain the ion balance, primarily of calcium and phosphorous. This balance is principally determined by the organic levels of parathyroid hormone and thyrocalcitonin, hormones that increase or decrease the activity of osteoclasts, triggering the indirect liberation of calcium ions into the bloodstream.

This storage function is important in bone surgery as it may influence the healing processes as well as the hardness of the tissue itself.

STRUCTURE

Bone tissue is a specialised type of connective tissue formed by cells and calcified extracellular material, making up the bone matrix.

The non-cellular connective tissue is formed by the osteoid matrix that constitutes 35 % of said tissue. This matrix, at the same time, is made up of 90 % collagen and 10 % proteins, lipids and proteoglycans. The remaining 65 % is formed by mineral substances, represented basically by calcium hydroxylapatite, distributed throughout the osteoid matrix, conferring the bone with its characteristic hardness.

There are three main types of cells that make up this tissue:

- **Osteocytes**: these are located in cavities or lacunae, in the interior of the matrix.
- **Osteoblasts**: producers of the organic portion of the matrix.
- **Osteoclasts**: giant, mobile and multinucleated cells that reabsorb bone tissue, participating in the remodelling processes of bones.

> *Osteocytes are largely responsible for bone healing, primarily that produced by first intention.*

Parts of the bone

Different parts of the bone can be differentiated from an anatomical perspective in long bones (Fig. 1).

- **Epiphysis**: portion of the bone located on the ends of the bone. Each bone has two epiphyses, one that is proximal (closer to the animal's trunk), and the other, distal.

- **Diaphysis**: largest, central portion of the bone where fractures most frequently occur.
- **Metaphysis**: transition area between the diaphysis and the epiphysis. This is where the bones grow lengthwise as they harbour the bone plates at young ages.

Each one of these parts is made up of different types of bone depending on the forces that they are subjected to (Fig. 1).

- **Periosteum**: a membrane of connective tissue that surrounds the diaphyseal area. Its thickness decreases with age and it is responsible for the growth of the diameter of the bone diaphysis. It is highly vascularised and possesses a large amount of pluripotent cells that are capable of differentiating themselves into osteoclasts and osteoblasts as needed.

  The periosteum is therefore fundamental in the first weeks of bone healing processes.
- **Endosteum**: a membrane similar to the periosteum but of less relevance, it is located covering the interior of the medullary cavity.
- **Nutrient canal**: found in the middle portion of the diaphysis, it is the point of entry and exit of the nutrient arteries and veins, responsible for intramedullary vascular supply.

Types of bone

There are basically two types of bone, cortical and cancellous.

- **Cortical bone**: this type of bone is the most abundant in the organism. Its structure (Fig. 1) is primarily designed for axial weight bearing, which is why it is the principal component of the diaphysis of long bones.

  The bone tissue is arranged in longitudinal columns that are attached to each other throughout the width of the cortical bone, creating a tube with an internal cavity called the medullary cavity. This structure is both resistant and light.

  In the diaphysis of the bones, the bone lamellae form haversian systems that can be circumferential, internal and external, and intermedial. Each haversian system is formed by one long cylinder, parallel to the diaphysis and made up by 4-20 concentric bone lamellae. The haversian canals are interconnected with the medullary cavity and the external surface of the bone through transversal or oblique conducts, which are known as Volkmann's canals that cross through the bone lamellae. The haversian and Volkmann's canals form the intraosseous vascular network.
- **Cancellous bone**: this type of bone is found primarily in the epiphyses of the long bone as well as in the interior of flat bones. It has a disorganised structure that looks similar to a sponge (Fig. 1). However, the bone trabecula is aligned creating reinforcing arches, similar to the architectural structures found in cathedrals and bridge spans, to more efficiently resist the forces that the epiphyses must bear. Unlike the diaphyses in which the forces are almost always parallel to the longitudinal axis of the bone, in the epiphyses, the forces can change.

  The direction of the forces that the joint condyles are subjected to vary depending on if the extremity is in flexion or extension, and thus the structure of the bone has been modified to be able to absorb this variation of loads (Fig. 2).

  The cancellous bone also serves as an area of protection for the haematopoietic cells.

VASCULAR SUPPLY

As a living tissue, the bone needs its blood supply (Fig. 3). The great difference between bone tissue and other soft tissues is the precariousness of its vascular supply and the slowness of its recovery after being damaged.

Bones present different blood supply routes:

- **Intramedullary vascular supply**: it comes from the nutrient artery, which enters the bone diaphysis through the nutrient foramen. The artery immediately divides into two branches, an ascending branch and a descending branch. When a diaphyseal fracture takes place, this blood supply is interrupted and takes approximately one week to re-establish itself. During this time period, the blood supply must be supplied from other sources.
- **Extraosseous vascular supply**: this includes the blood supply systems that the bone receives by means of the surrounding tissues. Within this type of vascular supply, two groups can be differentiated:
  - Periosteal supply: the periosteal vascular supply is that which the bone receives by means of the periosteum, forming what is called the periosteal plexus. Said plexus is formed by a network of small arterioles that come from the muscular insertions that irrigate the periosteum. Other vessels that provide the cortical bone with nutrients to maintain intraosseous vascular supply also originate in this plexus.

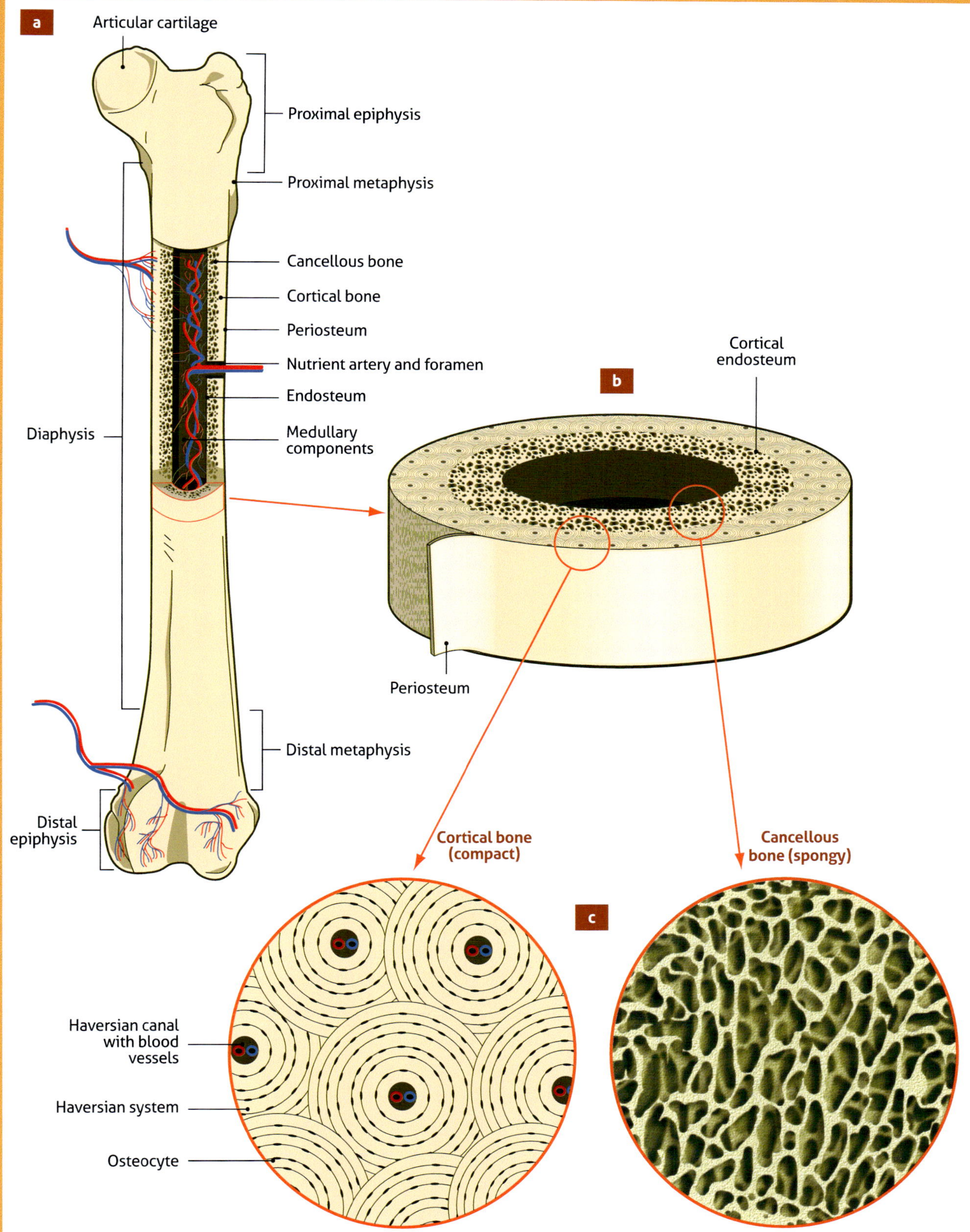

FIGURE 1. Different parts of the bone are shown in the image (a), the arrangement in layers of the two types of bones (b) and the characteristic structure of each type of bone (c).

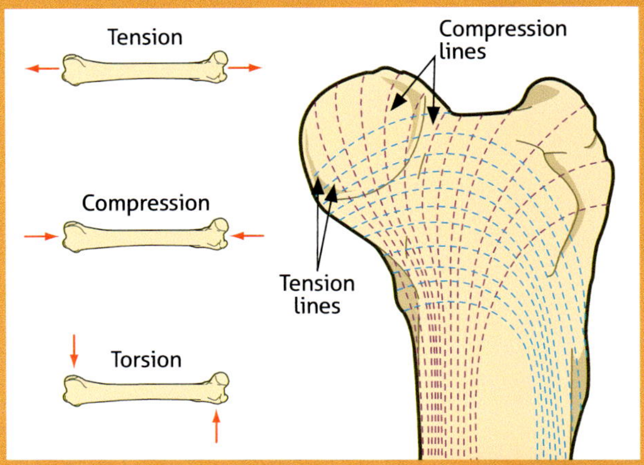

FIGURE 2. Representation of the load lines to which the cancellous bone is subjected, in this case, of the femur.

The preservation and care of the surrounding soft tissues to the area of the fracture are vital for the bone healing process. During the first weeks and up to the moment in which the intramedullary vascular supply is re-established, all nutrients are supplied through this plexus. During surgical interventions, all muscular anastomoses should be preserved, and especially the fragments that are found to be completely independent.

- Epiphyseal supply: the epiphyses of the bones receive their blood supply from a network of epiphyseal and metaphyseal vessels that substitute the periosteal supply. The vessels "drench" the cancellous bone; each trabecula constitutes a blood vessel in itself. The anastomoses are produced between each trabecula until they terminate in the intramedullary vein. That is, the cancellous bone can functionally be considered as "a large blood vessel". This is why the haematopoietic cells generate blood cells from the epiphyses and flat bones, releasing them into the bloodstream. For this same reason, in some cases, the cancellous bone can be used as a point of fluid supply to the vascular system.

  It is important to keep in mind that the extraosseous and intramedullary vascular networks are intimately related, namely, the blood flows from one network to the other through anastomoses and from the intraosseous network.

- **Intraosseous vascular supply**: the intraosseous vascular supply is located immersed in the thickness of the cortical bone. It is formed by the haversian and Volkmann's canals, which are anastomosed together forming a network to provide nutrients to the osteocytes located in the haversian lacunae (Fig. 4).

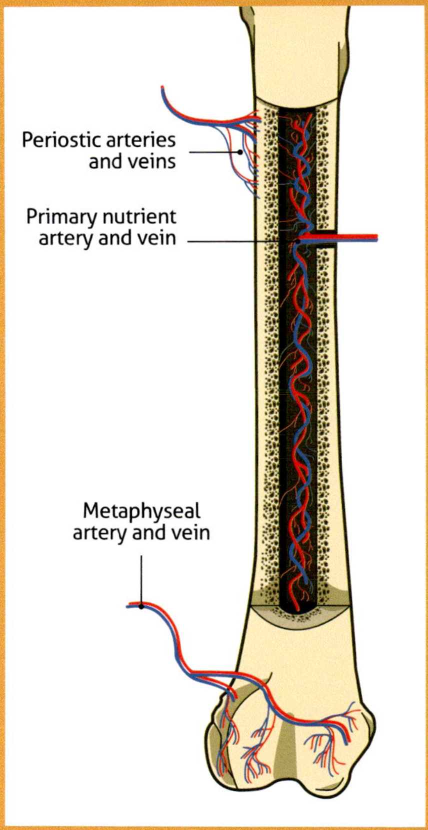

FIGURE 3. Vascularisation of the bone. The different types of blood supply that provide nutrients are shown in the illustration.

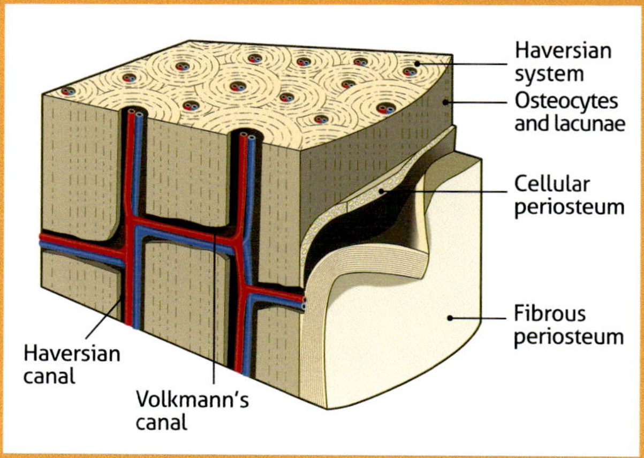

FIGURE 4. Intraosseous blood circulation.

The osteocytes are largely responsible for the healing process in bones, primarily that produced by first intention. When a fracture occurs, if the intramedullary artery breaks, the survival of the osteocytes depends on the blood supply from the intraosseous network, which in turn depends exclusively on the blood that arrives from the periosteum by means of its plexus. For this reason, it is important to remember the importance of not damaging the soft tissues surrounding the fracture site.

Bone growth and healing

2

BONE GROWTH

At birth, bones are formed mostly by a cartilaginous tissue that is progressively substituted by bone tissue. The substitution of one tissue by another starts from points found in the cartilaginous tissue that are activated, transforming themselves into bone. These points are called ossification nuclei (Fig. 1).

Each bone has a central nucleus located in the medial area of the diaphysis. This is called a primary ossification nucleus which is activated at birth. It is responsible for the transformation of the central part of the bone to become the diaphysis. Ossification takes place centrifugally from this point. The secondary ossification nuclei are found on the ends of the bones and are activated after birth. They are responsible for the transformation that takes place in the epiphyses. The number of secondary ossification nuclei is variable and depends on each bone. There are long bones that have no secondary ossification nuclei in one or both of their epiphyses; for example, the metacarpal bones only possess one secondary ossification nucleus in their proximal epiphysis. In other bones, such as the tibia, the proximal epiphysis has two secondary ossification nuclei, while there is only one on its proximal portion.

There is a thin layer located between the primary and secondary nuclei that is responsible for the longitudinal growth of the bone called the growth plate or cartilage (Fig. 2). Similarly, between these two secondary nuclei there are also remnants of cartilage that continue active for some time for the correct formation of the corresponding epiphysis.

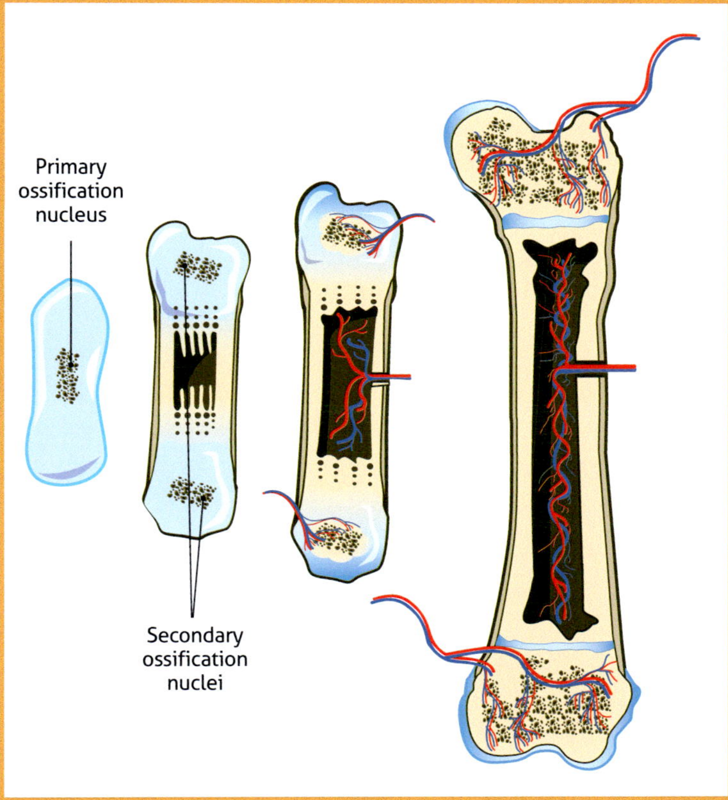

FIGURE 1. Representation of the ossification nuclei in a bone.

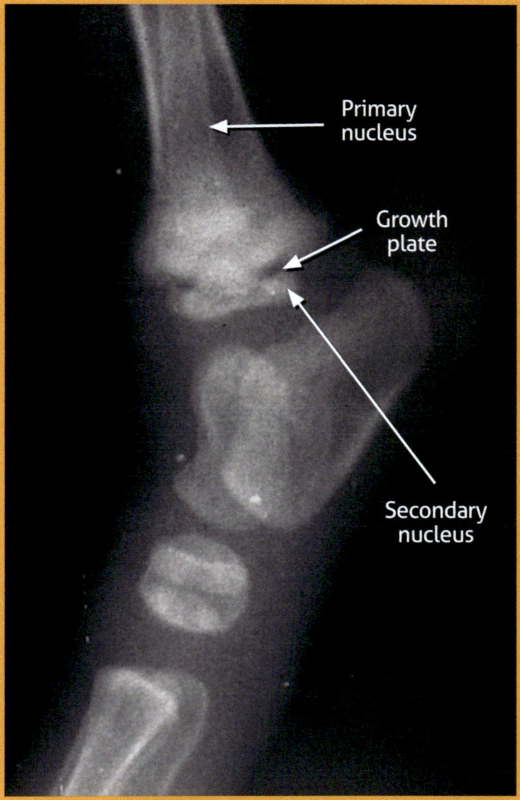

FIGURE 2. Ossification nuclei and growth lines in the tarsus of a young individual.

Understanding the peculiarities of each bone is important to avoid confusing the radiolucent appearance of the growth plates with fractures.

The process through which the cartilage transforms into bone is known as endochondral ossification. It is similar to that produced in the bone healing processes to transform an initial fracture callus into mature bone.

First, it must be taken into account that the epiphysis and the metaphysis of an immature bone possess different irrigation than that of a mature bone. In growing bones, the epiphysis and diaphysis are irrigated from two independent points. These two irrigation points are separated by the growth plate (Fig. 3). Although the epiphysis has a very complex vascular network, the growth plate is poorly irrigated. The nutrition of said plate takes place through penetration of the vessels and by diffusion of the nutrients through the cartilaginous matrix. Any interference in this source of nutrition may cause a decrease in the growth activity and multiplication, that is, resulting in less growth in the length of the bone. The metaphyseal irrigation is equally complex through the cancellous bone of the metaphysis. The vessels superficially penetrate the cartilage, favouring the transformation of the cartilaginous tissue into bone. Any interference in the metaphyseal irrigation can affect the growth plate, decreasing or impeding endochondral ossification.

Structure of the growth plate

The growth plate is stratified into various zones that are aligned in a parallel manner. The processes that take place in the different zones are shown in Figure 4: the reserve zone, the proliferative zone, the hypertrophic zone, the ossification zone and the metaphyseal zone.

- **Reserve zone**: this zone is found in close contact with the epiphysis and is formed by a small number of chondrocytes surrounded by a cartilaginous matrix. These cells have no mitotic capacity and their function is to store nutrients. The vessels that originate in the epiphysis pass through this layer to arborise in the proliferative zone. The partial oxygen tension in this zone is very low giving an idea of its low nutritional requirements.
- **Proliferative zone**: the proliferative zone is where cell growth actually takes place. The chondrocytes that are found in this layer have a high demand for oxygen due to their elevated mitotic activity. The germ cells are found forming columns of chondrocytes aligned parallel to the longitudinal axis of the bone. These cells secrete large amounts of proteoglycans and collagen that form septa which separate the columns. The longitudinal growth is produced as a result of active cellular division and the production of matrix.
- **Hypertrophic zone**: in the highest areas of the hypertrophic zone, the chondrocytes preserve their mitotic activity, however, the production of matrix is much lower. The chondrocytes become larger in size, storing calcium and lipids. As they grow, the columns become closer together, reducing the width of the septa. The oxygen tension in these zones is low as both the oxygen and the nutrients must be diffused through the capillaries of the proliferative zone.

  The previously stored oxygen is consumed due to the energy requirement of the chondrocytes. The energy needed for the metabolism and preservation of stored calcium is also reduced.

  As the distance with the proliferative zone increases, the delivery of nutrients is reduced, which leads to nutritional deficiencies. When the energy available to the cell is not enough, the cell must release the calcium accumulated in its interior. As a result, the cell membrane starts to degenerate and vacuoles appear in the cytoplasm. The lysosomal enzymes are released outside of the cell and begin to break down the matrix. In the uppermost area of this layer, the proteoglycan molecules begin to lose their merging capacity.

  At the same time, the calcium is deposited into the matrix, over the zones that were previously occupied by the chondrocytes. Most mineralisation takes place in the longitudinal septa, that is, between the cellular columns. The transversal septa that are found between the cells, remain unmineralised.

  In the zones where the mineralisation has taken place, the blood supply is practically cut off causing the chondrocytes to die.
- **Ossification zones**: the mineralisation of the matrix of the hypertrophic zone is essential for the correct formation of the bone. The mineralisation stimulates the new vascularisation coming from the metaphyseal zone. A network of capillaries is progressively formed that invade the lacunae, previously occupied by chondrocytes,

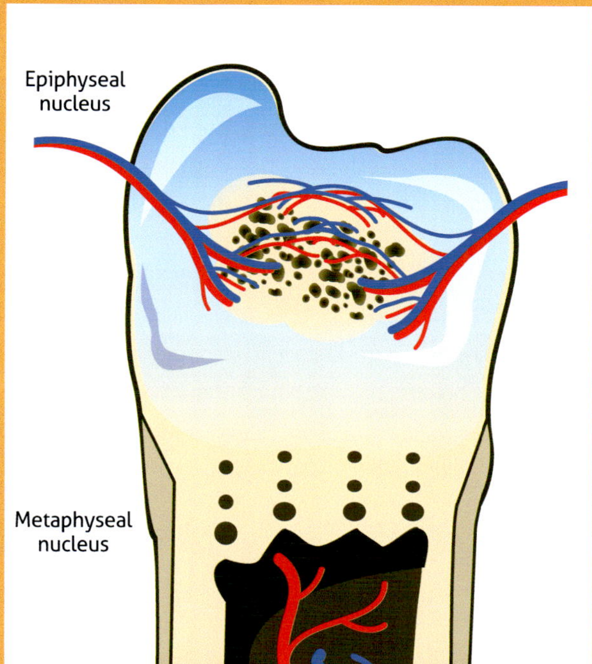

FIGURE 3. Epiphyseal blood supply during growth.

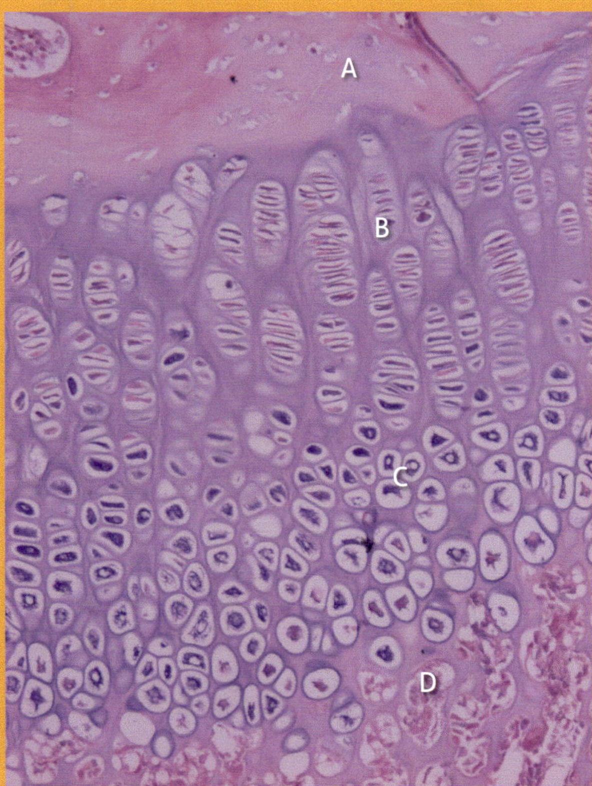

FIGURE 4. Histological section of a growth plate. Image courtesy of the Histology and Anatomical Pathology Unit of the *Universidad Complutense de Madrid*, Spain (UCM).

A. Reserve zone.
B. Proliferative zone.
C. Hypertrophic zone.
D. Ossification zone.

through which the osteoclasts and osteoblasts arrive. The lacunae and septa are broken down by perivascular cells through the liberation of enzymes. The osteoclasts reabsorb the septa in a longitudinal direction and the osteoclasts begin to secrete a matrix formed by proteoglycans and collagen (osteoid material) that is deposited on the remnants of mineralised cartilage. The osteoid matrix mineralises due to the depositing of calcium salts that form larger aggregates in the form of crystals of hydroxyapatite. The remnants of mineralised cartilage are surrounded by new bone, forming the primary cancellous bone. The osteoclasts will later break down this primary cancellous bone to form what will be the secondary cancellous bone.

- **Metaphyseal zone:** The ossification zone and the metaphyseal zone show no clear division. The metaphyseal zone is characterised by being the place where the remodelling of the primary and secondary cancellous bone takes place. The secondary cancellous bone is reabsorbed by osteoclasts through processes of phagocytosis. Later, the osteoblasts form the lamellar bone resulting in the haversian canals.

  Most longitudinal bone growth occurs through this plate. However, the epiphysis of an immature animal has another growth plate that contributes partially to longitudinal growth. The cartilage that covers the epiphysis is divided into two zones, a more external zone in charge of protecting the joint, and a more internal zone that corresponds with a transition zone in charge of epiphyseal growth. The radial zone has columns of chondrocytes that are comparable with the proliferative and hypertrophic zones of the metaphyseal growth line. The deepest part of the radial zone is the calcification zone where the remodelling process of the primary and secondary cancellous bone takes place.

In summary, the bone grows from the growth plates thanks to a process of mitosis in a longitudinal direction. The newly formed tissue goes through a process of death by anoxia and calcification that will later be the base for the formation of cortical bone. However, the growth in size of the joint epiphyses is produced in a similar manner in one of the layers of the subchondral bone.

BONE HEALING

To select the best osteosynthesis system for the correct stabilisation of a fracture, not only must the type of fracture be taken into account, but a series of other individual characteristics of the patient, habitat or type of owner. We believe that it is important to start with a brief summary of the phenomena that take place in the fracture site leading up to the healing of the bone tissue. Understanding said phenomena, as well as their influence on healing processes, is essential to selecting the right treatment.

First of all, it must be taken into account that the organism functions according to the "principle of least effort", and thus tries to invest the least amount of energy possible in said processes. Basically, the organism creates and prepares bone tissue according to its needs, depending on the direction and intensity of the forces a certain area is subjected to.

A clear example is the type of bone tissue that the organism creates for each part of a bone. The weight, that is, the amount of longitudinal pressure, requires that the femur be a hollow tube of compact tissue that is sufficiently strong to endure said forces. Nonetheless, the zones that are subjected to forces with no predominant direction, such as the epiphysis, are composed of a more elastic tissue (cancellous bone).

Bone healing is considered as the group of processes involved in the healing of a fracture. All healing processes have three phases: inflammatory, restorative and remodelling.

Inflammatory phase

When a fracture occurs, damage is caused to the bone structure as well as to the surrounding soft tissues. At a cellular level, the lysis of the osteocytes and of the cells of the dead soft tissues leads to the liberation of substances in the fracture site that attract inflammatory cells and macrophages in charge of "clearing away" all necrotic material (Fig. 5).

First, a blood clot is formed at the fracture site. This clot, although there are discrepancies between different authors, is important to the restitution of the neovascularisation to the fracture site.

Restorative phase

Two types of healing can be differentiated in this phase depending on the size of the bone callus that is formed during the process: healing by first intention with minimal bone callus formation and healing by second intention where the amount of callus formed is much greater. The quantity of newly formed tissue will primarily depend on the existing mobility in the fracture site. The two types of healing will be described below, starting with that which is produced more frequently.

Healing by second intention

Healing by second intention is the most natural and frequent type of healing. It consists of the union of bone fragments through scar tissue that will later undergo remodelling processes.

This type of healing is produced when the following circumstances occur:

- Late treatment.
- Deficient reduction of the fracture or loss of fragments.
- Poor blood supply.
- Infection.
- Absence of forces of compression.

It occurs when there is a certain amount of separation between the edges of the fracture or when the stabilisation system does not provide enough stability. In summary, this type of healing is fundamental in the formation of a succession of tissue of different characteristics that serve to temporarily stabilise the fracture to allow for complete bone recovery.

The first tissue generated is very similar to a hypercellular cartilaginous tissue. It is the most adaptive tissue given that its great elasticity allows for it to bear the deformations produced in the fracture site when the fragments are slightly displaced (Fig. 6). However, it is rigid enough to avoid excessive displacement of said fragments. Later, and through processes of endochondral ossification, this tissue will transform into bone tissue.

Initially, adjacent necrotic bone tissue on the edges of the fracture is reabsorbed. The quantity of tissue reabsorbed is of great importance as it increases separation between the edges of the fracture.

It must be taken into account that the blood supply in the first moments [after the fracture takes place] comes primarily from the periostium, and therefore, if surgery is needed, all soft tissues that surround the bone should be respected as much as possible.

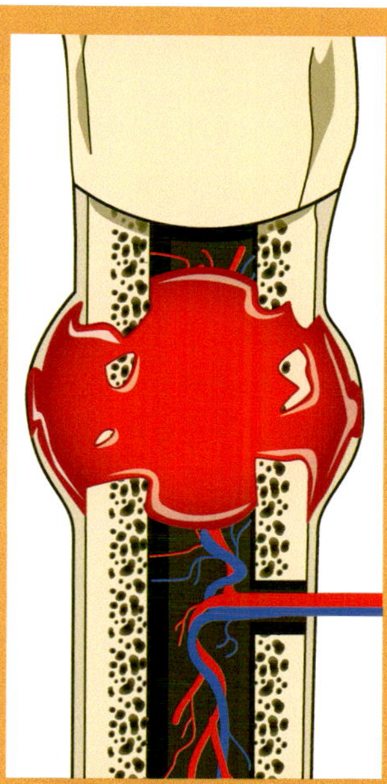
FIGURE 5. Inflammatory phase of the healing process.

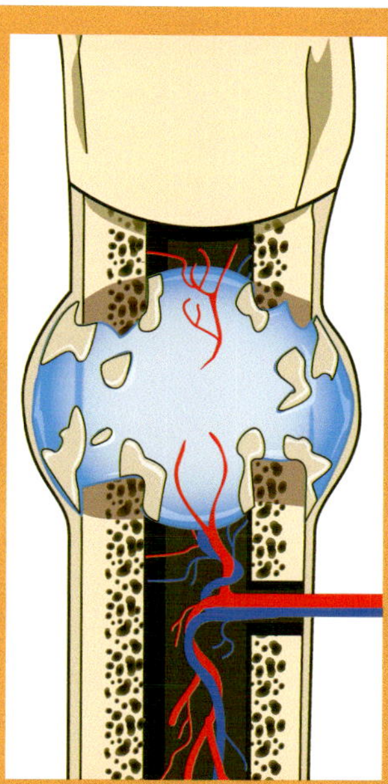
FIGURE 6. Soft callus formation phase.

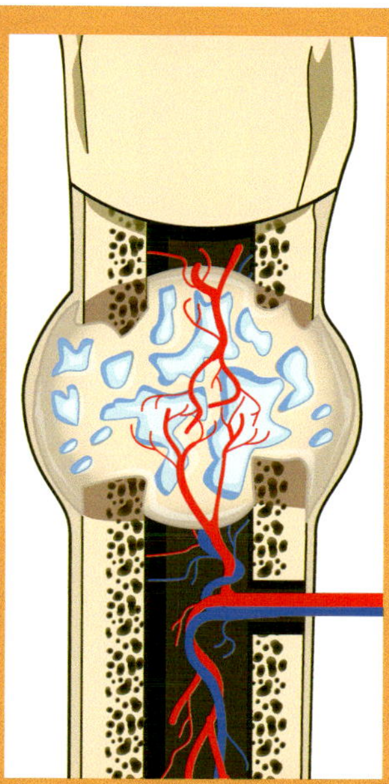
FIGURE 7. Hard callus formation phase.

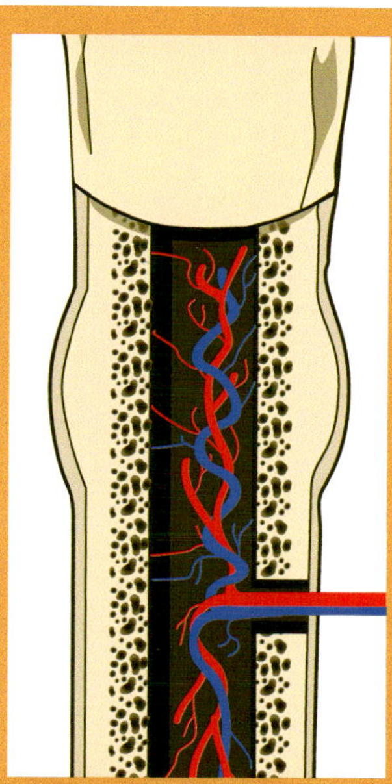
FIGURE 8. Remodelling phase.

The cells that travel to the fracture site rapidly begin to form the bone callus. This tissue is formed by fibrous tissue, cartilage and immature fibrous bone. The predominant type of tissue depends on different factors such as the stability, forces of pressure and partial oxygen tension in the fracture site. In environments with low oxygen tension, cartilaginous or fibrous tissue forms, whereas with high tensions, bone tissue is produced; hence the importance of respecting soft tissues.

As the fracture is stabilised and blood supply is restored, the newly formed cartilage is progressively substituted by bone tissue by means of a process that is similar to endochondral ossification (Fig. 7).

At the end of the process, the ends of the bones are enveloped by a fusiform mass, known as the bone callus, similar to scars found on skin after healing by second intention (Fig. 8).

Types of bone callus

There are different types of bone callus that vary depending on the different tissues that form the callus and its position within the fracture:

- **Medullary callus:** formed from cells of the medullary cavity and from osteoblasts originating in the endostium. This is the first union that takes place at the fracture site. They are not usually visible by X-ray. Vessels derived from the medullary cavity provide its blood supply.
- **Periosteal callus:** its formation begins at a small distance from the fracture line, just behind the necrotic tissue of the fracture edge. It serves to "hold" the fragments in place and its size depends on the possibilities of movement of these bone fragments. In the case of excessive movement at the fracture site, the callus involutions and the fracture does not heal. Its blood supply depends on the periosteal vessels and surrounding tissues, while it later is nourished through the intraosseous circulation.
- **Intercortical callus:** its size varies depending on the separation and reabsorption of the necrotic tissues on the edges of the fracture. The nature of its osteogenesis is variable and its irrigation depends on both the medullary as well as the peripheral circulation.

This leads to what is known as the clinical union, in which the fragments firmly unite and the bone is capable of bearing a functional level of weight.

Healing by first intention

Healing by first intention is characterised by the direct formation of bone tissue in a fracture line without the creation or production of bone callus. This is only achieved when the following conditions occur:

- Immediate stabilisation.
- Good blood supply.
- Perfect reduction of the fracture edges (reducible fracture).
- Absence of micromovements at the level of the fracture line.
- Interfragmentary compression (Roux Law): decreases the micromovements between the bone fragments, accelerating healing. This is achieved in several ways:
  - The patient's own weight when walking.
  - Application of osteosynthesis systems that compress the fracture lines.
  - Placement of osteosynthesis systems that redistribute the weight.
- Absence of infection.

It is very important that the blood supply is not excessively damaged, especially the intraosseous supply.

Within this type of healing, and regarding the ossification process, there are two subtypes of union depending on the space that exists at the fracture line:

- **Direct osteonal union**: this type of healing takes place in areas where there is already close contact between the edges of the fractures. Under these circumstances, an osteon that emerges from a Volkmann's canal directly crosses the fracture line until it comes into contact with the other healthy canal located in the bone of the other fragment. An osteon is basically a group of bone cells structured in one front line of osteoclasts that "perforate" the bone, followed by a line of osteoblasts that create bone as they go. A comparison could be made with a bulldozer that is used to construct long tunnels for trains.

  The healing takes place without the formation of bone callus, that is, no bone scar tissue is formed (Fig. 9).
- **Primary healing with separation**: this type of healing takes place in the areas of less contact. Although there is a certain amount of separation, the adjacent areas of close contact impede micromovements. The existing space is refilled with bone tissue. Depending on the distance between the fragments, lamellar bone is formed directly, or immature bone is formed that later transforms into lamellar bone. The orientation of the collagen fibres of the bone are initially aligned parallel to

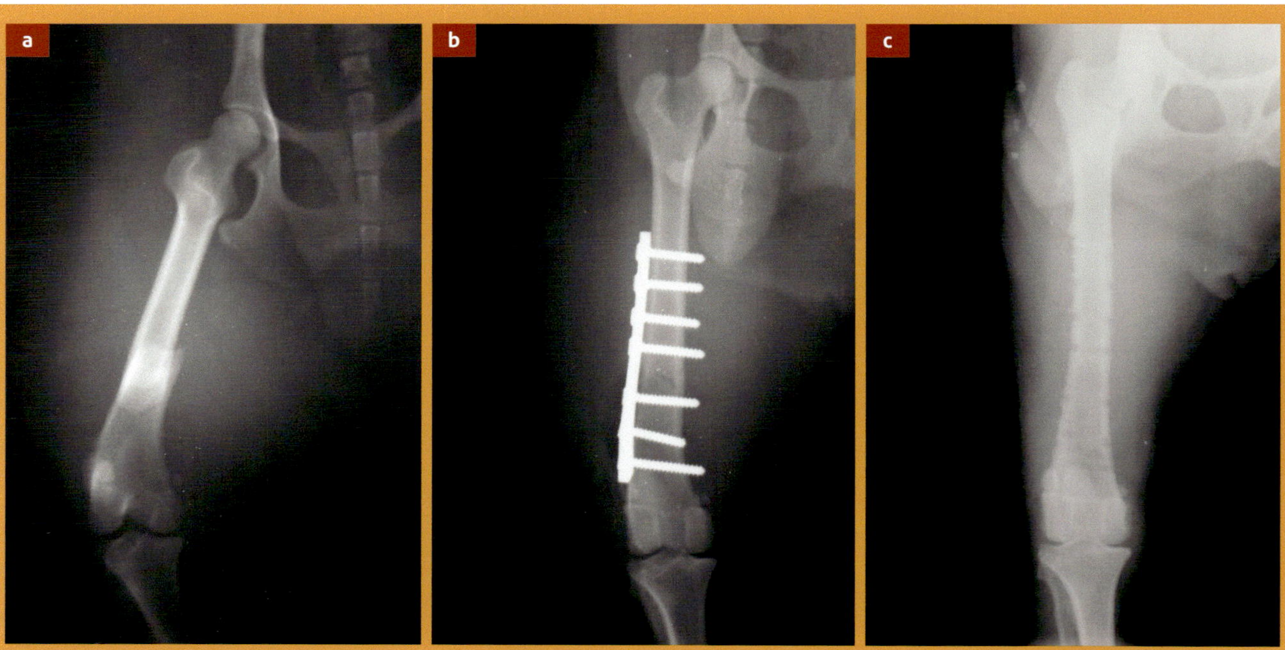

FIGURE 9. X-ray image showing the progress of a resolved fracture in which healing by first intention is produced. Note that there is no formation of bone callus.

the fracture line. Later, the structural remodelling of the compact bone creates new haversian canals, which are oriented in a direction that is longitudinal to the diaphysis of the bone.

The ossification by first intention takes place much faster than that by second intention. However, at first, the first type is not as stable as the second. This is due to the fact that there is no extra support provided by the bone callus and that the initial orientation of the bone is not physiological.

Remodelling phase

This phase is characterised by the reabsorption of the superfluous or misplaced bone material. That is, the organism eliminates all bone tissue that it does not need to bear the forces of pressure to which it is subjected (Fig. 8).

The mechanism of control is a consequence of a piezoelectric process. In the areas of the bone that are subjected to traction, an accumulation of electropositive charges is produced, while those that are subjected to pressure are charged with negative electrons. The osteoclastic activity increases in the electropositive areas, while the osteoblasts are predominant in the electronegative areas (Fig. 10).

It must be taken into account that neither of the two types of healing is better than the other. They are processes that are produced depending on the intrinsic conditions of the fracture, as well as the osteosynthesis system used, the age of the patient and even the resting period after surgery. The final result is the consolidation of the fracture, and this is achieved in both cases.

Laws of ossification

From the beginning of this study on osteosynthesis, we have tried to explain, through references to laws, a number of concepts that should be taken into account when assessing bone problems. All of these concepts can be summarised in the following core principal: if the mechanical conditions involving a bone are modified, the bone will adapt to its new situation using the minimum amount of energy possible.

Classically, there are three laws: Roux, Hueter-Volkmann and Wolf. The Roux laws describe the effect of forces (pressure, shearing or traction) on a fracture line.

It must be taken into account that a fracture is subjected to forces of pressure, traction and shearing depending on the direction of the bone flexion. This fact causes the formation of one kind of tissue or another in the fracture site depending on the predominance of the forces acting on

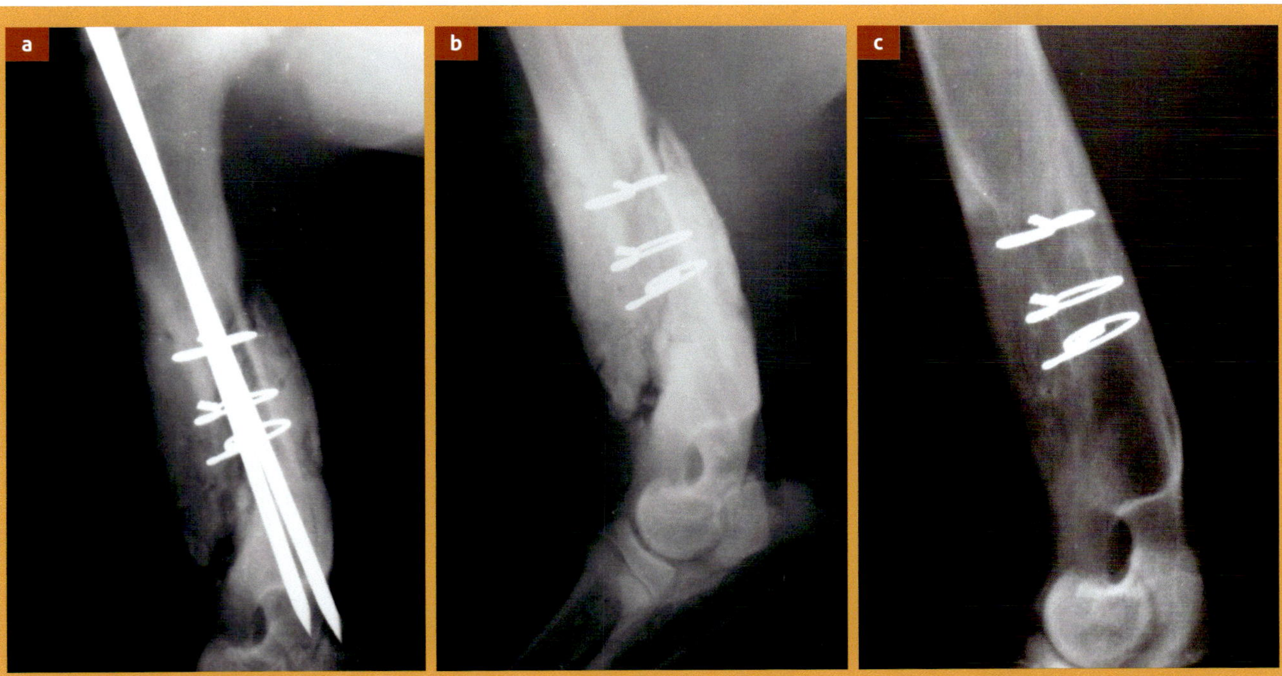

FIGURE 10. Progress of a fracture in a young animal treated with intramedullary pins and cerclages.

said site. This is especially significant in the case of forces of shearing, where the movements that cause the displacement of one fracture edge over the other induce the organism to cover them with a pseudo-cartilaginous tissue that leads to pseudoarthrosis (Fig. 11).

In bone surgery, the objective is always to favour forces of pressure while neutralising those of flexion, traction and above all, rotation.

On the other hand, the laws of Hueter-Volkmann describe the effect of forces on the growth cartilage.

When growth cartilage is involved, greater or lesser growth of a plate is not always a significant problem, unless it causes a decrease in the length of the bone or interferes with another bone, such as the case with the radius and the ulna (*radius curvus*, Fig. 12). The problem arises when the forces of traction and pressure on a plate are not

Roux laws

The Roux laws describe the effect of forces (pressure, shear strain or traction) on a fracture line.

- **Pressure:** the weight applied in a perpendicular direction on a fracture line favours bone healing. This is the base of interfragmentary compression in the treatment of fractures.

  The organism creates bone in response to the actions of external factors.
- **Shearing:** the movements that produce displacement of one fracture edge over another induce the organism to cover them with pseudo-cartilaginous tissue. This produces an undesirable effected called pseudoarthrosis.

  In this case, the organism protects itself from movements of flexion by fabricating a kind (pseudo) of joint (arthro) where previously there was no joint.
- **Traction:** the forces that attempt to separate one fragment from another induce the formation of a fibrous tissue that unites both fragments.

  The organism tries to avoid the separation of the fragments and attempts to unite them by means of a tendon (fibrous tissue).

Hueter-Volkmann laws

These laws describe the effect of the forces on the growth cartilage.

- **Pressure:** the weight applied in a perpendicular direction to a growth plate inhibits growth, and can even impede bone growth.

  The organism gives priority to the reinforcement of this cartilaginous area over its function of growing, leading it to ossify before it should.
- **Traction:** the forces that attempt to separate two ossification nuclei increase the growth velocity.

  In this case the organism responds to the requirements that come from the exterior.

Wolf laws

The effect of the forces are applied on the periostium.

- **Absence of pressure:** the areas of the periostium that are not subjected to weight tend to decalcify, losing bone mass.

  The organism has no need to sustain material located in areas where it is not needed (Law of the conservation of energy).
- **Pressure:** the areas of the periostium that are subjected to loads present greater growth and therefore the bone reinforces itself at these points.

  The organism provides bone mass to the compact bone that is subjected to forces of pressure of greater intensity.

symmetrical. When this happens, a curvature is produced in the bone similar to the one shown in Figure 13.

Regarding the Wolf laws, their postulates are related with the bone remodelling phase. As previously mentioned, this phase is characterised by the reabsorption of the superfluous or misplaced bone material. That is, the organism eliminates all bone tissue that it does not need to bear the forces of pressure to which it is subjected (Fig. 14).

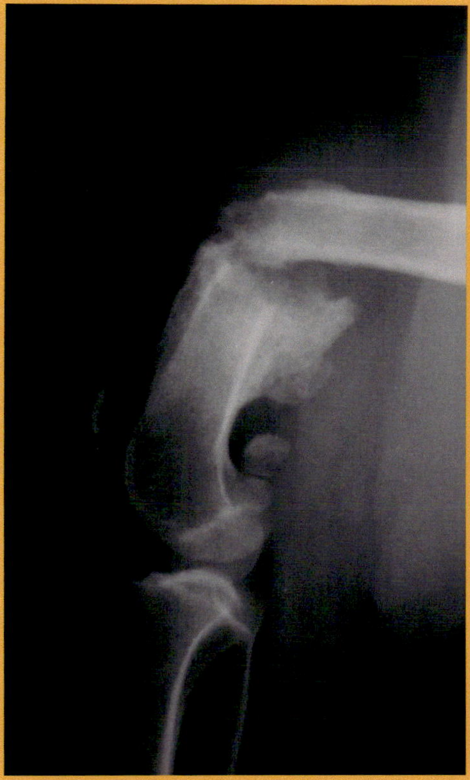

FIGURE 11. Pseudoarthrosis. Note the shape of the edges of the fragments that attempt to serve as a joint.

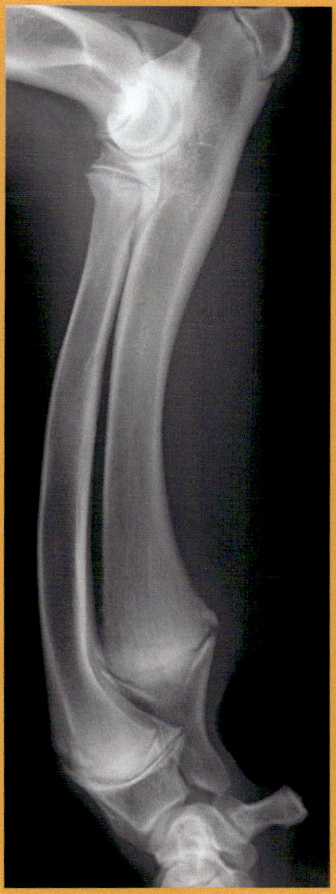

FIGURE 12. Curvature of the radius due to "candle-light" closure of the distal epiphysis of the ulna.

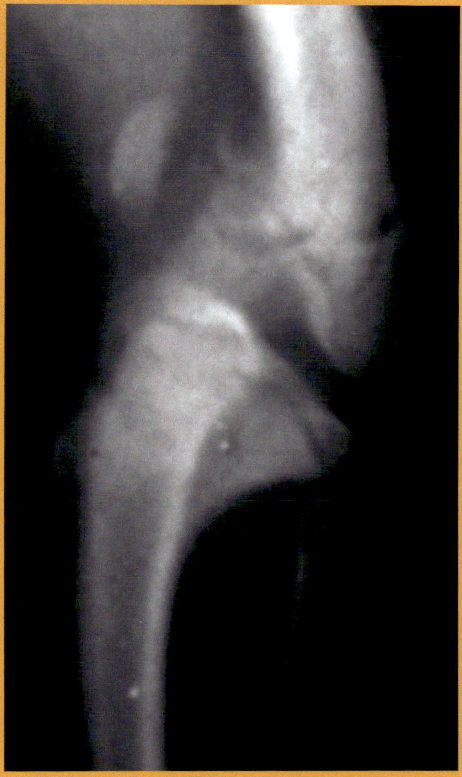

FIGURE 13. Curvature of the femur from asymmetrical pressure on the distal plate due to a medial patellar luxation.

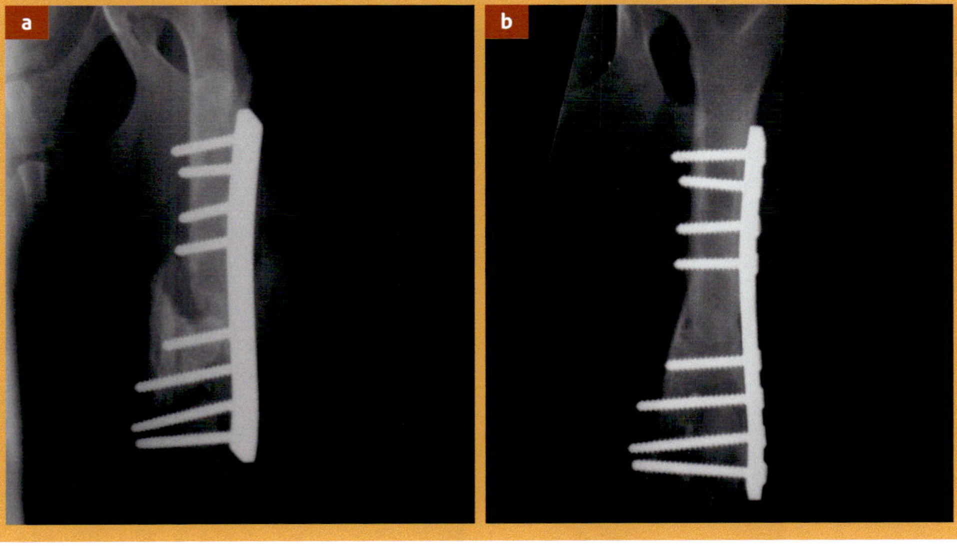

FIGURE 14. Bone remodelling of a pseudoarthrosis treated with a neutralisation plate one year after surgery.

3 Classification of fractures

There is no single current ideal classification system for fractures as they can be grouped by different aspects, each one providing information that can be relevant when applying one kind of treatment or another.

The most complete classification system may be the one proposed by a group of orthopaedic specialists of the AO (initials in German for *Arbeitsgemeinschaft für Osteosynthesefragen*), in which a great amount of information about the affected bone is provided using an alphanumeric system and, as its most relevant point, a subjective assessment of the difficulty regarding treatment is included.

Said classification system consists of the following:

- Each bone is assigned a number:
  - Humerus: 1.
  - Radius/ulna: 2.
  - Femur: 3.
  - Tibia/fibula: 4.
- Next, another number is included that corresponds with the segment where the fracture has occurred:
  - Proximal: 1.
  - Middle third: 2.
  - Distal: 3.
- Later, a letter is added that defines the type of fracture.
  - Simple fracture: A.
  - Multiple: B.
  - Complex: C.

Each group is subdivided in three subgroups depending on the difficulties of treating: from 1 to 3 from lesser to greater complexity, respectively (Fig. 1). This way, a transversal fracture of the femur would be classified as 32A1, whilst if it were a distal fracture, and difficult to treat, it would be 33C3.

This classification becomes even more complicated when epiphyseal fractures are added.

- Extra-articular: A.
- Partial articular: B.
- Complex articular fracture: C.

A series of fracture classification systems are presented below that may be of use as each one provides certain interesting characteristics regarding possible treatments.

SOFT TISSUE INVOLVEMENT

Depending on the affectation or involvement of soft tissues, the fractures can be classified as follows:

Closed fractures

There is no contact between the bone and the exterior, i.e. the skin is intact. This is the most frequent type of fracture. They are considered as sterile and do not usually present additional problems regarding vascularisation.

Open fractures

There may or may not be contact between one or more bone fragments and the exterior. The skin has been damaged, from the exterior or from the interior. This type of fracture is classified in three grades of severity:

- Grade I: one or more bone fragments (not visible) have perforated the skin, lacerating it from the inside.
- Grade II: there is slight exposure of one or more bone fragments (Fig. 2).
- Grade III: the fracture site is completely visible with loss of soft tissues and possibly bone fragments (Fig. 3).

In open fractures in which soft tissues are damaged, blood supply is affected to the extent that healing processes are slowed down. Evidently, this phenomena is accentuated when there is more exposure to the exterior.

When the loss of soft tissues is extreme, it may be impossible to completely cover the bone tissue. However, efforts should always be made to cover the periostium with this type of tissues to preserve its blood supply given that, as previously mentioned, it plays an important role in the first phases of bone healing.

If necessary, sliding skin flaps should be performed to protect the bone (Figs. 4 and 5). If this is not possible and

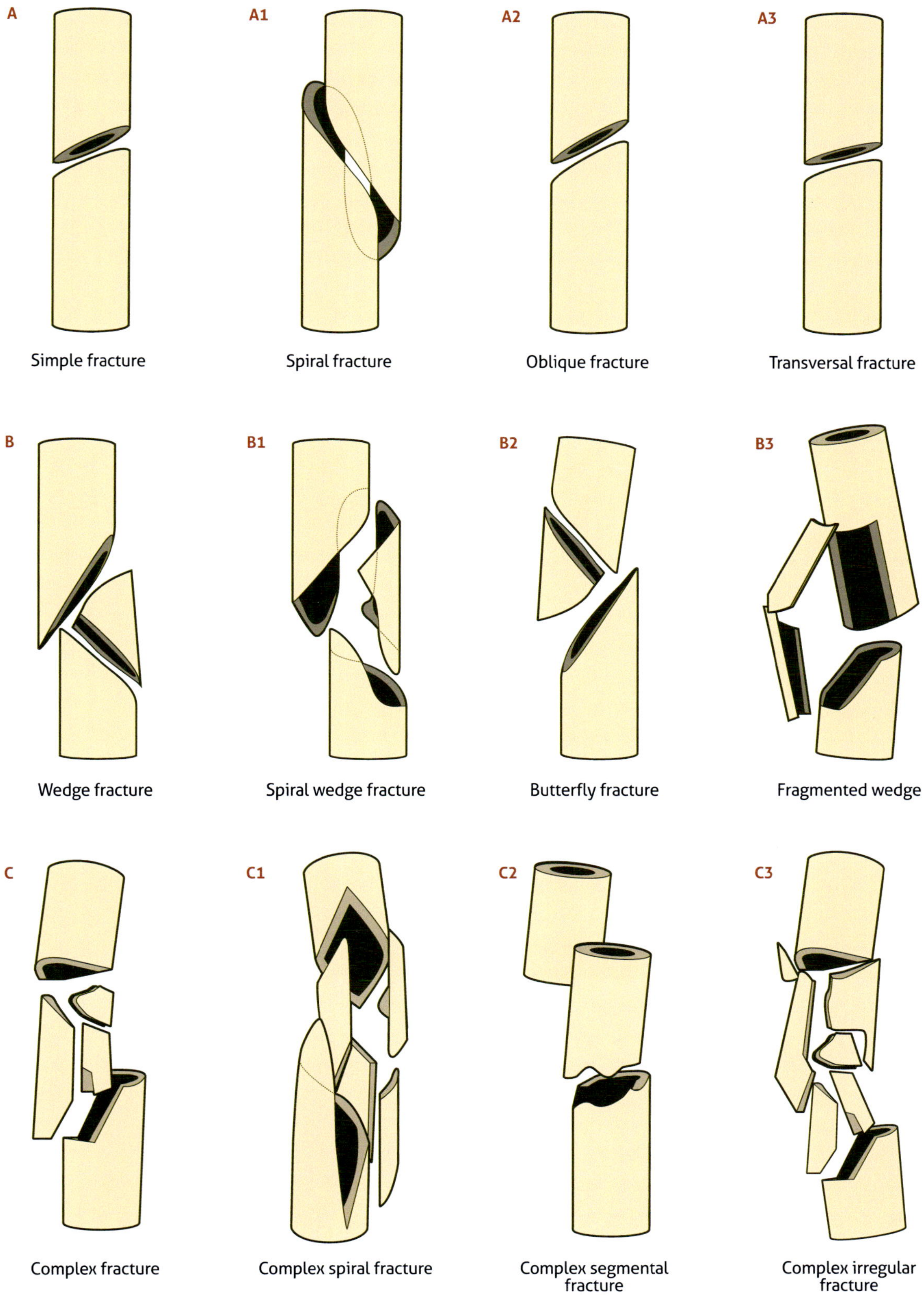

FIGURE 1. Name and classification of the fractures depending on their complexity and type.

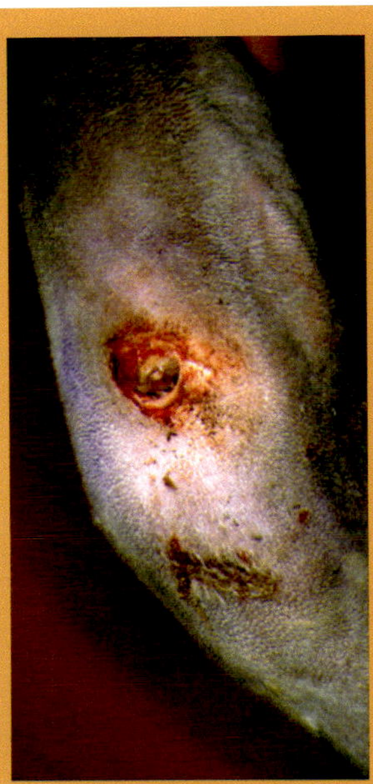

FIGURE 2. Open, grade II fracture.

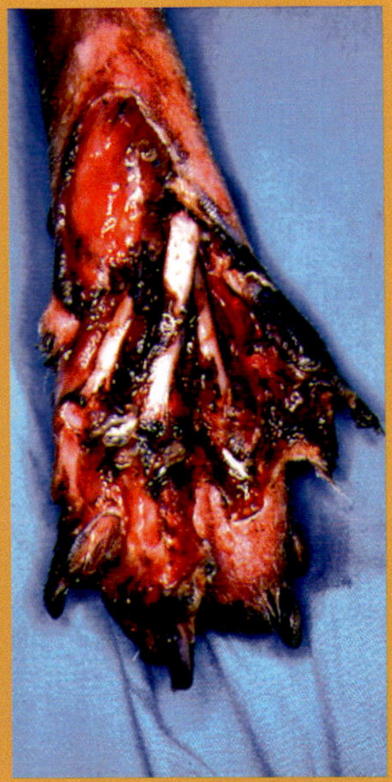

FIGURE 3. Open, grade III fracture.

until granulation tissue forms, the bone must be kept in adequate conditions of humidity by applying ointments and bandages.

On the other hand, the sterility of the bone is lost in open fractures as the skin has been damaged. Depending on the grade of infection of the structures, open fractures can be:

- Grade I: the fracture is considered to be sterile given the minimal exposure of the bone
- Grade II and III: these fractures are considered to be infected. Special actions should be taken in these cases to decrease the bacterial load.

Special interventions in grade II and III open fractures

- More aggressive antibiotic treatment with samples taken for antibiogram.
- Extensive rinsing with isotonic solutions ("flushing" effect).
- Cancellous bone transplant.
- Achieving absolute stability of implants in the fracture site or choice of osteosynthesis systems that do not invade the fracture site.

NUMBER OF FRAGMENTS

From this point of view, the number of fragments of the fractured bone must be taken into account as the stability achieved after reducing the fracture will depend on this, as will the possibility of applying compression. Depending on the number of fragments, fractures can be divided into three large groups:

Simple fracture

The bone has been fractured into two fragments (Fig. 6). This is the "typical" fracture in which there is only one fracture plane. The prognosis of these fractures is usually good and healing is simple, theoretically, and easy to treat. As there is only one plane, artificial forces of pressure can usually be applied on the fracture. The stability achieved is generally good, and therefore the implant is not subjected to excessive forces until the bone has healed.

Multiple fracture

The bone fractures into at least three fragments, two which are principal and one or more that are independent (Fig. 7). In these cases, as much as possible, the muscular insertions of these fragments must be maintained as the blood supply and survival during the first few weeks depend on them.

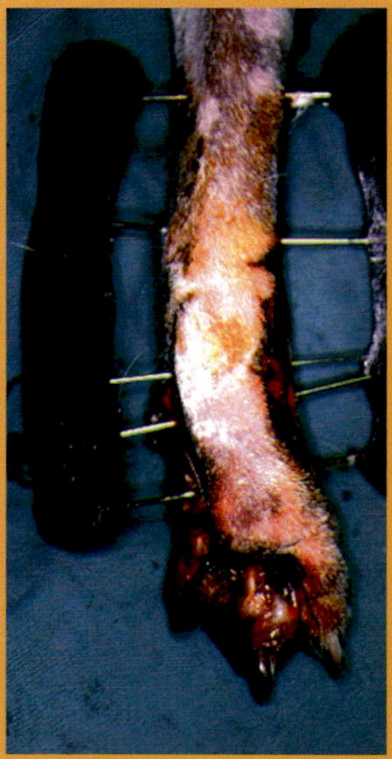

FIGURE 4. Skin flap performed in the treatment of a grade III open fracture.

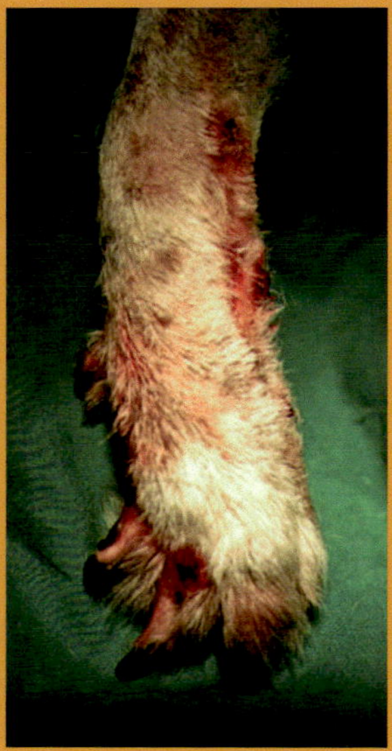

FIGURE 5. Result of the skin flap shown in Figure 4.

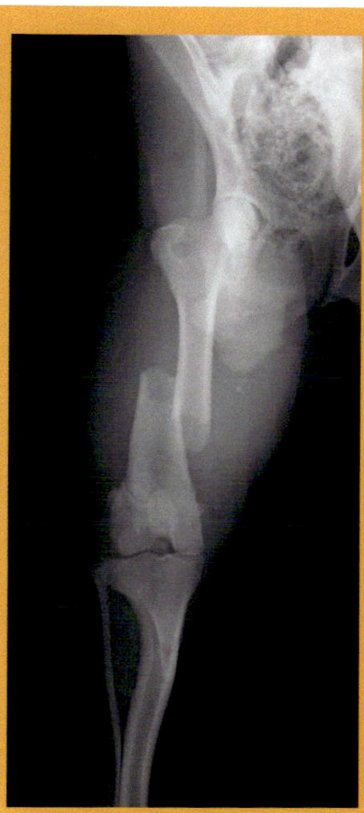

FIGURE 6. Simple femur fracture.

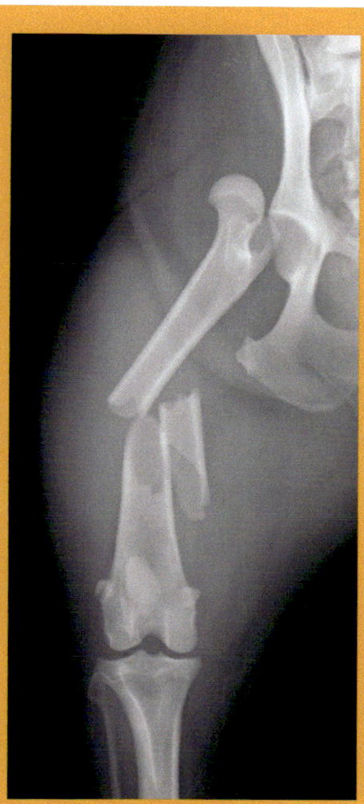

FIGURE 7. Multiple femur fracture.

On the other hand, the fragments can be reduced, that is, placed in their original position and stabilised. The "puzzle" can be put back together and the fragments can be fixed using osteosynthesis systems to maintain their position when bearing weight. If all the fragments can be reduced, the entire diaphysis can be reconstructed and therefore, there will be no errors in the bone alignment. Similarly, as the diaphysis can be reconstructed, the forces can be transmitted, partially, through its compact bone. The weight borne by the extremity while standing is transformed into forces of pressure that accelerate bone healing. As the implant does not have to bear all of the weight, the intensity of the forces that it has to neutralise and, therefore, the risk that the fixation systems loosen or bend, decrease.

Comminuted fracture

The bone breaks in various fragments, but unlike multiple fractures, due to its small size and its shape, it cannot be properly stabilised in its anatomical position (Fig. 8). Like multiple fractures, the insertions of the soft tendons must be respected to preserve blood supply.

In these cases, the orientation of the bone axis is found using the bone protrusions as anatomical references and the direction of the joints when flexing and extending.

As there is no continuity in the diaphyseal compact bone, forces cannot be transmitted directly from the distal fragment to the proximal fragment. The forces are passed through the osteosynthesis system until the fracture site ossifies. This means that more resistant implants or configurations must be selected that are capable of withstanding great forces of flexion. The *débricolage* is more probable than in anterior fractures.

DIRECTION OF THE FRACTURE PLANE

The direction of the fracture plane is important as it determines if the weight borne will transform with greater or lesser intensity in displacement from one direction or another from the fracture site.

Regarding comminuted fractures with total instability, the direction of the fracture lines is irrelevant. Instability is also complete in multiple fractures, but the direction of the fracture lines must be taken into account if reducing the fragments is a priority.

Taking into account their direction, fractures can be classified as:

Transversal fracture

The fracture plane courses more or less perpendicular to the longitudinal axis of the bone (Fig. 9).

This fracture can be compared with a column formed by two cylinders. When the fracture is reduced, that is, with one of the cylinders over the other, it can easily support the forces of pressure in a parallel direction from the longitudinal axis of the bone. It is not an especially stable structure against forces of flexion, although it can tolerate them up to a point.

The biggest problem is that it does not resist forces of rotation. When this type of movement is produced, the edges of the fracture lines slide over each other, making healing more difficult.

Oblique fracture

The fracture plane forms a more or less closed angle with respect to the longitudinal axis of the bone (Fig. 10). Depending on the amplitude of said angle, they can be:

- Short oblique fractures, if the angle tends towards perpendicularity (Fig. 11).

- Long oblique fractures, if they tend to be parallel with the longitudinal axis of the bone (Fig. 12).

Concerning the resolution of the oblique fractures, they can be compared to an inclined plane. Once the fracture is reduced (in the case of forces of pressure, i.e. forces that are parallel to the longitudinal axis), both fragments slide over the other as if it was a "playground slide". This displacement, aside from destabilising the reduction, impedes healing.

In this sense, the closer the fracture line is to the longitudinal axis of the bone, the easier the displacement will be; and on the contrary, the more it resembles the plane of a transversal fracture (short oblique), the more stable it is.

Regarding movements of rotation, it is slightly more stable than transversal fractures.

Spiral fracture

Spiral fractures are similar to long oblique fractures but the fracture line encircles the cortical bone making a spiral (Fig. 13).

It is typical in puppies due to the thinness of the compact portion of their bones. It occurs from forces of rotation under an axial load, a common movement in these patients.

Due to the fact that the fracture line resembles a long oblique fracture line, its response when faced with axial loads is very similar. On the other hand, its spiral component makes it an unstable fracture when faced with forces of rotation.

The closer the fracture is to the longitudinal axis of the bone, the easier it is for the fragments to slide over each other. On the contrary, in perpendicular fractures, the longitudinal axis, movements of rotation are more probable.

METAPHYSEAL AND EPIPHYSEAL FRACTURES

Although most fractures are produced at the diaphyseal level of the bones, a large number are located at the meta- and epiphyseal level, primarily in growing patients, in which the process is complicated due to the possibility of the growth plates being affected. Different classifications fit within this

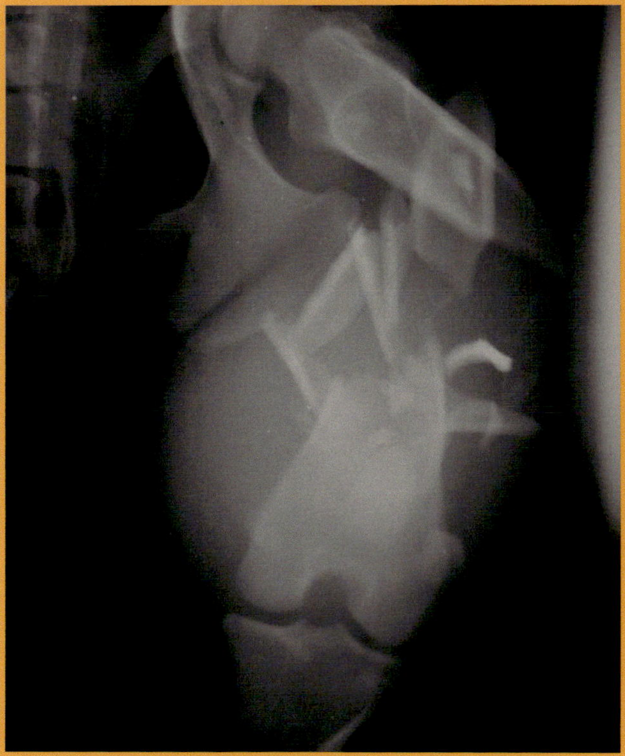

FIGURE 8. Comminuted femur fracture.

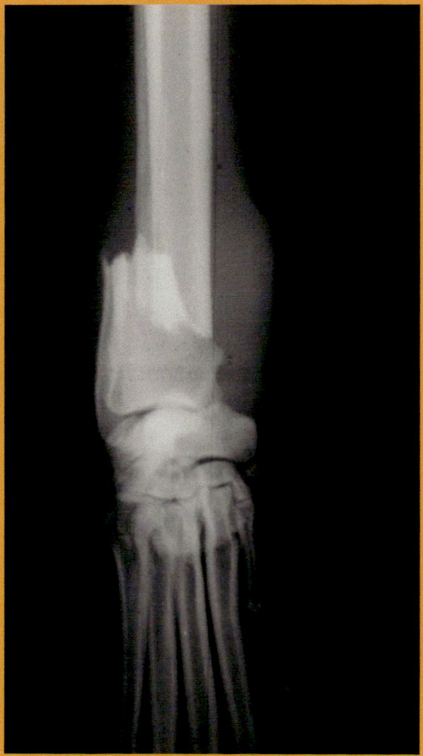

FIGURE 9. Transversal radius fracture.

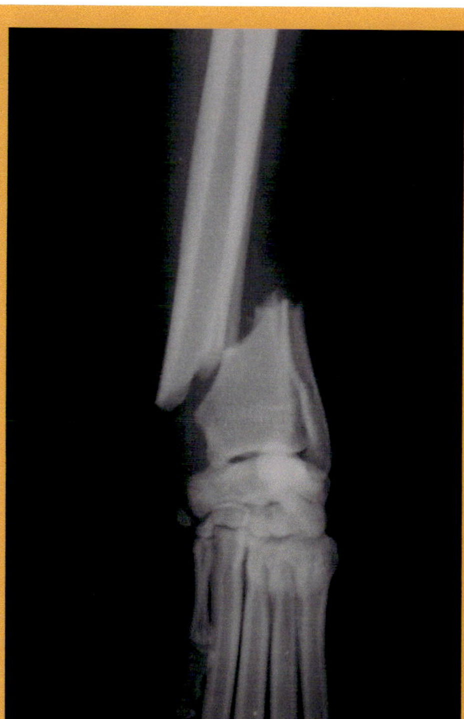

FIGURE 10. Oblique radius fracture.

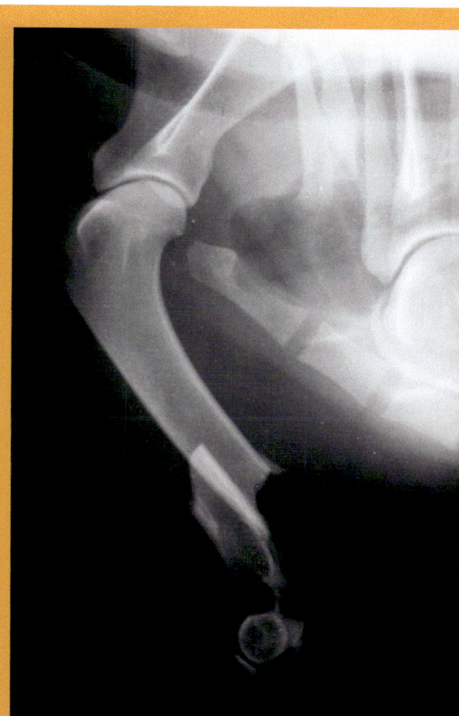

FIGURE 11. Short oblique fracture of the humerus.

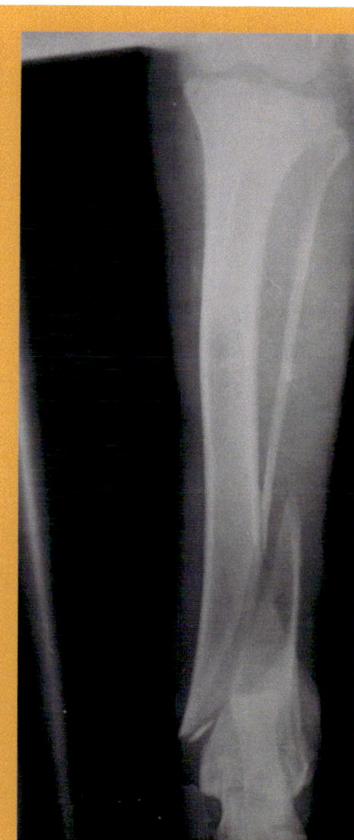

FIGURE 12. Long oblique fracture of the tibia.

group that allow for the rapid identification of the characteristics of a fracture:

Salter-Harris classification

This is a classification system in human medicine created by Salter and Harris that is also applicable in veterinary medicine for fractures that affect growth plates in young patients. There are five types:

- **Type I:** this fracture is produced all along the growth plate affecting the hypertrophic zone, which is the weakest zone.

  The fracture is therefore a net separation of the epiphysis and metaphysis (Fig. 14). It is produced more frequently in the distal epiphysis of the radius, and the head of the femur and the humerus. The germ cells of the proliferative zone stay in the fragment located in the epiphysis and thus the growth potential is not excessively damaged.

  On numerous occasions, the displacement of the epiphysis is hardly noticeable as the fibres of the periostium stay intact. If the germ cells have not been damaged and the vascular supply of the proliferative zone remains intact, the prognosis of the fracture is good.

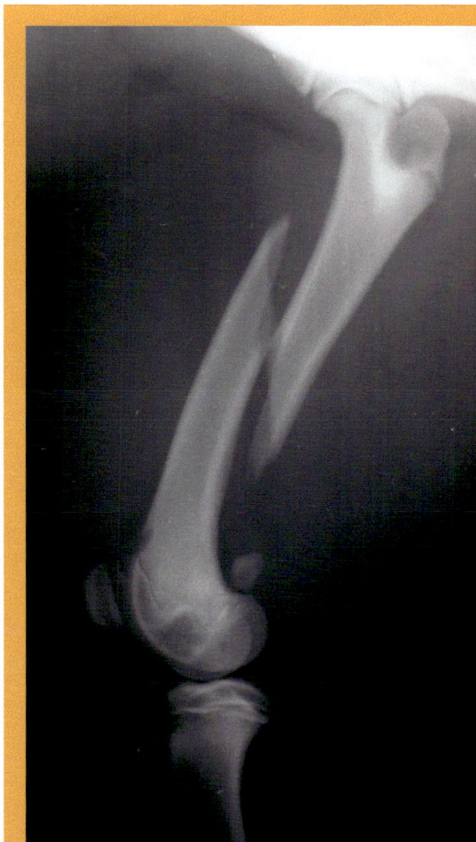

FIGURE 13. Spiral femur fracture.

One specific type of these fractures is produced as a consequence of the forces of traction produced by tendon or ligament insertions that uproot the bone portion at their insertion point.

- **Type II:** this fracture is produced through the hypertrophic zone of the growth plate associated with a fracture that is directed at the metaphysis (Fig. 15). This is the most common fracture in pets and is primarily found in the distal epiphysis of the femur.

  The prognosis is similar to a type I fracture although it varies depending on the integrity of the germ cells and that of the metaphyseal vascular support.

- **Type III**: this fracture partially affects the growth plate, but instead of prolonging itself towards the metaphysis, as in the previous case, it extends towards the joint surface (Fig. 16). It is rare in veterinary medicine and is primarily found in the distal epiphysis of the femur in cats and some cases in the distal epiphysis of the radius.

  The prognosis of this fracture is more severe than the previous cases, given that it is an intra-articular and epiphyseal fracture. Its healing primarily depends on the reaction time and whether it can be reduced, as well as the damage suffered by the germ cells.

  The possibility that the growth line closes prematurely is relatively probable as the epiphyseal irrigation is affected.

- **Type IV**: this fracture does not actually occur in the growth plate, rather it extends from the joint surface to the metaphyseal area of the bone (Fig. 17).

  This type of fracture is primarily produced affecting the lateral condyle of the distal epiphysis of the humerus. Logically, it is an intra-articular fracture and its prognosis is reserved as it depends on the anatomical reduction of the joint surface and the damage produced to the blood supply.

  The growth plate may prematurely close due to the same reasons as those for type III fractures.

- **Type V**: this "fracture" is not technically a fracture but a group of micro-fractures that affect the structure of the growth plate. The lesion can decrease or even nullify the essential function of this bone area, that is, growth.

  Although no areas of growth can avoid suffering from this pathology, it usually affects the distal area of the radius and the ulna. This is due to the fact that the lesion is usually a consequence of a strong impact in the longitudinal direction of the bone, a phenomena that occurs in the front legs when a patient falls from high heights. Another reason for the appearance of this type of lesions is the deviation of muscular forces that increase pressure on certain areas of a plate, such as in the case of high grade patellar luxations.

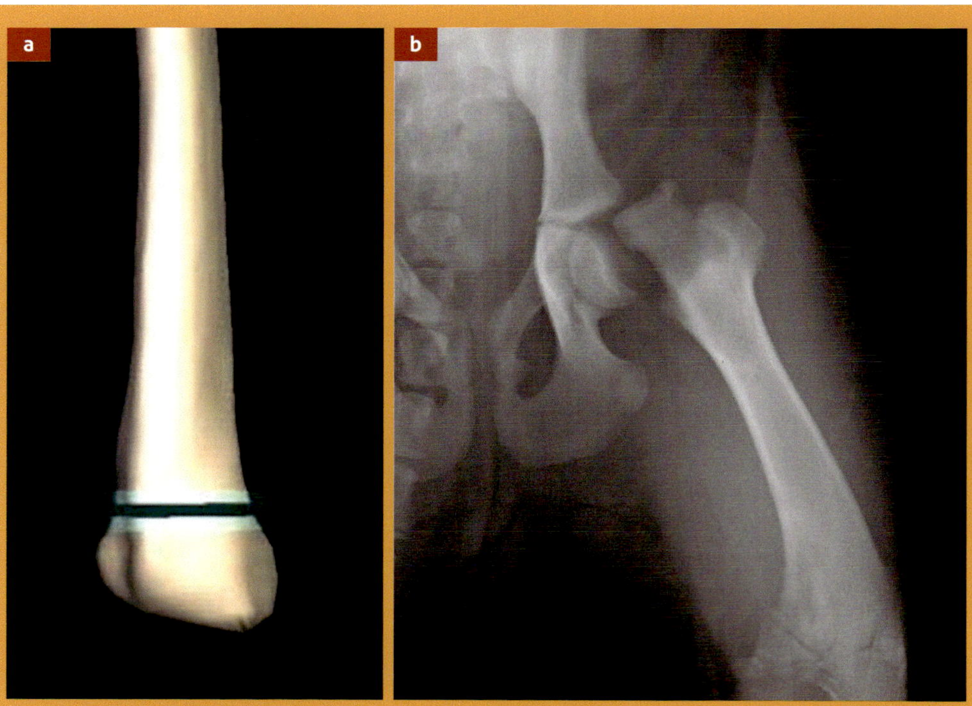

FIGURE 14. Type I Salter-Harris fracture that affects the head of the femur. In Figure 14a, the theoretical trajectory of this fracture is graphically represented.

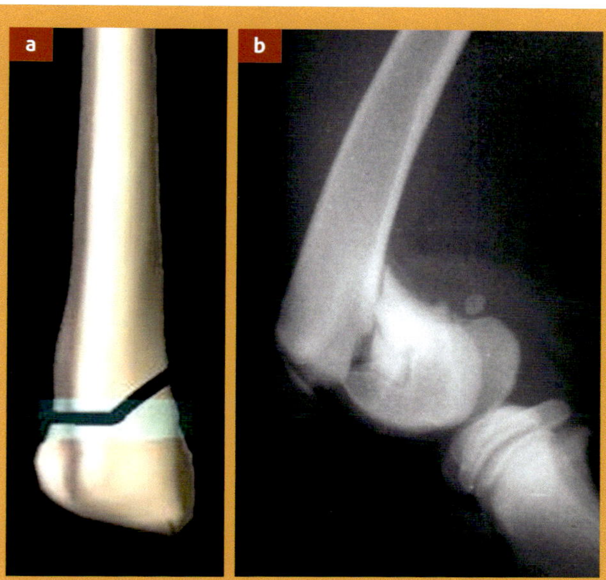

FIGURE 15. Type II Salter-Harris fracture of the distal epiphysis of the femur. The fracture line used to classify this fracture is represented in Figure 15a.

This type of fracture is always accompanied by damage to both the germ cells as well as the epiphyseal vascular supply.

The prognosis depends on the intensity of the trauma and the time passed from the moment of the injury. It must be kept in mind that growth is always reduced in the affected limb in this type of fracture.

One of the most serious consequences of the type V Salter-Harris fracture is the asymmetrical interruption of growth. This not only causes shortening of the limb in question, but also a curvature in its longitudinal axis with the respective repercussions on the joint surface (Figs. 18 and 19).

Type V Salter-Harris fractures, and sometimes type III and IV fractures, imply an alteration of the vascular supply of the growth plate that may be the cause of the shortening of the affected limb.

- **T and Y fractures:** this type of fracture is not included in the human classification systems due to its low frequency in said species. However, it is not uncommon in veterinary medicine. They are actually bicondylar fractures that primarily affect the distal epiphysis of the humerus and, occasionally, the distal epiphysis of the femur. The fracture is a combination of type III and IV Salter fractures and its name comes from the image that the fracture lines make when a cranio-caudal X-ray is taken of the affected epiphysis. Two juxtaposed type III Salter fractures form a T (Fig. 20), while two type IV Salter fractures form a Y (Fig. 21).

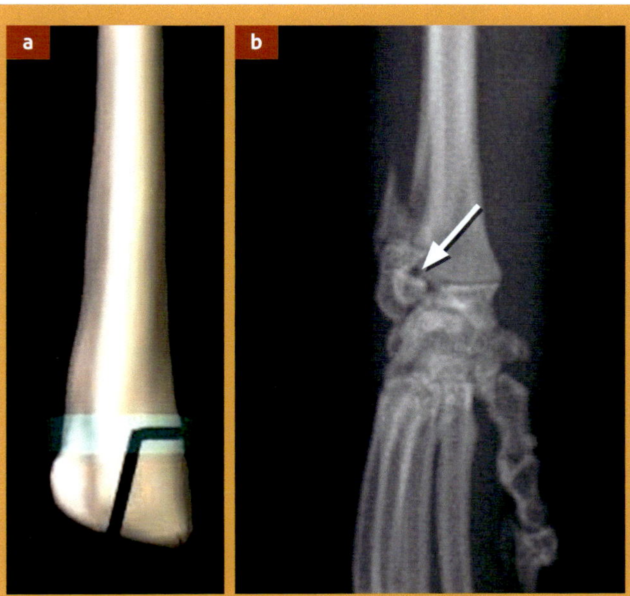

FIGURE 16. Type III Salter-Harris fracture of the distal epiphysis of the radius.

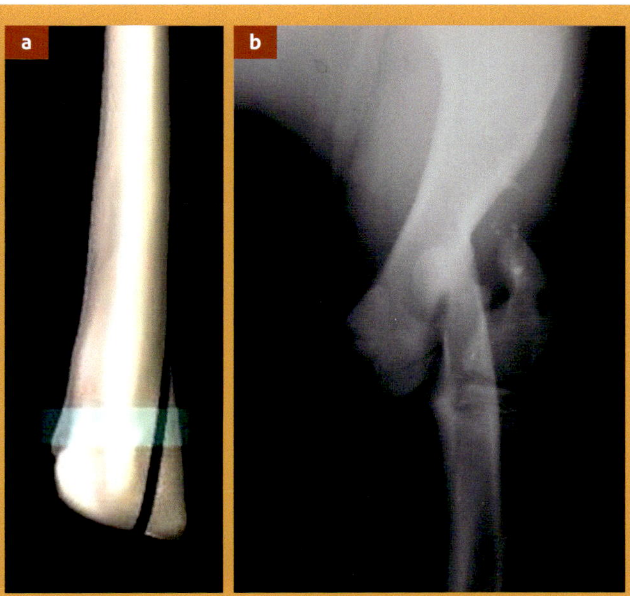

FIGURE 17. Type IV Salter-Harris of the lateral condyle of the humerus.

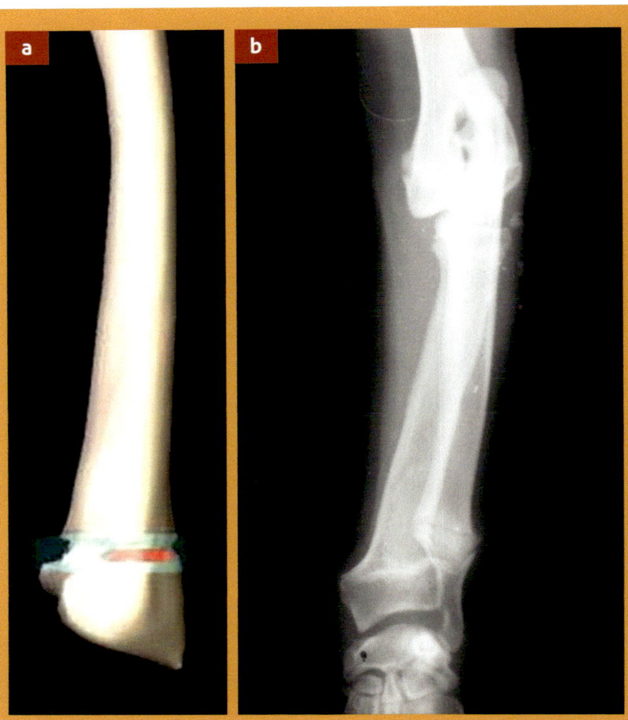

FIGURE 18. Symmetrical type V Salter-Harris fracture of the distal epiphysis of the radius.

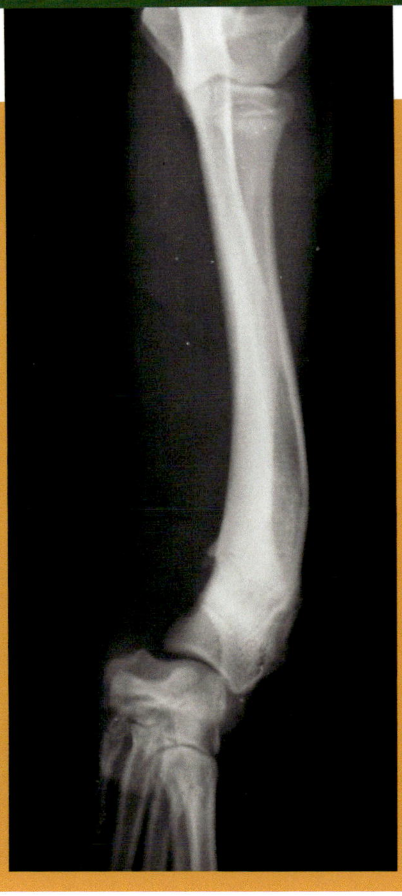

FIGURE 19. Type V Salter-Harris fracture of the distal epiphysis of the radius. Note the curvature in the longitudinal axis of the bone in respect to the image of Figure 18, caused by the asymmetry of the fracture.

The Salter-Harris classification system has been generalised and extrapolated to other fractures and, although this is not the case in young patients, if the fracture lines coincide with any of the previously described models, the corresponding name is adopted in an orthodox manner.

Affectation of the joint surface

Another way of classifying fractures that affect the meta-epiphyseal area of a bone is based on whether the joint area is affected or not.

Following this criteria, two types are established:

- **Non-articular:** the fracture line, even if it is intra-articular, does not affect the joint surface.

  These fractures are hard to reduce due to the presence of tiny fragments as they cannot be stabilised by any type of implant.

  Type I and II fractures, supracondylar fractures and most fractures by avulsion or tearing are included in this group.
- **Type I and II Salter fractures:** previously described.

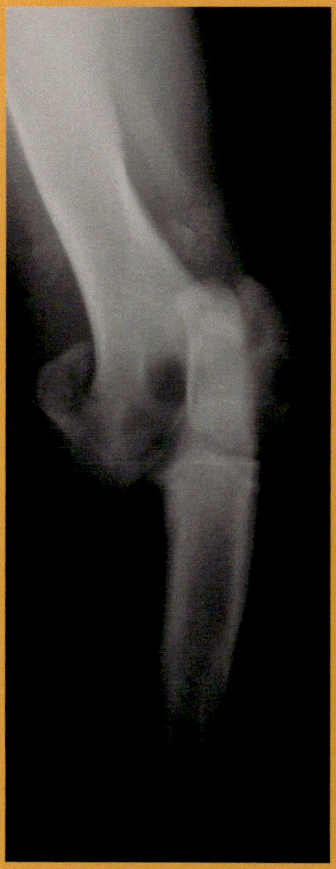

FIGURE 20. T fracture that affects the distal epiphysis of the humerus.

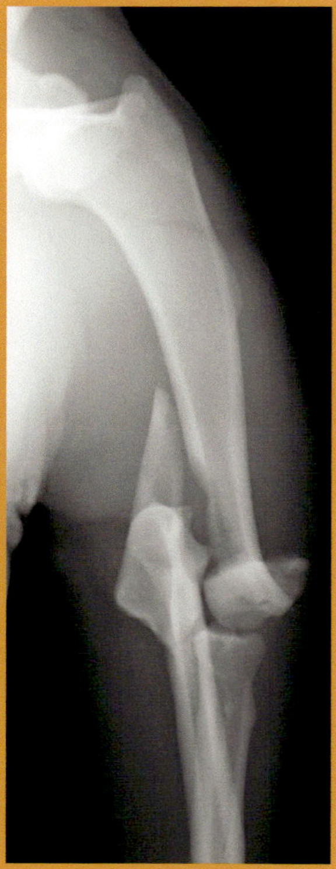

FIGURE 21. Y fracture of the distal epiphysis of the humerus.

- **Supracondylar:** supracondylar fractures are located just above the condyles (Fig. 22). They are actually metaphyseal fractures that, due to their aetiology, it is likely that they progress to a type I or II Salter-Harris fracture if they occur in growing patients.

  The largest problem in reducing this kind of fracture is the lack of space to correctly anchor implants to provide adequate stabilisation of the fracture without interfering with joint movement.

> *The primary difficulty in the treatment of joint fractures is properly reducing the joint surface without interfering with joint movement.*

Avulsion fractures

This type of fracture has been mentioned when discussing the type I Salter-Harris fractures. Classification of this type of fracture is complex given that it possesses a series of special characteristics that cannot be compared with any other types of fractures.

In avulsion fractures, the fracture line tends to separate itself (unlike most fractures, in which the fracture site tends to collapse when the limb bears weight, i.e. the fragments get closer together).

This is due to the fact that this type of fracture occurs as a consequence of a sudden traction caused by a ligament or a tendon at its insertion point. Type I Salter-Harris fractures are frequently caused, given that most bone protrusions that serve as the point of insertion to the tendons originate in a secondary ossification nucleus. In the case of sudden traction of the tendon, this fragment will more likely separate from the rest of the metaphysis from its corresponding growth plate. The mechanical resistance of the cartilaginous tissues that form said plate is inferior to the resistance of the fibrous tissues of the tendons and ligaments.

The most frequent avulsion fractures are produced in the tibial crest, at the patellar tendon insertion point (Fig. 23), and in the olecranon, from the triceps tendon.

In adult patients, as they have no growth cartilage, the fracture occurs in the weakest zone of the bone. The tibial crest is rarely injured in adult patients. However, the olecranon is frequently fractured in its narrowest zone of the semilunar notch (trochlear notch) of the ulna (Fig. 24). In these cases, the problems of joint fractures are added to those of the avulsion fracture.

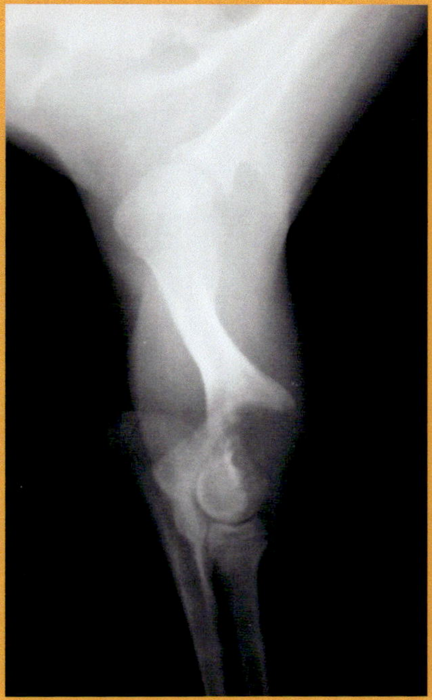

FIGURE 22. Supracondylar fracture of the distal epiphysis of the humerus.

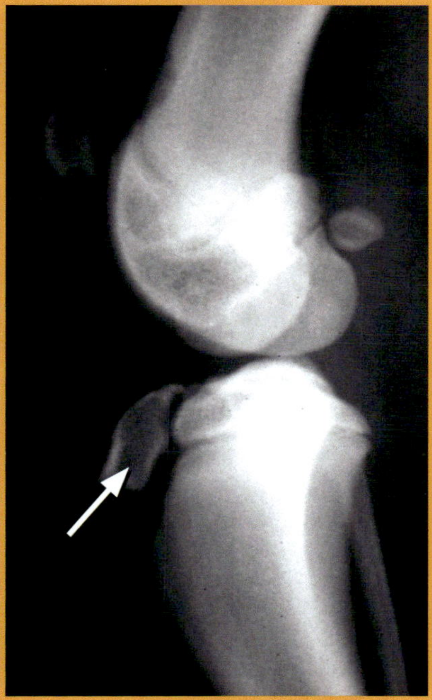

FIGURE 23. Avulsion of the tibial crest. Note how the fragment appears detached.

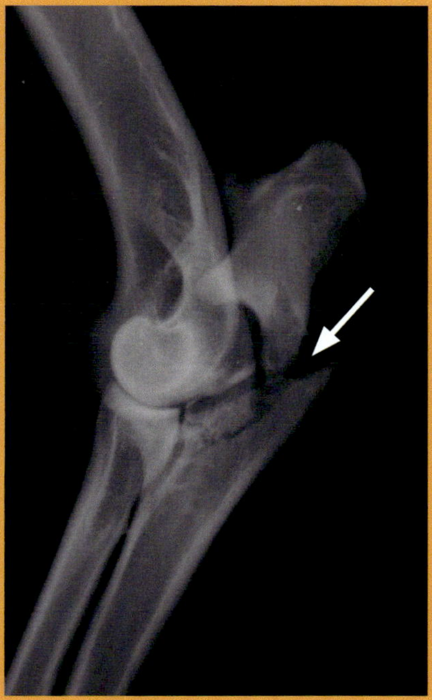

FIGURE 24. Fracture from avulsion of the olecranon in an adult patient.

JOINT FRACTURES

Joint fractures, fortunately, are not very frequent in bone surgery in small animals. Fractures of the lateral condyle of the distal epiphysis of the humerus in canines, during growth, is probably the most frequent.

When a joint fracture takes place, the surgeon is faced not only with the normal problems of all fractures, but also with a series of added difficulties that are described below:

- Difficult healing of the cartilage. This kind of fracture affects the joint surface that is covered by cartilaginous tissue, logically. This tissue has unique characteristics that should be taken into account when treatment is established.

  Cartilaginous tissue is a tissue that has no healing capacity of its own. Cartilage does not contain blood vessels. Its nutrition depends on the subchondral bone and the synovial fluid. If cuts were made on the cartilaginous surface of a joint without reaching the subchondral bone, and the joint was opened again after a few months, the cuts would remain unhealed.

  The healing of cartilage depends fundamentally on the cells of the subchondral tissue. That is, healing by second intention is always produced. During the process, cells from the edges of the lesion cover the defect with fibrous connective tissue (Fig. 25). This tissue, depending on the forces of pressure that its subjected to, transforms into a fibro-cartilaginous tissue that in turn progressively transforms into hypercellular cartilaginous tissue (it is not a proper cartilaginous tissue, but it is completely functional).

  As is the case with all lesions in which healing is produced by second intention, the speed of the repairing process depends on the size of the defect. In the case of cartilaginous tissue, a lesion of approximately 2 mm (diameter) takes approximately three months to be covered by functional tissue.

  In the particular case of cartilaginous tissue, forces of pressure play an important role in the transformation of the connective tissue into functional articular tissue. The lesions in areas of pressure are covered by hypercellular pseudo-cartilaginous tissue, while in areas with no pressure they are covered by dense connective tissue, which is much less physiological. In other words, for the ideal healing of cartilaginous lesions, the surface should be subjected to forces of pressure.
- The optimal reduction of the joint surface is indispensable. Another added problem of joint fractures is the need to perfectly reduce the joint surface, especially in the areas of contact with the adjacent bone surface. If the reduction of a fracture is deficient, a certain amount of inconsistency will be formed in the area of the fracture (Fig. 26). When the joint moves, this inconsistency will cause abnormal wearing of the surface of the other bone, which in the long term will cause problems of secondary joint degeneration.
- Other causes that complicate treatment and lead to a worse prognosis are:
  - Small size of fragment which makes stabilisation of the fracture more difficult.
  - Sufficient stability is needed to tolerate joint movements as soon as possible.

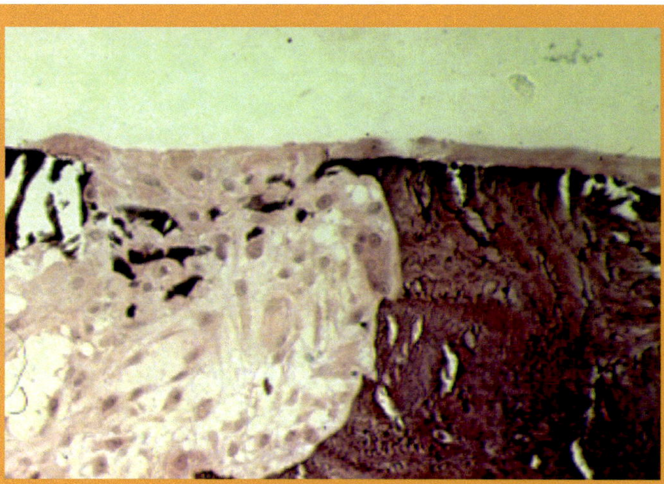

FIGURE 25. Bone tissue covered by fibrous tissue from the adjacent joint cartilage.

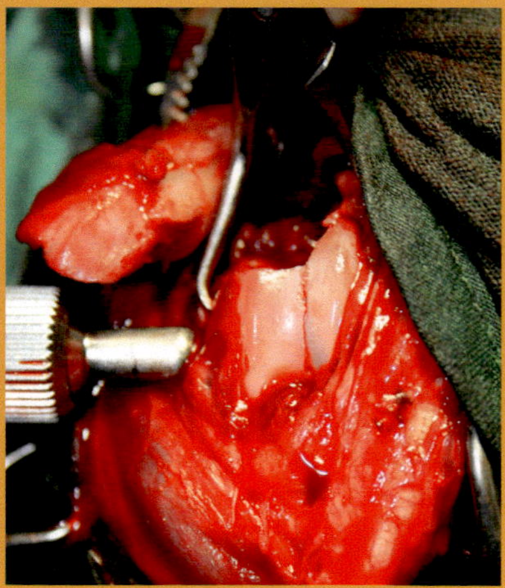

FIGURE 26. Proper reduction of a joint fracture.

Perhaps, to mention at least one advantage of this type of fracture compared to those produced in bone diaphyses, is that they occur in areas of the bone that are fundamentally made up of cancellous bone. As mentioned in the corresponding chapter, bone healing in this type of bone is much faster than if it were compact bone.

To conclude, all of these characteristics of the cartilaginous tissue imply certain particularities that must be taken into account when planning the treatment of a joint fracture.

Joint fractures must be treated as surgical emergencies as a delay in surgery could hinder the correct reduction of the joint surface.

First of all, in order to achieve perfect functional recovery of the joint, these fractures must be treated almost as if they were a surgical emergency. A delay in treatment would imply greater difficulty in achieving a perfect reduction. Especially if it is taken into account that in the epiphysis, the healing process starts soon as it is made up of cancellous bone.

To administer prompt treatment, the joint fracture must be diagnosed right away. In most cases, these kind of fractures are easily detected by routine X-rays. However, there are certain fractures that due to their direction or in the case that they are overlapped by other joint structures, they can be difficult to identify. When in doubt, stress X-rays should be taken, forcing the joint to the point where the ligament structures displace the fragments, thus making them visible by X-ray. In other cases, X-ray series must be taken in infrequent projections, to make the fracture lines visible (Fig. 27).

Diagnosis by means of CT scan may be equally useful as it allows for radiographic cross-sections in any necessary directions.

Treatment

Treatment of most joint fractures basically includes reduction of the joint surface and stabilisation using compression screws.

In certain cases, when the fracture occurs, fragments may be produced that are too small to be stabilised. In these cases, removing said fragments is preferable to taking the risk of them getting loose and circulating freely inside of the joint.

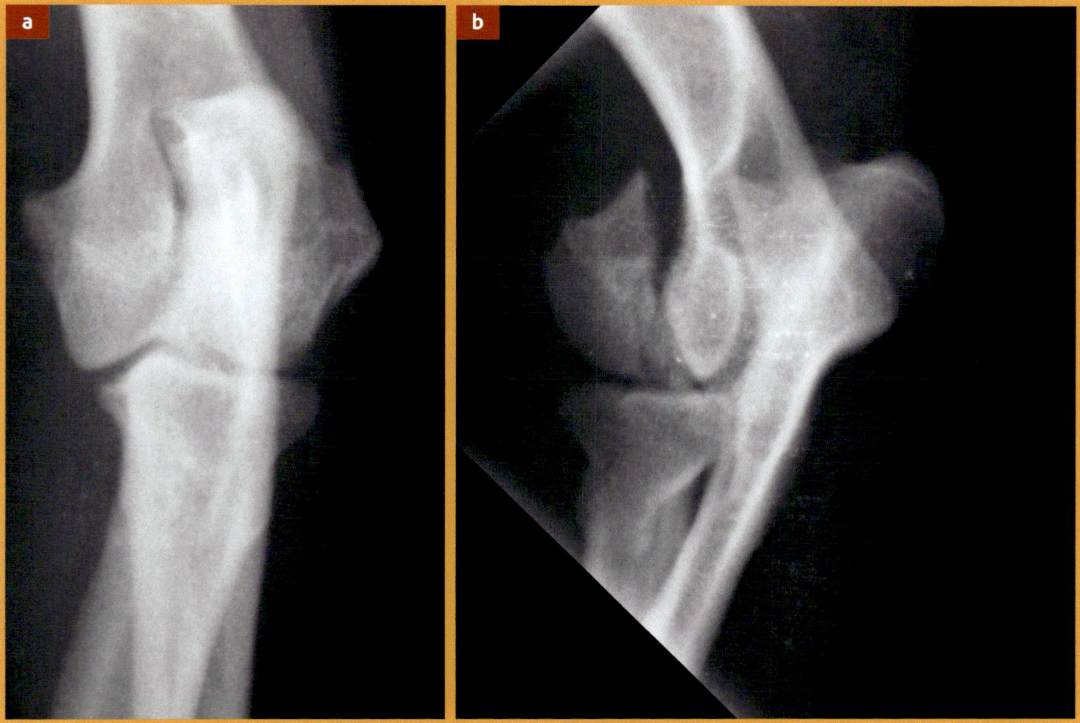

FIGURE 27. Cranio-caudal X-ray (a) and oblique X-ray (b) of a joint fracture. Note how the bone lesion is easier to see in the oblique view.

It is recommended that the small fragments that cannot be stabilised be removed to avoid them from moving freely in the joint where they can cause secondary joint degeneration.

When certain fragments must be removed, the clinician may be faced with a situation where the primary fragments do not fit together adequately. If this is the case, preserving the overall anatomical shape of the joint is preferable, sacrificing the perfect continuity of the cartilaginous surface (Fig. 28). The defect of the removed fragment will heal by second intention and be covered by functional pseudo-cartilaginous tissue.

On the other hand, premature joint movement after a surgical intervention is fundamental to avoid what is known as "joint disease". Joint immobility for a long period of time leads to the progressive loss of range of movement. This phenomena is the result of a loss of elasticity of the tissues surrounding the joint that can eventually be irreversible. In these cases, the joint can partially lose its function with the respective repercussions in the patient's quality of life.

Similarly, an optimal supply of nutrients from the synovial fluid is necessary to preserve the elasticity of the cartilaginous tissue itself. For this to happen, the intra-articular circulation of the synovial fluid must be correct, and this depends, primarily, on the joint movement.

It is possible that in some joint fractures, the small size of the bone fragments requires the use of minimal osteosynthesis systems that do not guarantee proper stability. In these cases, an accessory stabilisation system must be added to protect the implants. Depending on the location of the fracture, external bandaging or a temporary transarticular external fixation system will be necessary. Of course, these immobilisation systems must be removed as soon as possible, always taking into account the stability achieved, the complexity of the fracture, and the patient's age. Normally, a joint should not remain rigidly immobile for more than three weeks as it could cause ankylosis with loss of joint movement.

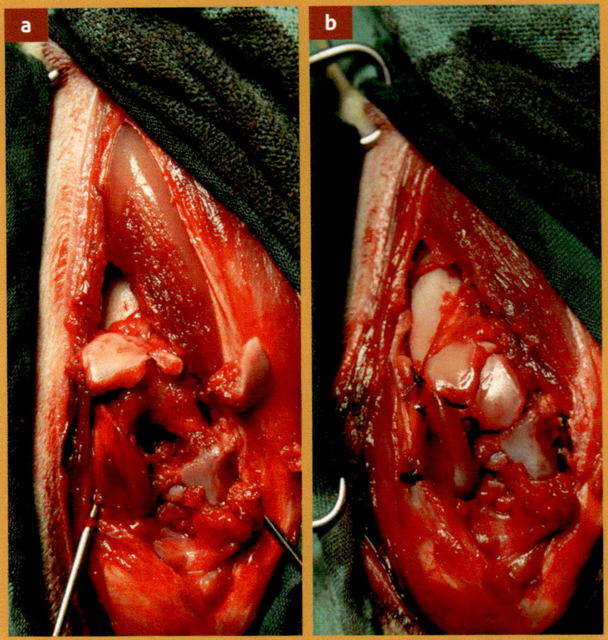

FIGURE 28. Comminuted fracture of the femoral trochlea before (a) and after being reduced (b). In spite of the lack of fragments, an attempt has been made to maintain the anatomical form.

Bone stimulation

4

Techniques used to improve the treatment of fractures by stimulating normal bone consolidation when there is a delay or when said consolidation is absent will be studied in this chapter. The objective of bone transplants and bone stimulation with platelet-rich plasma (PRP) or with substances that stimulate bone morphogenetic proteins (BMP) is to achieve faster bone formation to accelerate healing.

BONE TRANSPLANTS

A bone transplant consists of a bone tissue graft from a donor to a recipient. It can be done using bone from a donor, which is called an allograft, or from bone from the same patient, which is called an autograft.

Functions of the graft

There are three functions of a bone transplant: osteogenesis, osteoinduction and osteoconduction.

Osteogenesis

This process consists of the formation of new bone from the cellular elements that survive the transplant process.

After performing the autograft, approximately 95 % of the cells are destroyed. In this case, the surviving cells are differentiated in osteoblasts, which form new bone in approximately 8 days with a posterior mononuclear infiltration that destroys it. However, by that point, neovascularisation of the fracture site has taken place as well as the formation of a new bone matrix on which new bone can quickly form.

Osteoinduction

This process consists of stimulating the pluripotent cells of the tissues found at the fracture site, transforming them in osteogenic precursor cells, by means of the effect produced by a series of substances found in the transplanted bone. These substances are bone morphogenetic proteins, known as BMP. The osteoinductor effect is only produced around the transplanted tissue in a radius equal or lesser than 150 μm. This implies that when a cancellous bone transplant is performed, efforts should be made to distribute the material to all areas where ossification will take place. All of the cancellous bone should not be concentrated in one single point.

> *The osteoinduction effect of the graft has an action radius of 150 μm, and therefore the material must be distributed to all of the ossification areas.*

Osteoconduction

This is the process by which the grafted material acts as a guide to the structure of the new tissue formed. It also serves as a passive source of support for the newly formed blood vessels.

In osteoconduction, the osteoclasts begin to form tunnels in the graft, forming the Howship's lacunae. Later, these lacunae are invaded by new vessels through which the osteoblasts arrive. The newly formed bone deposits in concentric layers, destroying the tunnels, except for in its most central part where an arteriole is located. This way, the osteon is formed. All of the transplanted bone is substituted by new bone by a process that lasts for several years. It has been calculated that one year after the transplant, approximately 60 % of the bone material will have been substituted. At that moment, the bone will have acquired a level of mechanical resistance similar to that of a normal bone.

TYPES OF BONE TRANSPLANTS

Taking into account the type of bone being grafted, there are two types of bone transplants:

- Cancellous bone transplant.
- Compact bone transplant.

Cancellous bone transplant

Its function is to stimulate the formation of new bone. This is achieved by supplying viable osteoblasts to the fracture site, as well as the protein that stimulates bone formation (BMP). That is, its functions include osteogenesis and osteoinduction.

As previously mentioned, the cancellous bone is rich in undifferentiated mesenchymal cells with a high survival capacity, given that it can induce the formation of new vessels. This bone material is obtained from bone areas rich in trabecular bone (flat bones and the metaphyses of long bones). The areas where cancellous bone is typically obtained for transplants are the greater tubercle of the humerus and the iliac crest, given the easy access to said areas as well as the relatively high quantity of material that can be extracted (Figs. 1 and 2). In certain cases and due to the coincidence with the approach that has already been carried out to treat the fracture, small quantities can be obtained from the greater trochanter of the femur and the proximal metaphysis of the tibia.

When considering a transplant of cancellous bone, it is important to keep in mind that, as previously mentioned, it is a living tissue. This fact imposes two conditions: first, obtaining the tissue must be done in conditions of absolute sterility; and second, the viability of the cells must be preserved. Ideally, the cancellous bone should be extracted and directly transplanted in the fracture site (Fig. 3a). If this is not possible, the graft must be kept as little time as possible outside of the organism, storing it wrapped in moistened sterile gauze in some type of isotonic medium. A good alternative is to use gauze soaked in the patient's own blood (Fig. 3b).

Cancellous bone transplants are applied in:

- *Non-unions.*
- *Arthrodesis.*
- *Comminuted fractures.*

Compact bone transplant

The functions of the compact bone transplant are to serve as a structural base and orient the bone healing process. Also, the transplant provides stability to the osteosynthesis system impeding movements in the fracture site. The essential functions are osteoconduction and mechanical fastening.

Two basic types of compact bone can be differentiated depending on their origin, if they are autologous (obtained from the same patient) and heterologous (obtained from a donor).

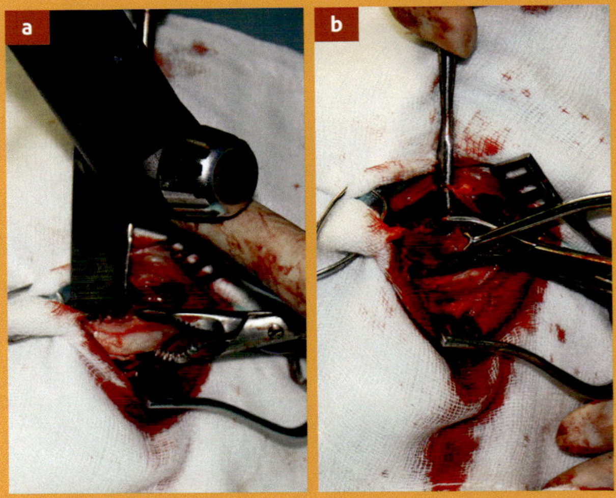

FIGURE 1. Obtaining cancellous bone from the iliac crest.

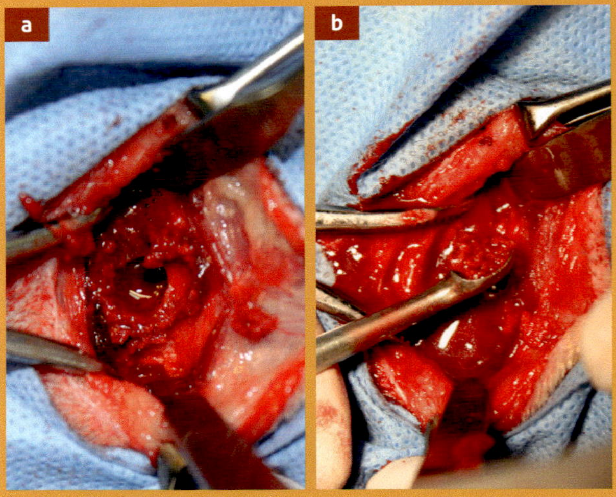

FIGURE 2. Obtaining cancellous bone from the proximal metaphysis of the humerus.

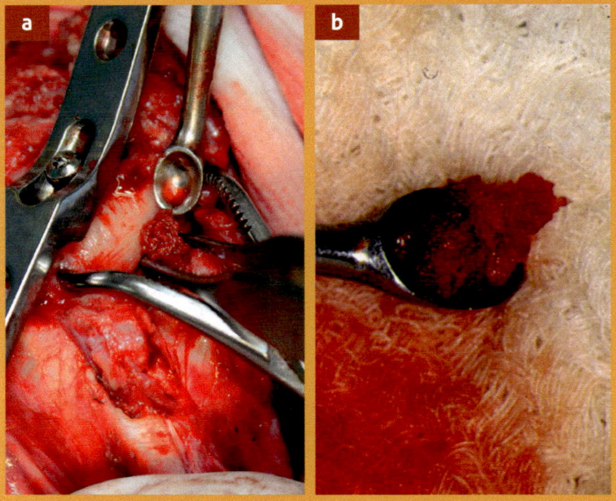

FIGURE 3. Handling the graft. Cancellous tissue deposited in the fracture site (a) and bone tissue preserved in gauze soaked in the patient's own blood (b).

Autologous transplant

An autologous transplant must be obtained, logically, from areas that will not cause any harm or discomfort to the animal. Consequently, they are normally taken from the ulna (Fig. 4), iliac crest (Fig. 5), or the patient's ribs. When performing this type of transplant, there is also certain osteoinduction as a consequence of the supply of immune-compatible live cells.

Heterologous transplant

This transplant is of poorer quality, given that there is a possibility that it be rejected. Extreme measures of asepsis must be followed when obtaining the material. The bone fragment, obtained from a patient that will later be euthanised, is usually taken from the same bone as that of the recipient bone, which will be transplanted. Given that donors are not always easily available, one solution is to create a bone bank.

Once the bone material has been obtained in the previously mentioned manner, all adhered soft tissues must be removed from the bone along with the periostium. The clean bone must be introduced in a sterile plastic bag where it will be stored until it is used.

One of the most used storage systems, given that it is not expensive, is freezing.

A bone that has been correctly extracted can be stored for at least half of a year at a temperature of -20 °C.

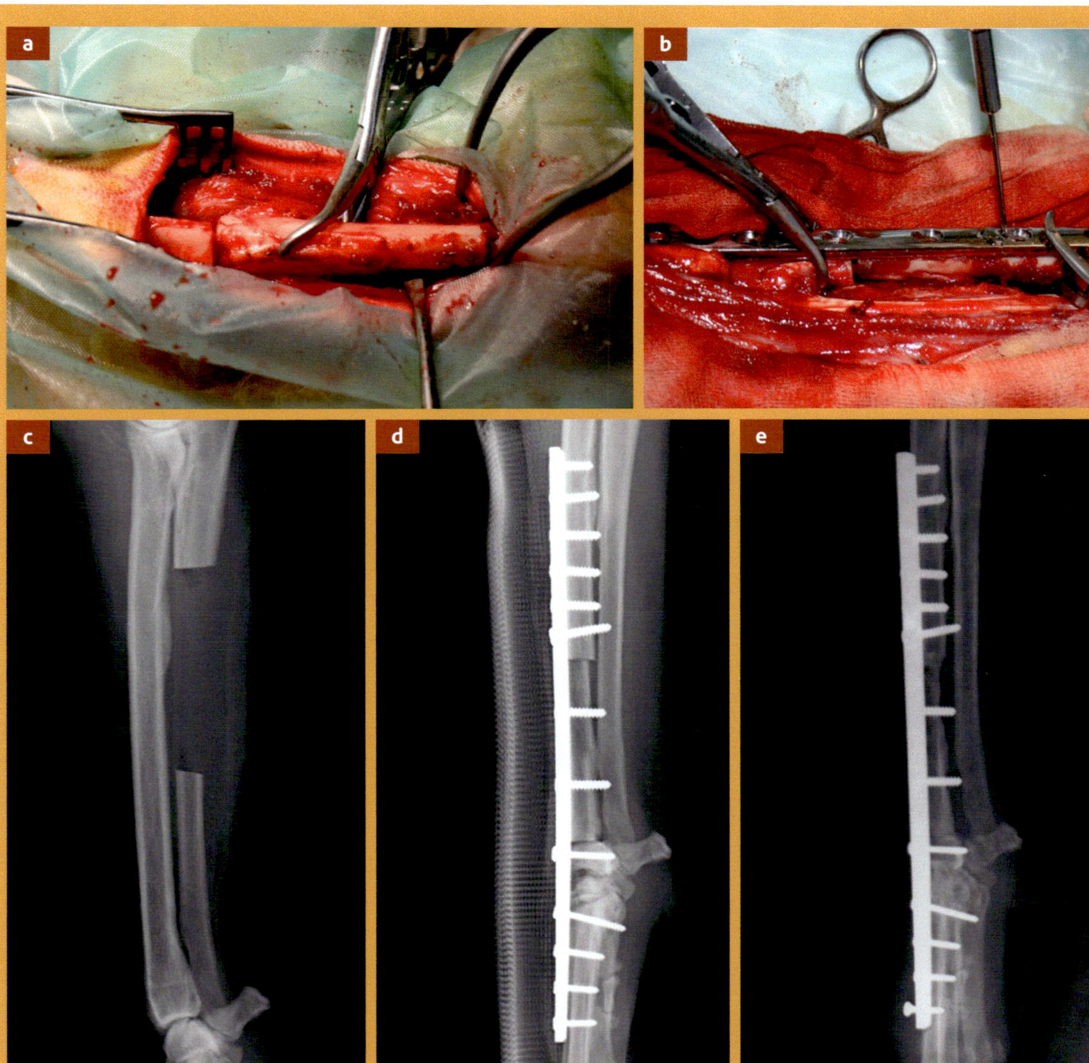

FIGURE 4. Extraction (a) and placement (b) of an autologous ulnar transplant in an osteosarcoma of the radius. The areas of extraction and osteointegration of the bone fragment are observed in these X-rays (c, d and e).

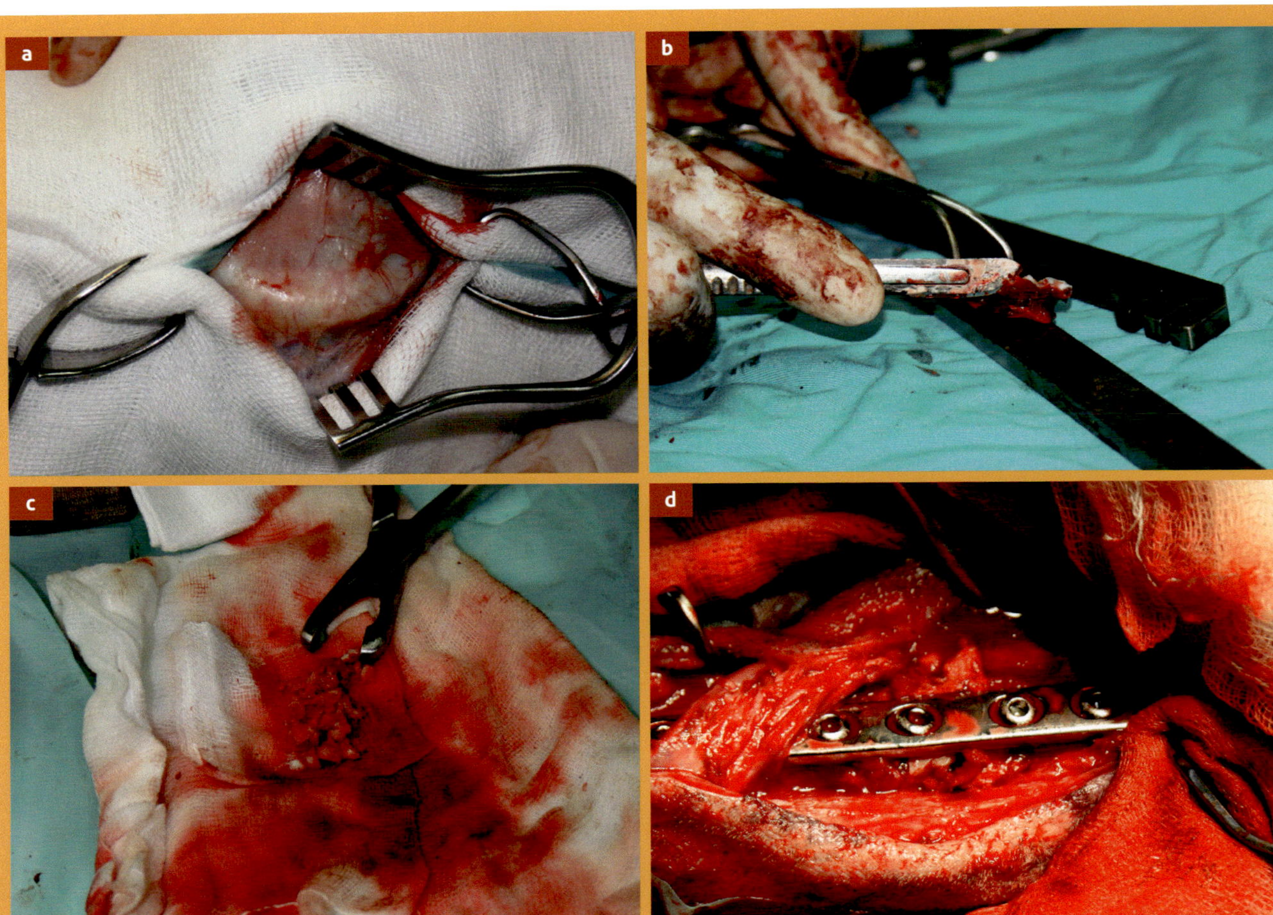

FIGURE 5. Performance of a autologous transplant from the iliac crest. Iliac wing approach (a), removing muscle remnants and fragmentation of the distal portion of the wing (b and c) and the graft of the cortico-spinal tissue in the fracture site from the same individual (d).

There is another type of heterologous compact bone available on the market that is formed by small fragments that are commercialised in different sizes to be used in bone defects. They are called bone "chips" (Fig. 6). They are usually used mixed with cancellous bone to increase the volume of "filling" material, as well as to act as support for neovascularisation (osteoconduction function, Fig. 7).

Their use is limited to:

a. Replacing a fragment of compact bone (serving as support and direction).
b. Filling the defect using bone chips (serving as a guide).

Due to the lack of osteogenic function of this type of graft, a cancellous bone transplant must always be performed on both fragment edges. Similarly, proper stability is essential. Given that the edges of the graft will be subjected to processes of

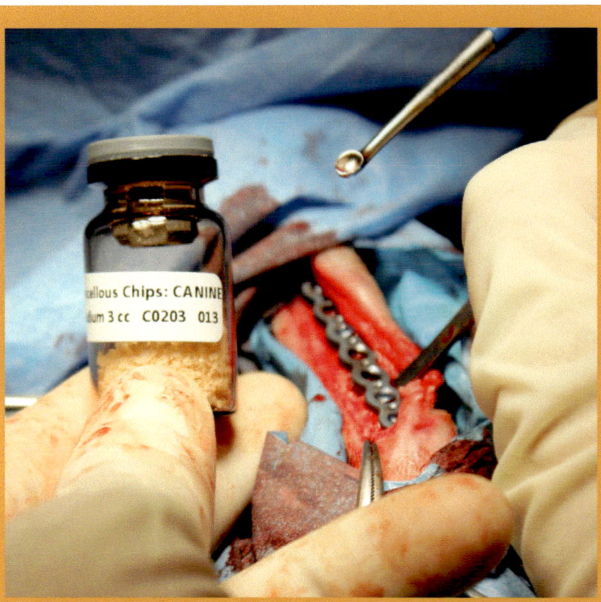

FIGURE 6. Use of bone chips to fill bone defects.

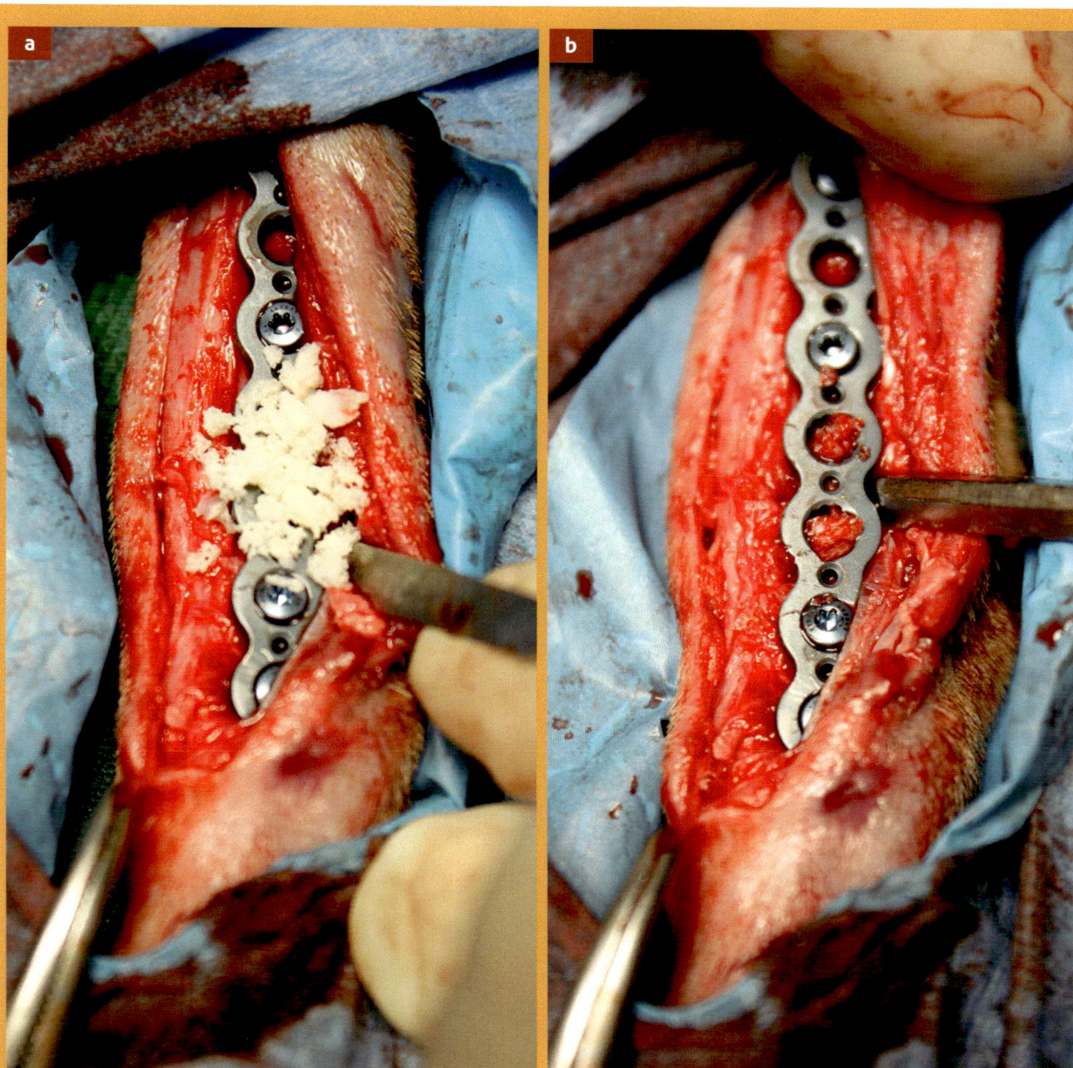

FIGURE 7. The bone chips are deposited on top of the fracture, once the plate has been placed (a) and they are mixed with cancellous bone (b).

reabsorption, which are more accentuated when dealing with non-vascular tissues, avoiding micromovements is of utmost importance. For this reason, axial compression should always be applied from the healthy bone towards both edges of the compact bone graft, which is achieved using dynamic compression plates (DCP).

BMP OR PRP GRAFTS

Also called artificial osteoinduction, this refers to a stimulation technique for bone consolidation through the application of substances that simulate the BMP, such as the dibotermin alfa (rhBMP-2). The use of this substance in veterinary bone surgery is very recent and its function is to stimulate bone healing. The rhBMP-2 can be used in cases of non-union or as a preventive measure in comminuted fractures to accelerate healing. It is a liquid that once soaked in a substrate, similar to a compress, it can be placed in contact with the edges of the primary fragments (Fig. 8). BMP strengthen healing phenomena and therefore accelerate bone formation (Fig. 9).

> *Substances should never be used in infected fracture sites as they would have no affect whatsoever.*

Another possibility to accelerate healing processes is to deposit platelet-rich plasma in the fracture site (PRP)

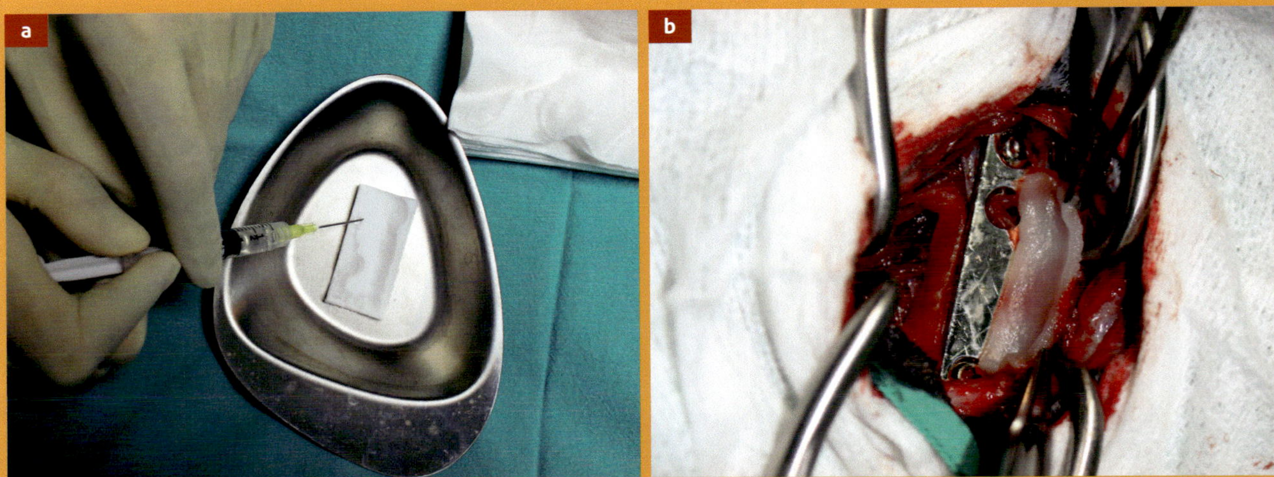

FIGURE 8. Process to soak the compress with dibotermin alfa (rhBMP-2) (a). Once the indicated time has passed, the compress is placed in contact with the edges of both fragments (b).

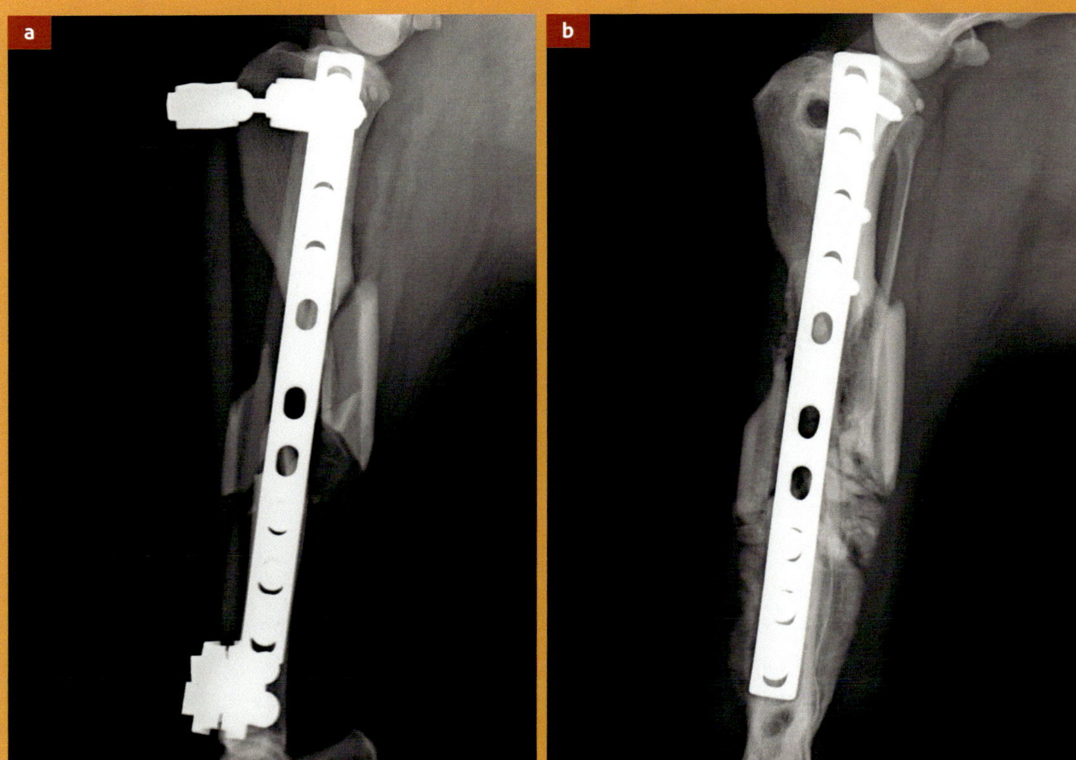

FIGURE 9. Exuberant consolidation of a comminuted tibia fracture treated using BMP

(Fig. 10). It has been observed that platelet-rich blood extract possesses substances that favour revascularisation and the activation of healing phenomena of the tissues. When these substances are deposited in the fracture site, healing phenomena are accelerated (Fig. 11).

The PRP can be mixed with cancellous bone to prevent possible complications that are inherent to comminuted fractures even if the fracture site is infected. In the case of delayed healing, they can also be inoculated percutaneously without having to intervene once again on the patient.

The effect of the PRP and BMP should never substitute deficient stabilisation of a fracture, they are supporting systems.

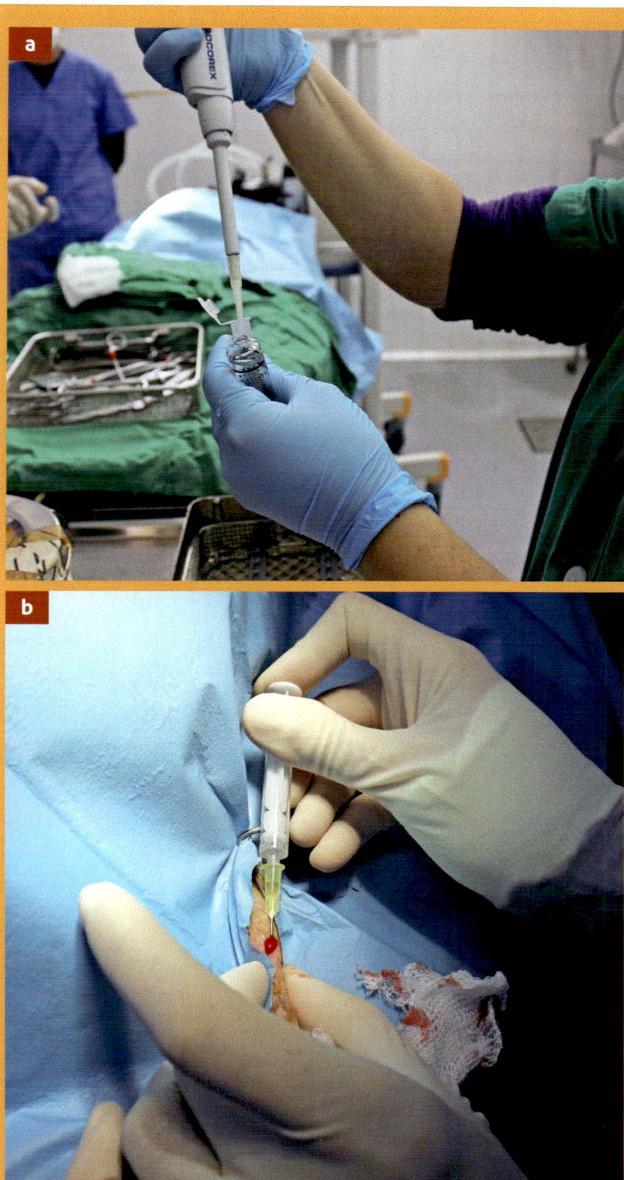

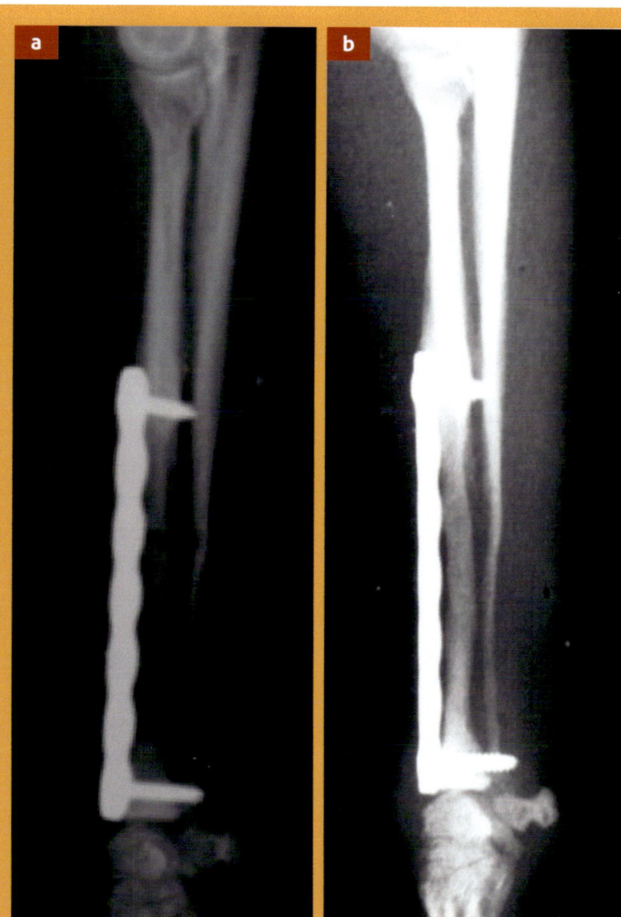

FIGURE 11. Previous case before (a) and after treatment (b). Note the increase in bone density under the graft.

FIGURE 10. Activation of PRP with calcium bicarbonate (a) and percutaneous injection in an area of loss of bone density caused by the overprotection of the graft (protection stress) (b).

5 Osteosynthesis systems and biomechanics

BIOMECHANICS AND THEIR APPLICATION IN DIFFERENT OSTEOSYNTHESIS SYSTEMS

Pins

The intramedullary fixation system is the first internal stabilisation system that was developed to treat fractures. Basically, this system consists of introducing a metal rod through the medullary cavity of a fractured bone to impede any excess movement at the level of the fracture site. This way, time is given for bone to form around the fracture through specific healing processes.

Intramedullary fixation is done using nails or pins. Both implants are made of surgical metal rods (steel or titanium), and their only difference is their diameter (Fig. 1). Implants with a diameter greater than 2 mm are called Steinmann pins while those that are thinner are called Kirschner pins.

The stability provided by this type of implants is primarily due to their resistance to flexion (Fig. 2). That is, as long as the forces of flexion to which a bone is subjected when bearing weight does not surpass the flexibility of the implant, it will continue to perform its function (Fig. 3). It is a dynamic system given that it allows for certain bending movements of the bone. The forces of pressure on the fracture site vary depending on the direction in which the implant curves.

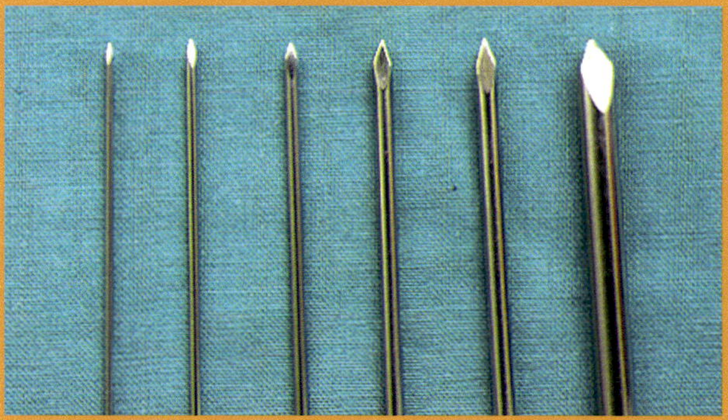

FIGURE 1. Sample of pins with different diameters.

The resistance of the pins is directly proportional to their diameter. Using the largest implant possible (as long as there is enough space in the intramedullary cavity) is the best option.

The resistance of the implant is directly proportional to the diameter of the pin, increasing exponentially with its thickness. Therefore, using the largest implant possible (as long as there is enough space in the intramedullary cavity) is the best option.

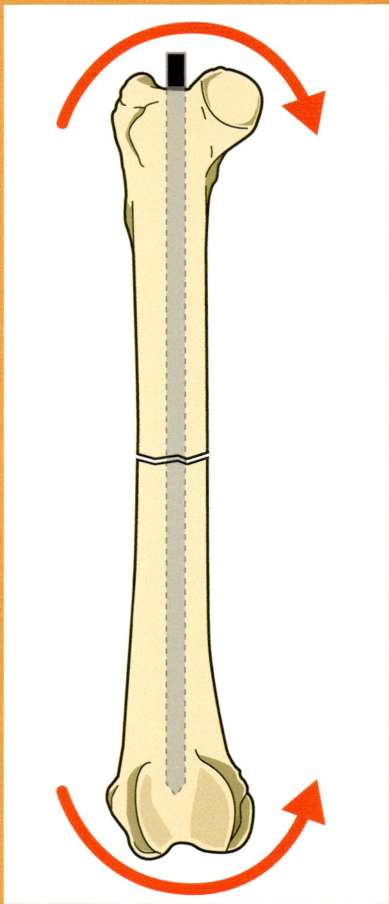

FIGURE 2. Representation of the forces of flexion that a bone may be subjected to and that must be compensated by the implant.

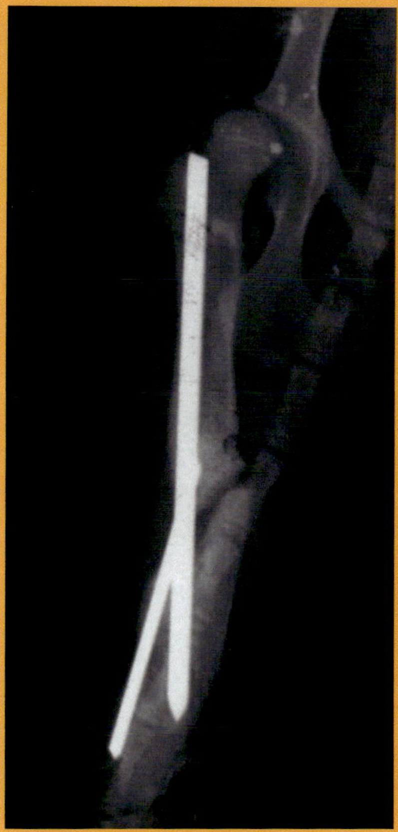

FIGURE 3. X-ray image of an implant bent from forces of flexion. The implant is too thin.

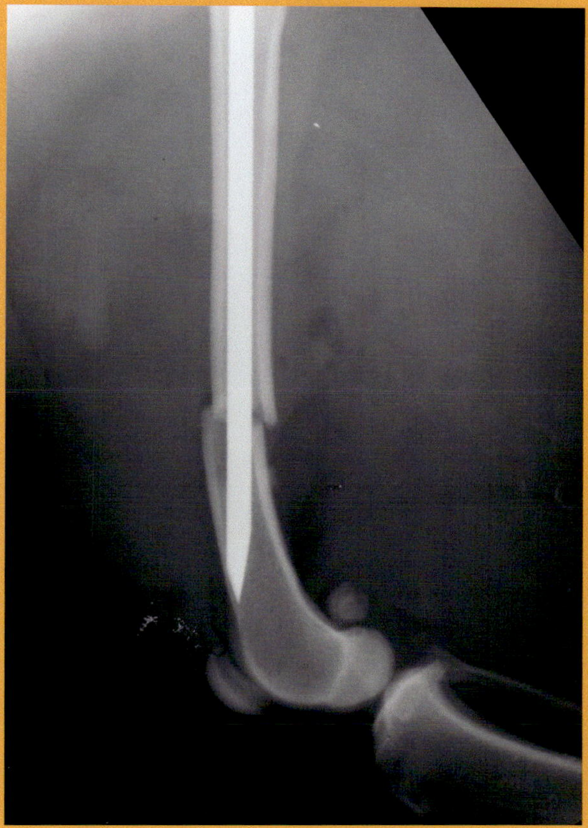

FIGURE 4. The contact of the pin with the compact bone impedes shearing movements.

Interrupting the bone's intramedullary blood supply should not be a concern if the medullary cavity is completely filled by the implant. There are experimental studies that demonstrate that even though 95 % of the section of the medullary cavity is occupied, neovascularisation will still take place correctly.

Intramedullary pinning impedes shearing movements of the fracture site, that is, strictly lateral displacement of both of the primary fragments. The pin acts as a block against this type of movement as the implant is trapped between the internal portion of the compact bone of both of the primary fragments (Fig. 4). The capacity of the intramedullary fixation system to neutralise this type of displacement depends, once again, on the relationship between the diameter of the pin and that of the medullary cavity. The lesser the space between the compact bone and the pin, the sooner the lateral displacement of the fragments will be blocked. However, the stability of this implant against displacement is relatively poor.

The primary problem of this type of fixation system is its complete ineffectiveness to neutralise movements of rotation and separation-approximation of the primary fragments as shown in Figure 5. The displacement of the edges (one over the other) in the fracture site delays healing processes given that parallel displacement of both compact bone portions is caused (Fig. 6).

More than one pin can be inserted into the medullary cavity in an attempt to stabilise movements of rotation. It should be reiterated that, although this technique partially avoids the "hinge" effect, it does not guarantee good stability against movements of rotation.

Similarly, and following the hinge simile, both fragments can be separated just as a door is unhinged by lifting it up.

In practice, pinning does not counteract the forces of traction that fracture lines are subjected to. It also is incapable of counteracting axial loads for the same reason, and thus, if the fracture site is not stable against forces of pressure, the system will fail (Fig. 7).

When a fracture site is subjected to movements of flexion, the fracture line area located in the compact bone portion near where the flexion is produced, is subjected to forces of compression, while the other portion is subjected to forces

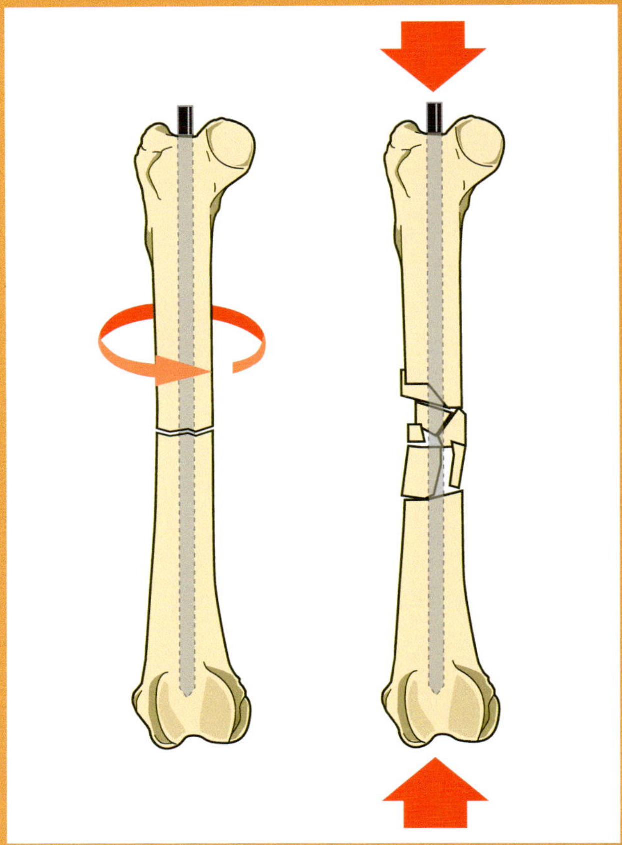

FIGURE 5. Representation of the movements of rotation and collapse that a fractured bone may suffer. The implant inside of the medullary cavity would act as a "rod" inside of a "tube", both fragments could freely turn like a hinge of a door.

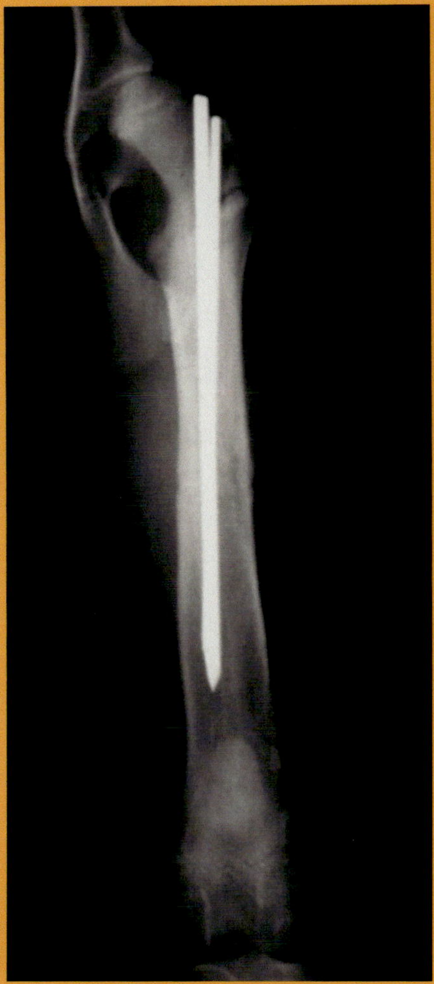

FIGURE 6. X-ray image of a fracture with an intramedullary implant. This femur, in spite of the instability caused by movements of rotation in relation with the axial axis, has healed.

of traction. This movement is produced in all directions of the space. Due to the fact that intramedullary fixation is not capable of completely stabilising the bone fragments, the fracture callus that forms acquires the shape of a spinning top, bulging more where there is greater instability (Fig. 8).

This movement pushes the pin softly but consistently towards its ends. If the movement is intense enough to surpass the force with which the pin is fastened to the bone tissue, it will loosen and come out of where it was introduced. This is known as implant migration. When this happens, all stability is lost (Fig. 9).

The stability that this type of fixation system gives also depends on the length of the primary fragments. When one of the bone fragments is short, the portion of the implant that is introduced into the medullary cavity may not be able to provide the stability needed to keep the fragments from moving. With shorter fragments, side-to-side movements will be less compensated and thus possibilities of migration will be greater. Highly distal fractures can never be stabilised with an intramedullary fixation system alone (Fig. 10).

Diaphyseal fractures that are located very proximal to the epiphyses cannot be stabilised with an intramedullary fixation system alone.

It must be taken into account that the intramedullary pins almost always stick out on one end of the bone where they are inserted. This limits the number of bones in which they can be used as an osteosynthesis system given that by sticking out from one end, they will invade and damage the

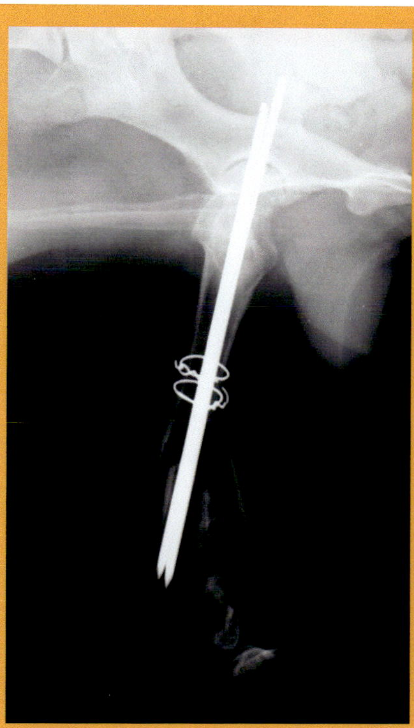

FIGURE 7. X-ray showing a collapsed fracture site improperly treated with intramedullary fixation.

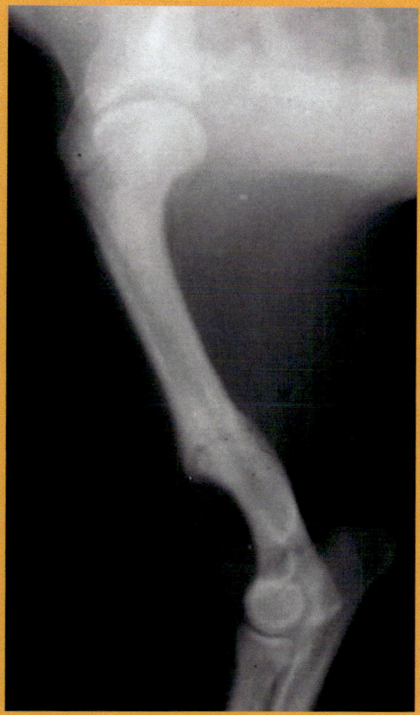

FIGURE 8. X-ray image showing a bone callus that originates in a fracture treated with an intramedullary implant as a consequence of forces of flexion.

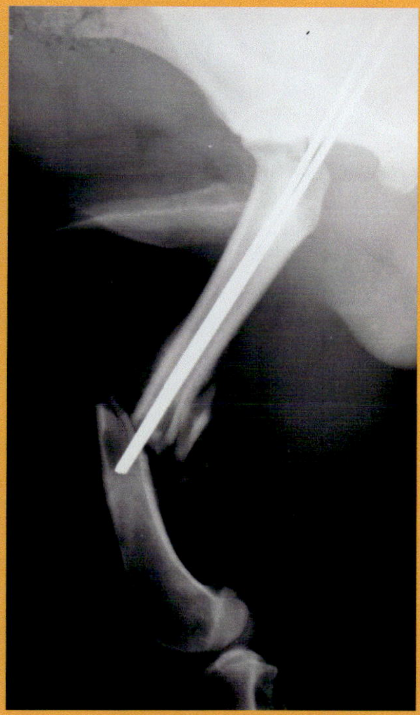

FIGURE 9. X-ray image of a case of migration and loss of stability. Note how the implants stick out proximally.

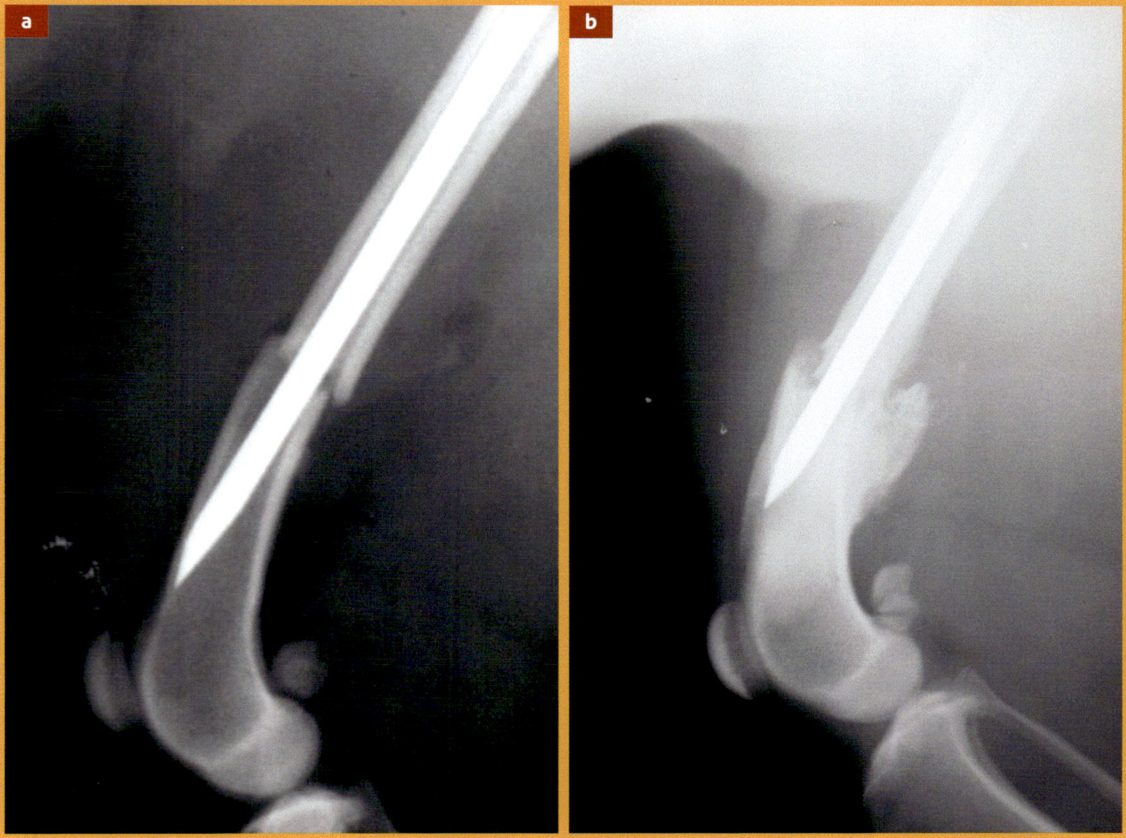

FIGURE 10. X-ray images of one patient that experienced migration and failed intra-medullary fixation.

respective joint. This happens, for example, in the proximal and distal epiphyses of the radius, and in the distal epiphysis of the femur (Fig. 11).

The point where the implant is anchored, which is responsible for keeping it inside of the medullary cavity of the bone, is precisely the epiphyseal zone where it will emerge. The friction index between the implant and the compact bone is what provides the fracture with stability. This coefficient of friction depends on the thickness of the compact bone, the hardness of the bone, the diameter of the pin and even the system chosen for its insertion. The insertion of intramedullary pins can be done in two different ways:

a. **Normograde insertion**: this consists of inserting the pin from one end of the bone towards the fracture site, introducing it through the medullary cavity of the opposite fragment until it comes into contact with the intramedullary metaphyseal zone (Fig. 12).
b. **Retrograde insertion**: the pin is first inserted from the fracture site towards the bone epiphysis that can be crossed through without causing any joint damage. It is pushed until the tip of the implant is evened with the edge of the fracture line. The fracture is reduced and the pin is inserted, pushing it from the end from which is sticks out until it hits the opposite metaphysis (Fig. 13).

This system is simpler given that, for normograde insertion, the clinician must possess extensive anatomical knowledge to successfully introduce the implant from one of the epiphyses so that it enters correctly into the medullary cavity of the other fragment. However, on a positive note, its anchoring provides more stability as the implant only has to "pass" through the compact bone that it is fastened to once. Regarding retrograde insertion, the pin passes through the epiphysis twice, once when exiting, and again when being reinserted. The fit of the pin is not as tight in this case and it is more likely that it will migrate.

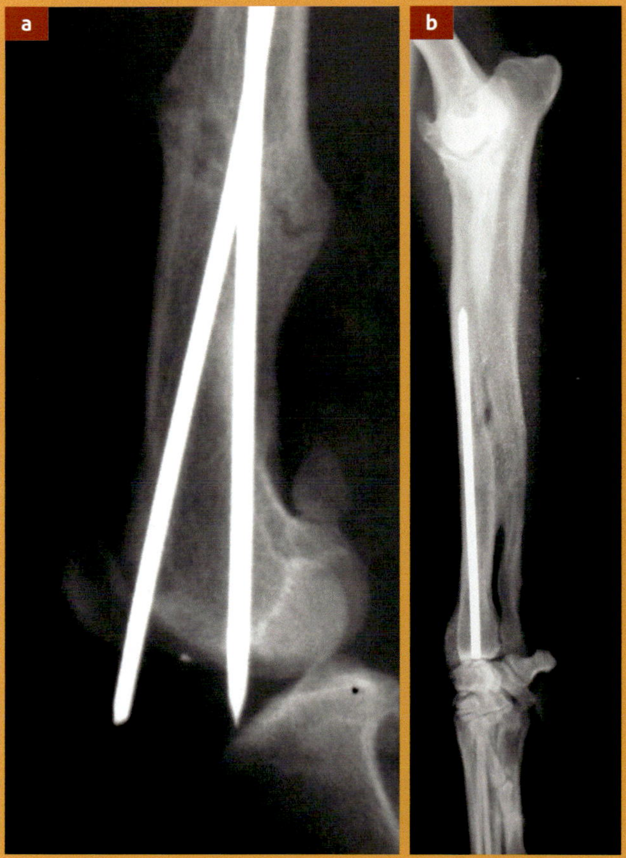

FIGURE 11. X-ray image showing how the pins come into contact with and damage the nearby joint. Stifle joint (a). Radius-ulna joint (b).

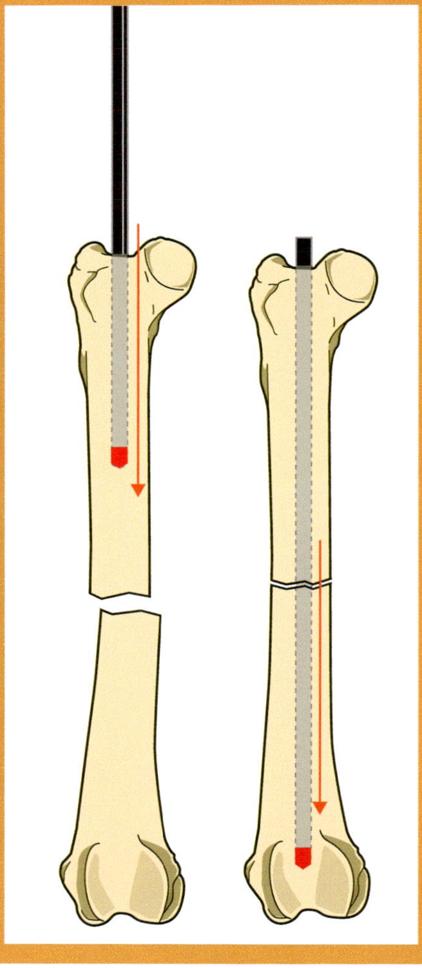

FIGURE 12. Representation of the insertion of a pin in a normograde manner. Note that the pin is inserted through the epiphysis of the bone (arrow).

One possibility to avoid the pin's tendency to migrate is to bend the tip that sticks out from the bone. When bent, it is less likely that the tip will pierce the soft tissues that it comes into contact with. This way, they also impede its movement (Fig. 14). If the clinician wants to remove the pin, it will also be easier to pull it out.

If more than one pin are inserted, the first one can be inserted in a retrograde manner, and the others can be inserted in a normograde manner, using the first as a guide.

To conclude, this system is not usually the best surgical option to be used alone. It is usually associated with other implants that correct its shortcomings (cerclages, external fixation or plates).

Rush pins

Rush pins are a variety of this osteosynthesis system. They are actually found somewhere between intramedullary fixation and other types of systems.

They were originally intramedullary pins, but as osteosynthesis systems have evolved, they are currently grouped under this name (Rush pins as well as fixation systems using pins).

> ***Rush pins constitute the only fixation system capable of stabilising fractures that affect growth plates.***

This system is the only possibility existing to stabilise fractures that occur at the growth plate level. As previously mentioned, this type of fractures present the peculiarity that they cannot be stabilised with any system that joins both fragments using a rigid bridge. That is, they must be stabilised without interfering in the longitudinal growth processes of the bone. On the other hand, they are fractures that are always located on the bone metaphyses, which means

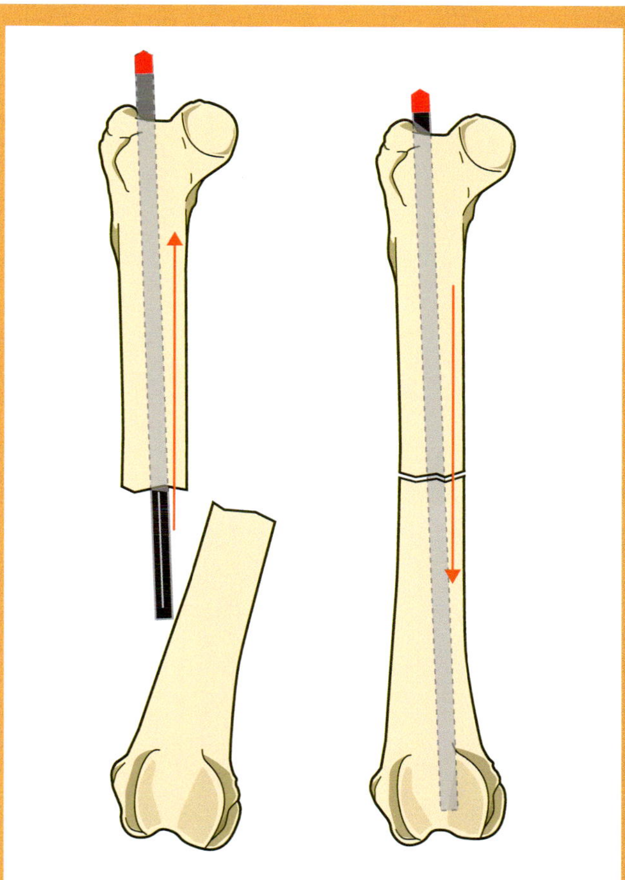

FIGURE 13. Representation of the insertion of a pin in a retrograde manner. Note that the pin is introduced through the fracture site (arrow).

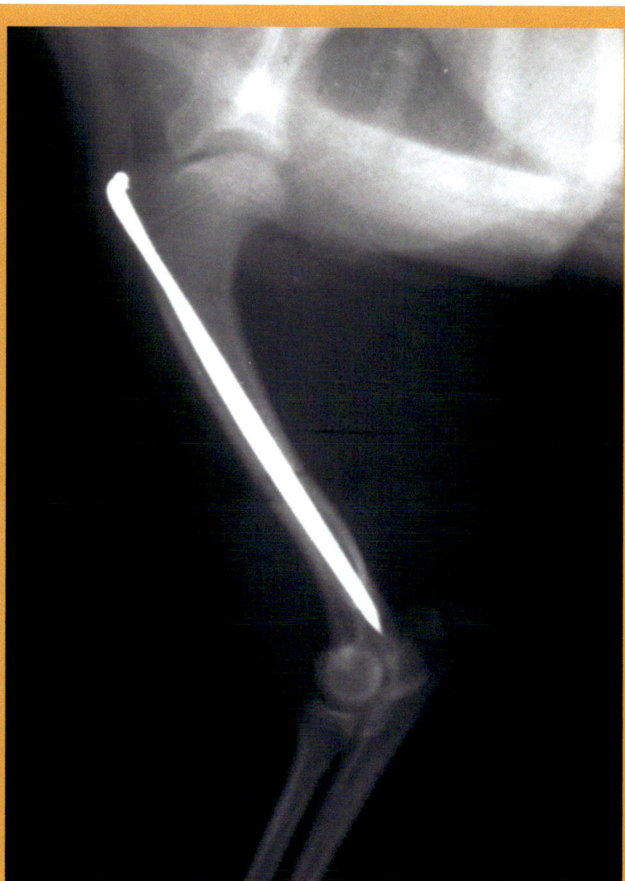

FIGURE 14. X-ray image showing the bending of the proximal end of the pin to avoid it from moving and damaging the surrounding tissues.

that one of the fragments is always small. There is almost always a joint nearby.

Obviously, the osteosynthesis material should never invade the joint areas that directly come into contact with the cartilaginous surface of the adjacent bone. The implant is frequently located inside of a joint, but it should never be placed in a position that could interfere with the joint's movement.

When faced with these circumstances, the only possibility is to stabilise the smaller fragment, the epiphysis, fastening it using pins that cross the growth line perpendicularly. Perforations with a diameter of less than 2 mm, performed perpendicularly to the growth plate, do not significantly interfere with its growth.

In the past, the Rush pins were smaller than 2 mm and their tip was similar to the front portion of a ski (Fig. 15). Once the fracture was reduced, perforations were made using a drill with an angle that was adequate for the pins (after their insertion) to slide over the endostium of the medullary cavity. Later, the pins that were fixated when their tip exerted pressure from the inside of the medullary cavity were introduced (Fig. 16).

As the bone grew in length, the pins slid over the endostium of the medullary cavity. This way, they preserved their stabilising function without interfering in the bone's growth.

Kirschner pins

Currently, Rush pins are hardly commercialised. Kirschner pins are now used in their place (Fig. 17). Once inserted, the tip that sticks out is bent using a bender, forming a "hook" that will serve as leverage, dragging the pins as the bone grows (Fig. 18).

It is best to impact and adapt the "hooks" into the compact bone to avoid harming the joint, as well as avoiding migration as much as possible (Fig. 19).

The growth potential varies with the age of the patient and the younger the patient, the less they should be interfered with. As the Rush pins are not firmly anchored in the

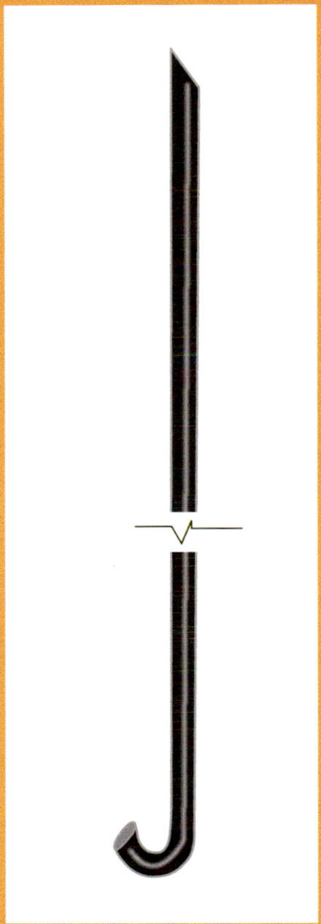

FIGURE 15. Graphic representation of a Rush pin, note the ends.

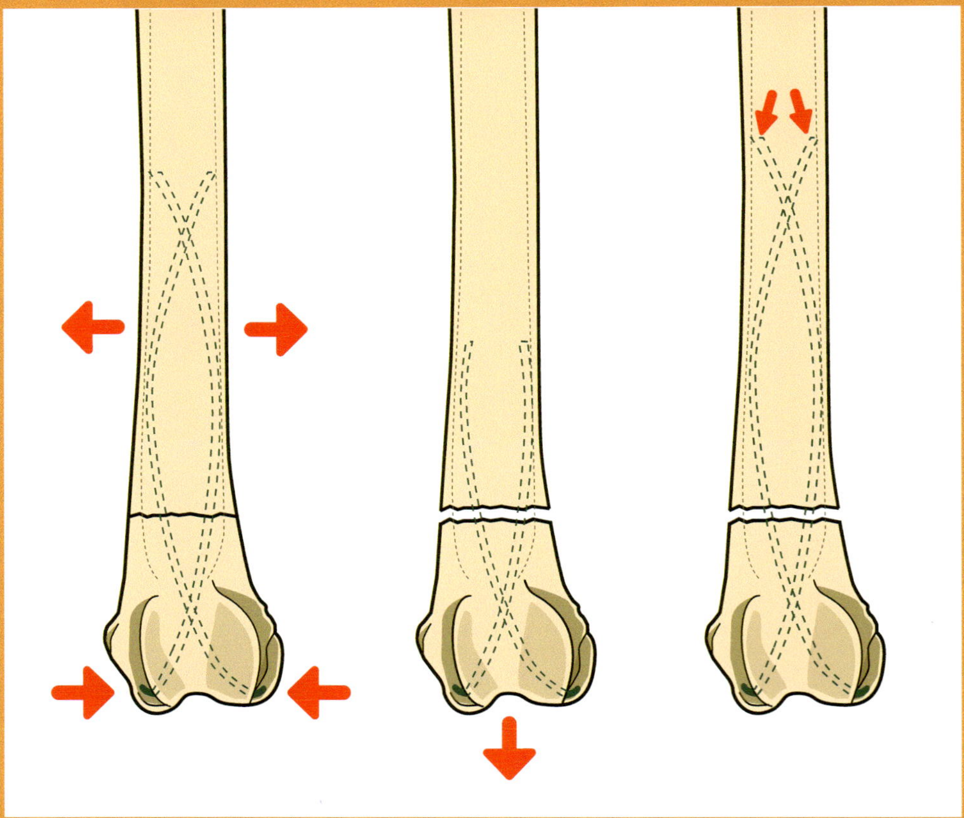

FIGURE 16. Graphic representation of fixation using Rush pins.

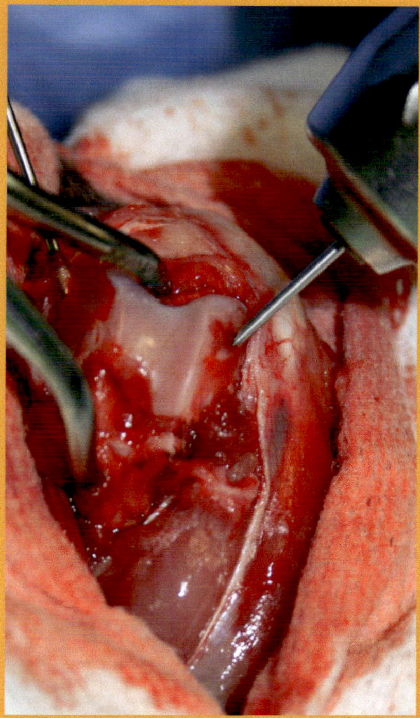

FIGURE 17. Reduction and insertion of the pins.

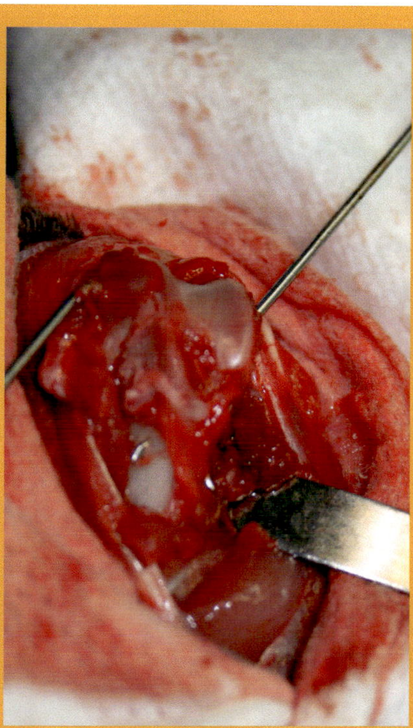

FIGURE 18. Bending the pins.

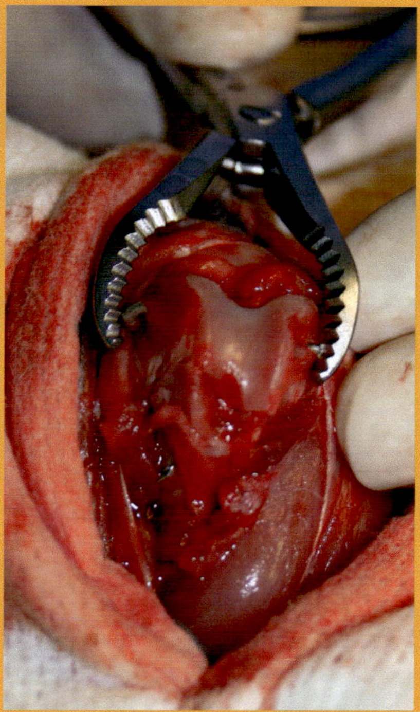

FIGURE 19. Pins cut and adapted to the bone surface.

Kirschner pins

Before inserting the Kirschner pins, they should be cut to the same size so that one of them serves as a reference to know how far the first one has been inserted (it is placed outside of the compact bone with the same orientation). When the second pin is inserted, the portion that sticks out of the first inserted pin is used as a reference.

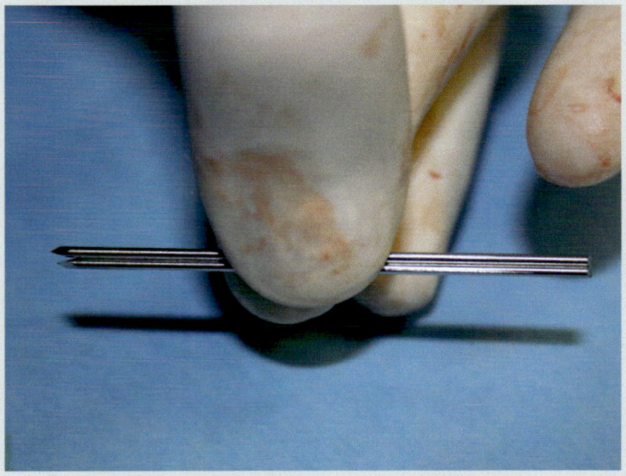

Rush pins cut to the same length.

diaphyseal fragment, their stability depends greatly on the initial equilibrium of the fracture site. If the Kirschner pins are inserted with the tip oriented somewhat more than perpendicular to the longitudinal axis of the bone, they will perforate the metaphysis. More stability is gained, but the growth preference is interfered with (Fig. 20).

There is an option that is somewhat more difficult to perform and that cannot be used in all fractures, it consists of inserting the pins from the metaphyseal area (Fig. 21). The pins are inserted in a direction perpendicular to the growth plates without, of course, invading the joint. This way, the pins are firmly anchored in the metaphyseal area. By arranging them parallel to the plates, growth is not altered (Fig. 22).

Regarding the procedure to insert the pins, it depends primarily on the patient's age (the younger the patient, the less the growth plate should be interfered with, logically), on the stability of the fracture and, of course, on the surgeon's skill and preferences.

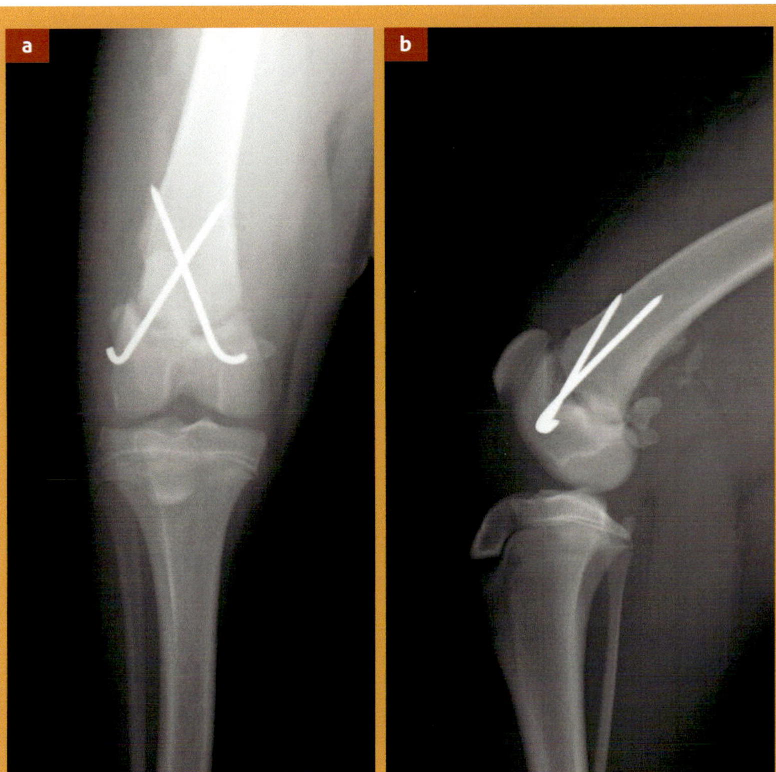

FIGURE 20. X-ray images that show the bent distal ends of the pins to avoid their displacement. Cranio-caudal view (a); latero-lateral view (b).

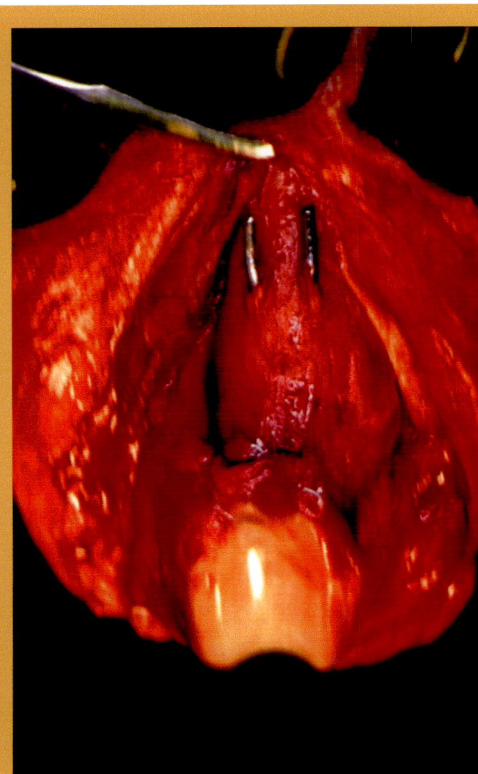

FIGURE 21. Image of a Salter-Harris II fracture in the femur, stabilised with pins introduced through the metaphysis.

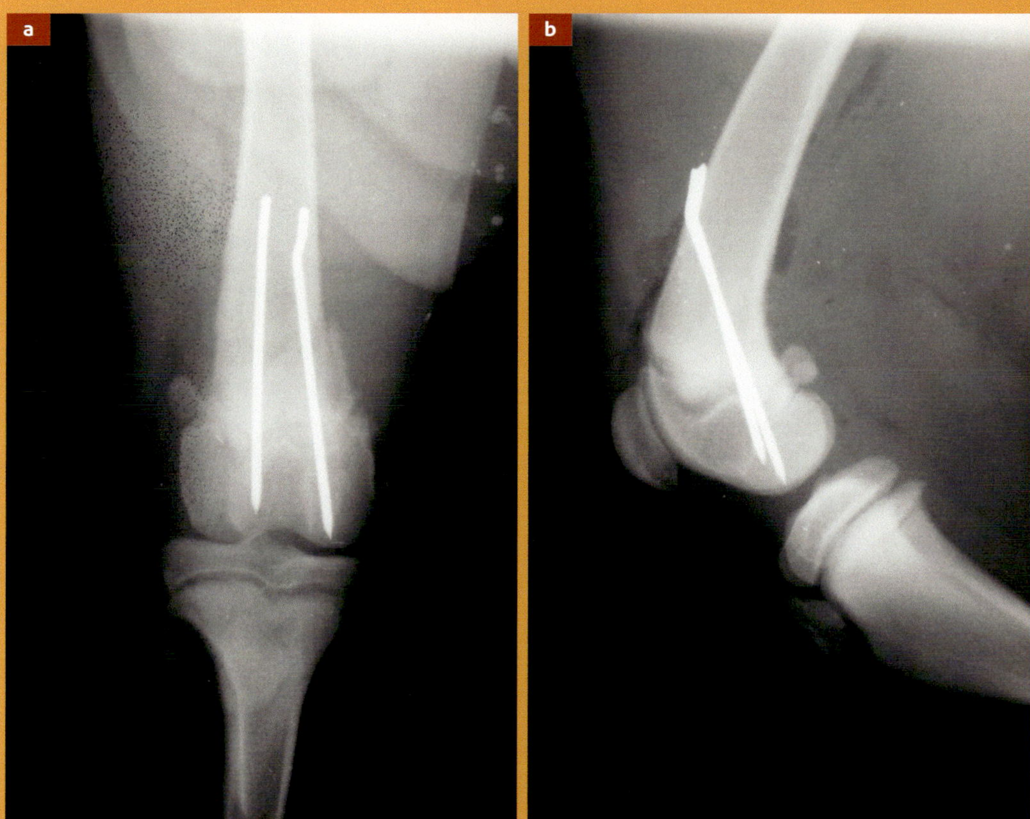

FIGURE 22. X-ray images of the stifle join. Note the placement of the pins in a parallel manner. Cranio-caudal view (a); latero-lateral view (b).

CERCLAGES

Cerclages

Cerclages are steel surgical wires that are typically used around the diaphysis of long bones to stabilise and compress fracture lines (Fig. 23).

This system functions like the hoops around a barrel, that is, a metal circumference that surrounds wooden staves that when pressed together, they maintain their lateral position forming a tube. When applied to the resolution of a fracture, by reducing the perimeter of the wire, it applies a force from the compact bone in a centripetal direction that pushes and keeps all of the fragments together (Fig. 24).

It is of utmost importance to keep in mind that this osteosynthesis system is not capable of stabilising a fracture when used alone. It is an interfragmentary compression system that must always be associated with other stabilisation systems.

Cerclages should never be considered as a system that can stabilise a fracture when used alone. Their use should always be associated with other fixation systems.

To apply the cerclage first the fracture lines to be compressed must be properly reduced. As previously mentioned, this system requires that the fragments fit together perfectly. If not, when pressing one against the other, they could move out of place. The fragments must be perfectly set in place and all must be present to reconstruct the entire perimeter of the bone. If this is not the case, when tightening the wire, the pieces will tend to gather together in the centre of the medullary cavity, causing the fracture site to collapse. The same will happen if we remove one of the staves that make up a wooden barrel (Fig. 25).

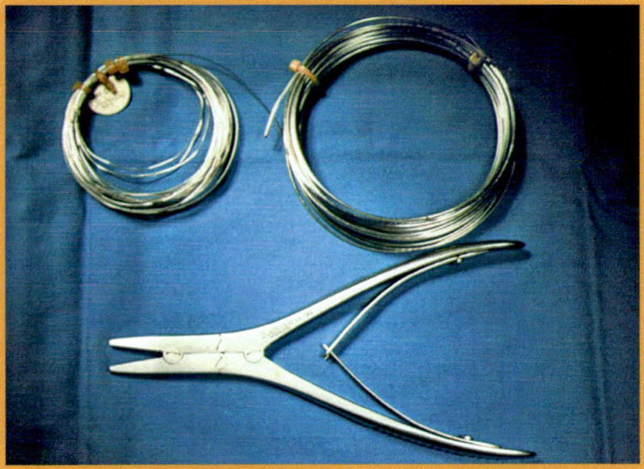

FIGURE 23. Cerclage wires of different diameters next to the pliers used for their insertion.

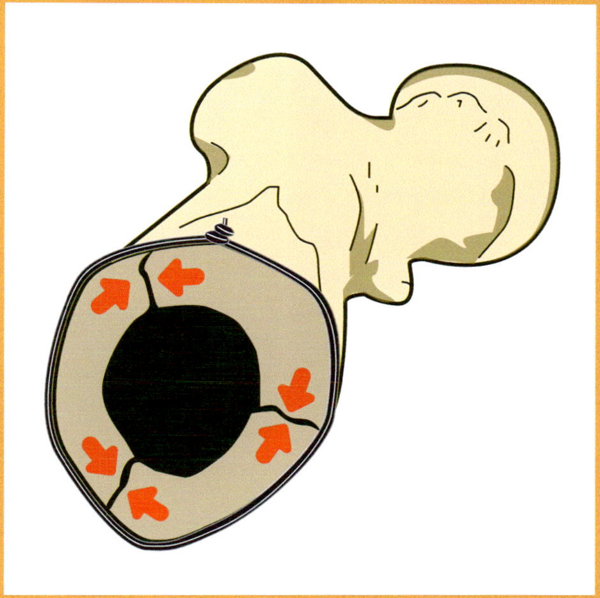

FIGURE 24. Action of a cerclage on fragments of a fracture.

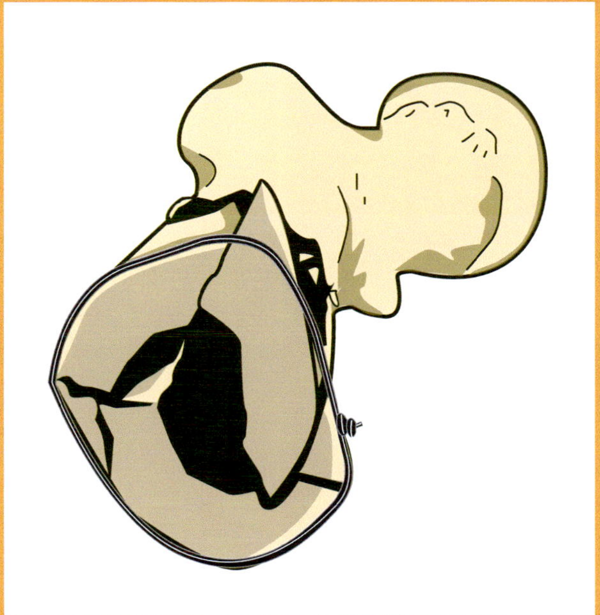

FIGURE 25. Collapse of the fracture site due to inadequate reduction.

To summarise, cerclages cannot be used if the fracture line cannot be properly reduced or if the compact bone perimeter cannot be completely reconstructed (Fig. 26).

> *If the fracture line cannot be properly reduced and the compact bone perimeter cannot be completely reconstructed, cerclages cannot be used or the medullary cavity would collapse.*

The selection of the wire calibre depends on the diameter of the bone, the patient's weight and the forces that the implant will presumably have to counteract. Normally, a cerclage of 1.2 mm is used in patients that weigh more than 30 kg, of 1.0 mm in those that weigh between 10 and 30 kg, and of 0.8 mm in animals that weight less than 10 kg. As a general rule, the tighter the wire, the more difficult it is to adapt it to the bone's shape. The wire may thus be too loose and not perform its function.

Metallic materials, polyfilament or other types of non-metallic sutures should never be used to perform cerclages unless they are specifically designed for said use. These materials are not resistant enough and due to their elasticity, they quickly lose tension (Fig. 27). Currently there are plastic cerclages that imitate the clamps used to hold cables.

Cerclages are the ideal fixation system to resolve long oblique fractures in the diaphysis of circular sectioned bones. The fracture must be thoroughly assessed as this system should generally not be used in fractures whose length is not at least double the diameter of the bone (Fig. 28).

Once the fracture is reduced, the fragment must be temporarily stabilised using reduction forceps, to keep it stable until the cerclage has been tightened. The best option is to use two-pointed reduction forceps in such a position that an imaginary line is formed that joins both points by perpendicularly crossing the fracture plane. This way, the force exerted by the forceps is transferred in this direction, avoiding displacement (Fig. 29).

When temporarily reducing the fracture, only one side of the bone can be observed as the other compact bone surface is not visible. This is important given that the structures located between the fracture and the cortical bone can be damaged when tightening the cerclages (blood vessels, nerves, etc.).

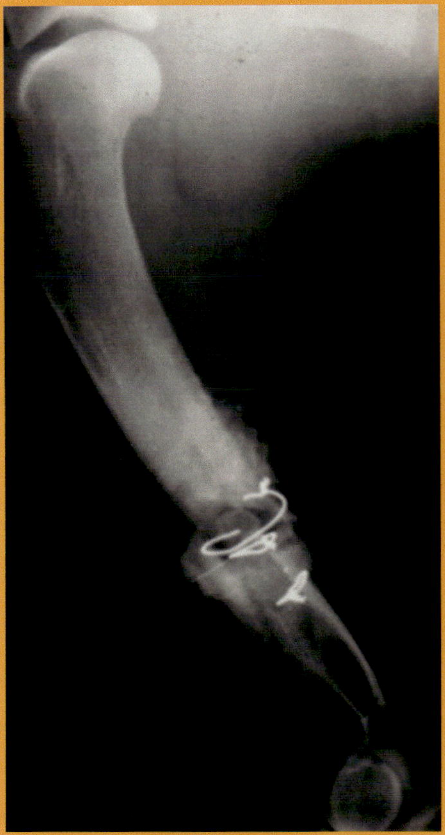

FIGURE 26. Once the implants to be associated with the cerclages are implanted, their stability must be tested. If they can be moved, even slightly, they should be substituted, or, if possible, removed.

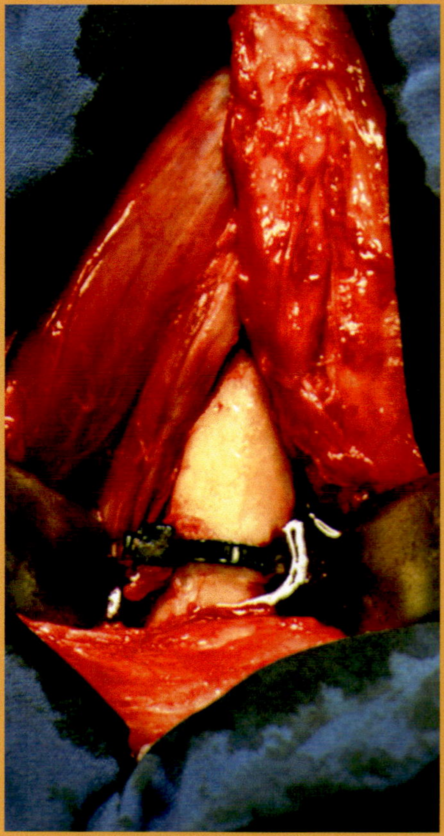

FIGURE 27. The use of inappropriate materials that are not apt to perform cerclages can cause them to loosen prematurely. Note how a plastic tube has been used in this case.

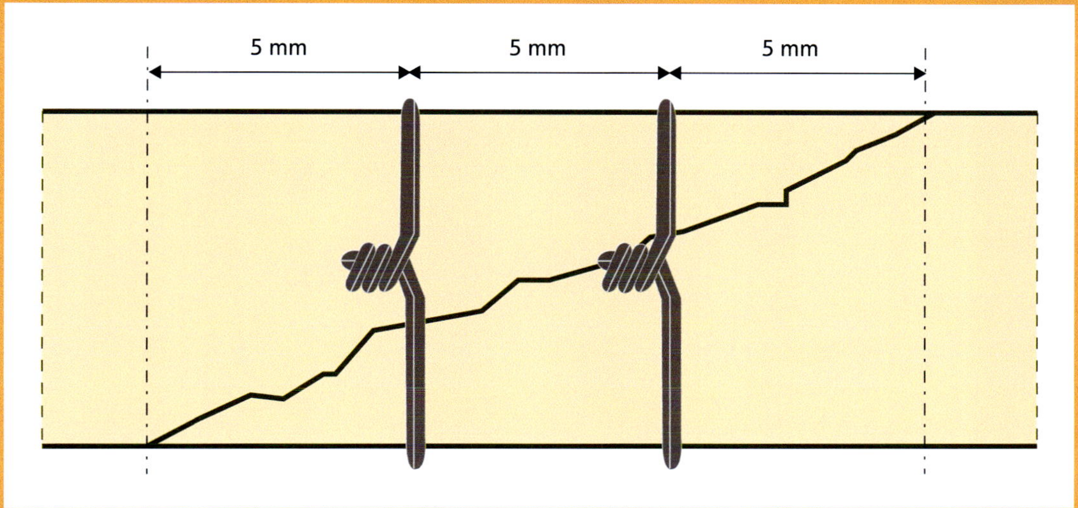

FIGURE 28. Length and safety margins that should be taken into account when inserting a cerclage.

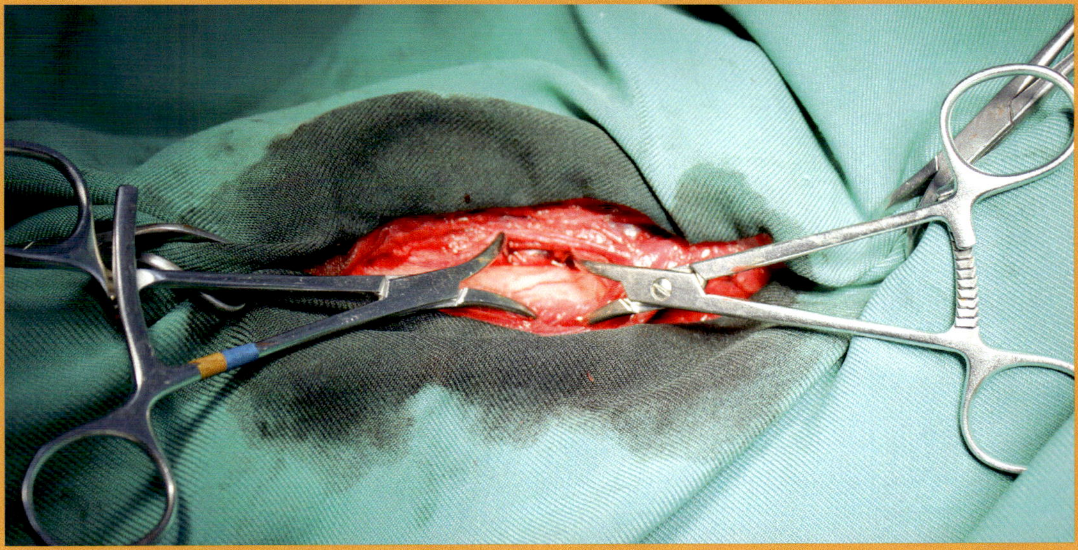

FIGURE 29. Oblique fracture stabilised using two-point reduction forceps.

Cerclage passer

This instrument is basically a thin curved tube with a bevelled tip with its most prominent part located in the concave portion.

How to use the cerclage passer

The passer is inserted into the area where the cerclage will be placed, making its tip slide by pressing on the cortical bone. Due to its rigid nature, the tip "lifts" the soft tissues and, consequently, avoids damage caused by the wire. When the tip of the passer reaches the other side of the bone, the cerclage is placed inside of it. Once this is done, the passer can be removed and the cerclage can be tightened.

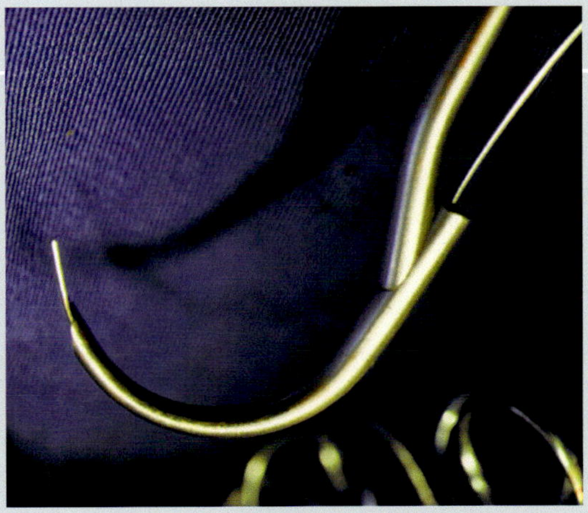

Cerclage passer.

To avoid this problem, there are cerclage passers and other possibilities as explained below:

Procedure to apply a cerclage

a. Use a cerclage passer.
b. Bend the cerclage wire in the shape of a hook (Fig. 30) and insert it while noting how its tip slides over the cortical bone.
c. Introduce a curved haemostat clamp underneath the bone. Hold the tip of the cerclage and while tractioning the haemostat clamp, pull the wire out on the opposite side.
d. Put the cerclage wires in place before reducing the fracture.

Once the wire is in place, the only thing left to do is twist its ends together to reduce the diameter of the ring formed, and apply a centripetal force that is transformed into compression. To perform this operation, the simplest method is to use pliers or a strong needle holder to hold and twist the ends. There are specific instruments available for tightening cerclages.

Tightening of cerclages using pliers

For proper functioning of this system, each end should be twisted around the other, similar to the wire twisted around the cork in a bottle of champagne. If only one of the ends is twisted around the other, a slipknot is formed and the cerclage's function is lost due to loosening as soon as the fragments start to move (Fig. 31).

To achieve a proper knot, both ends of the wire must be tractioned and the tension maintained when the pliers are twisted. (Fig. 32a). One finger should be placed on the bone to avoid its displacement in the direction of the traction (Fig. 32b).

Another frequent error is pulling in the wrong direction. To avoid this, the pliers must be placed in a direction that corresponds with an imaginary line that divides the circumference formed by the cerclage in two equal parts.

Once the cerclage is tightened as much as possible, the twisted end is cut leaving at least three turns; we then bend it around the cortical bone to avoid harming the soft tissues (Fig. 32c).

To avoid losing tension when the tip is bent, a turn should be made in the same direction as that used for tightening, while simultaneously bending said tip towards the cortical bone.

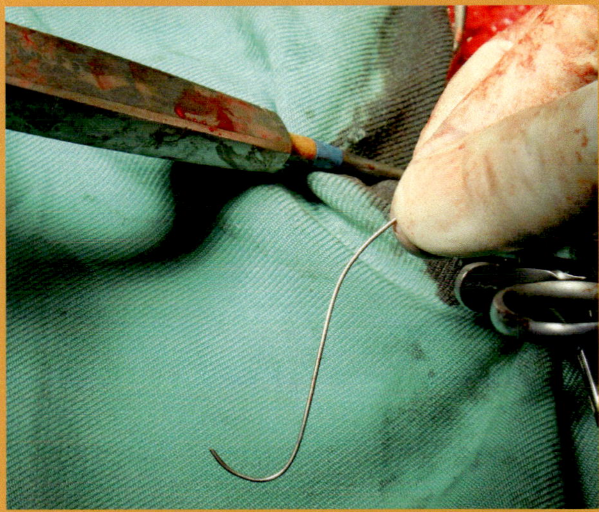

FIGURE 30. Take note of the curvature of the cerclage wire needed for its correct placement.

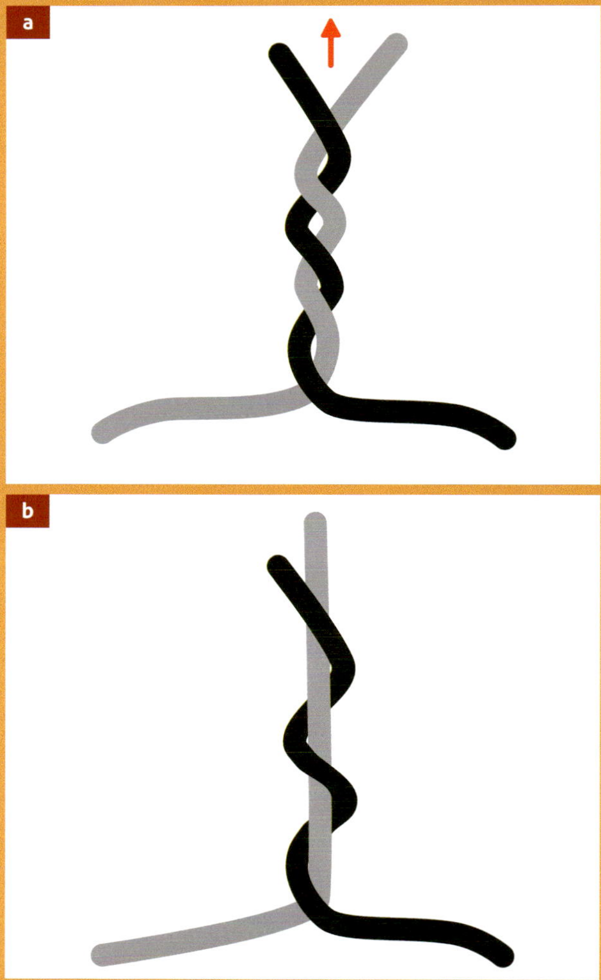

FIGURE 31. Twisting of the cerclage wire. Correct. The two ends must be twisted together (a). Incorrect. If only one is twisted over the other, a slipknot is formed that provides no stability (b).

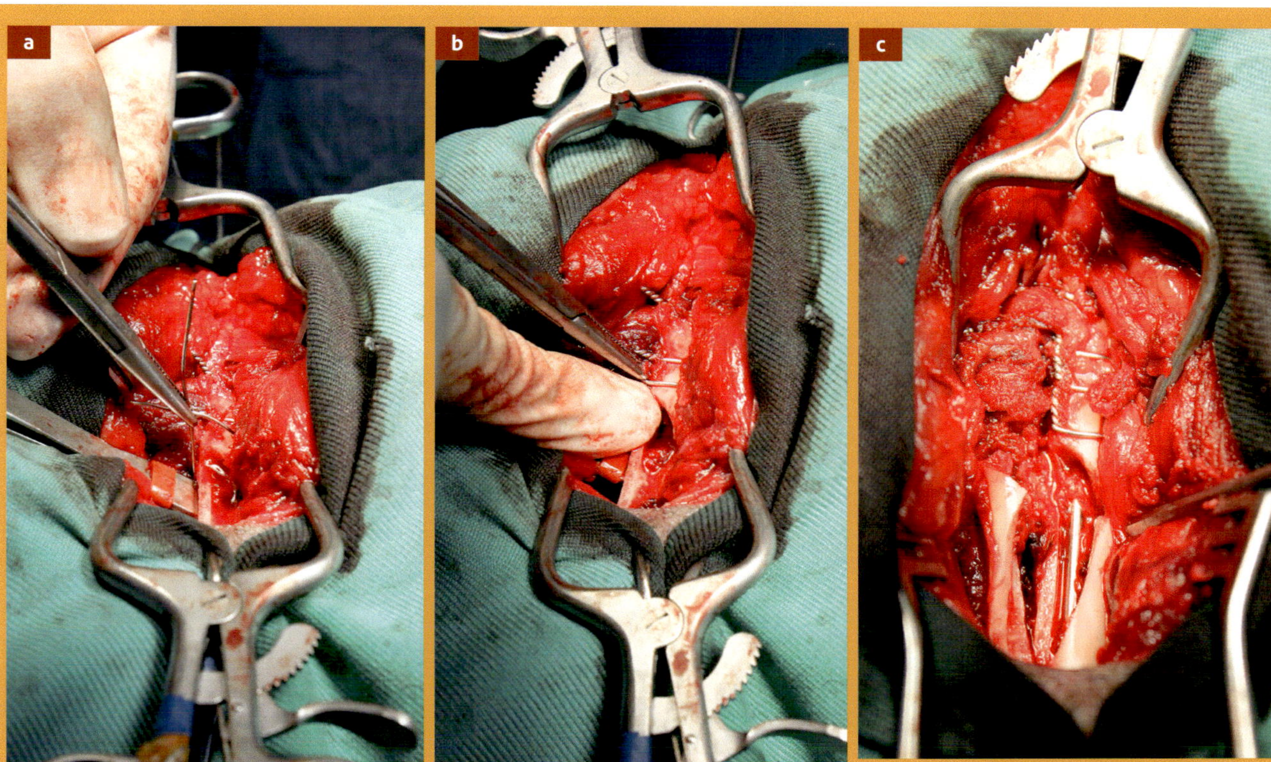

FIGURE 32. Correct cerclage placement procedure. Traction both ends of the wire at the same time and maintain the tension when twisting the pliers (a). To avoid the bone from moving while the cerclage is tightened, it is immobilised with the help of a finger (b). Cut the ends leaving three turns and bend them so that they lay closely on the bone (c).

The cerclage will be slightly more stable if the end is bent towards the cerclage instead of perpendicular to the wire. However, its loosening will hardly depend on the direction in which the bending is made, but on the technique used for tightening.

Tightening using cerclage tighteners

Given that one of the primary problems is the insufficient tightening of cerclage wires, specific instruments have been created for use when following the traditional tightening method.

There are different models available, however, the most used due to its simplicity is one that consists of a key similar to the old system employed in tin openers (Fig. 33).

A cerclage wire with an eyelet hole on one of its ends should be used with said model. Wires can be purchased that are already prepared for this system, although they can also be easily made. A small cerclage must be formed on one of the ends around a nail with a diameter of approximately 2 mm, taking special care to tighten it as much as possible, that is, making the spiral as compact as possible (Fig. 34).

Once the wire has been wrapped around the bone, the free end is introduced into the eyelet hole and the first is pulled manually until it comes in contact with the cortical bone. Next, the free end of the cerclage is introduced into the sharp part of the tightener and then pulled out of its upper part. When making the cerclage, the length needed for a few centimetres to project from said end must be taken into account.

The end is then introduced in the key hole and displaced until it fits into the tightener (Fig. 35a). The key is then turned so that the free end twists, pulling on the wire. While this operation is being carried out, the cerclage will tighten around the bone, compressing the fragments (Fig. 35b). When the tension applied seems adequate, without releasing the key, the cerclage is bent over the eyelet hole, forming a hook which impedes loosening (Fig. 35c). The key must then be turned in the opposite direction to separate the cerclage tightener enough to cut the wire and adjust it to the cortical bone (Fig. 35d).

The cerclage with the eyelet hole is the most stable type due to the pressure that it is capable of exerting.

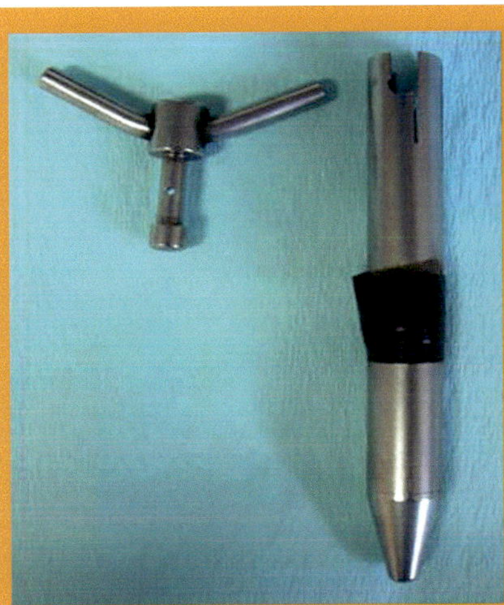

FIGURE 33. Cerclage tightener.

FIGURE 34. Loop cerclage.

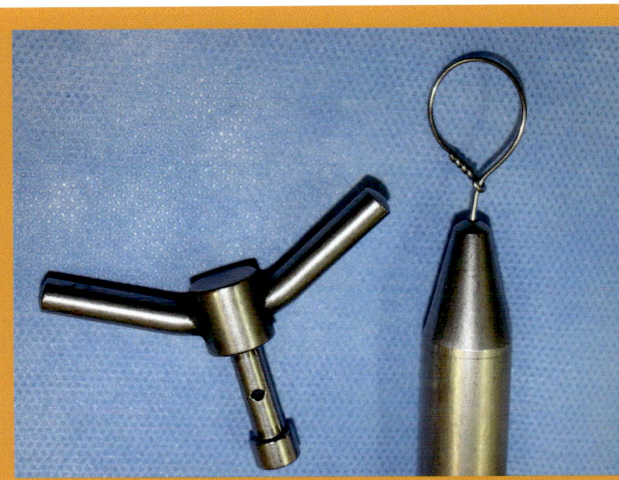

Contrary to the traditional cerclage system, it does not depend on the surgeon's experience or technique.

Once the cerclage and complementary osteosynthesis systems are put in place, and before finalizing the intervention, its stability should be tested. To do so, the knot is pulled on using pliers or needle holders, attempting to move it in all directions. If any instability is perceived, it should be substituted or removed. Another possibility is to tighten it again, but this solution is not highly recommended as it could place strain on the material.

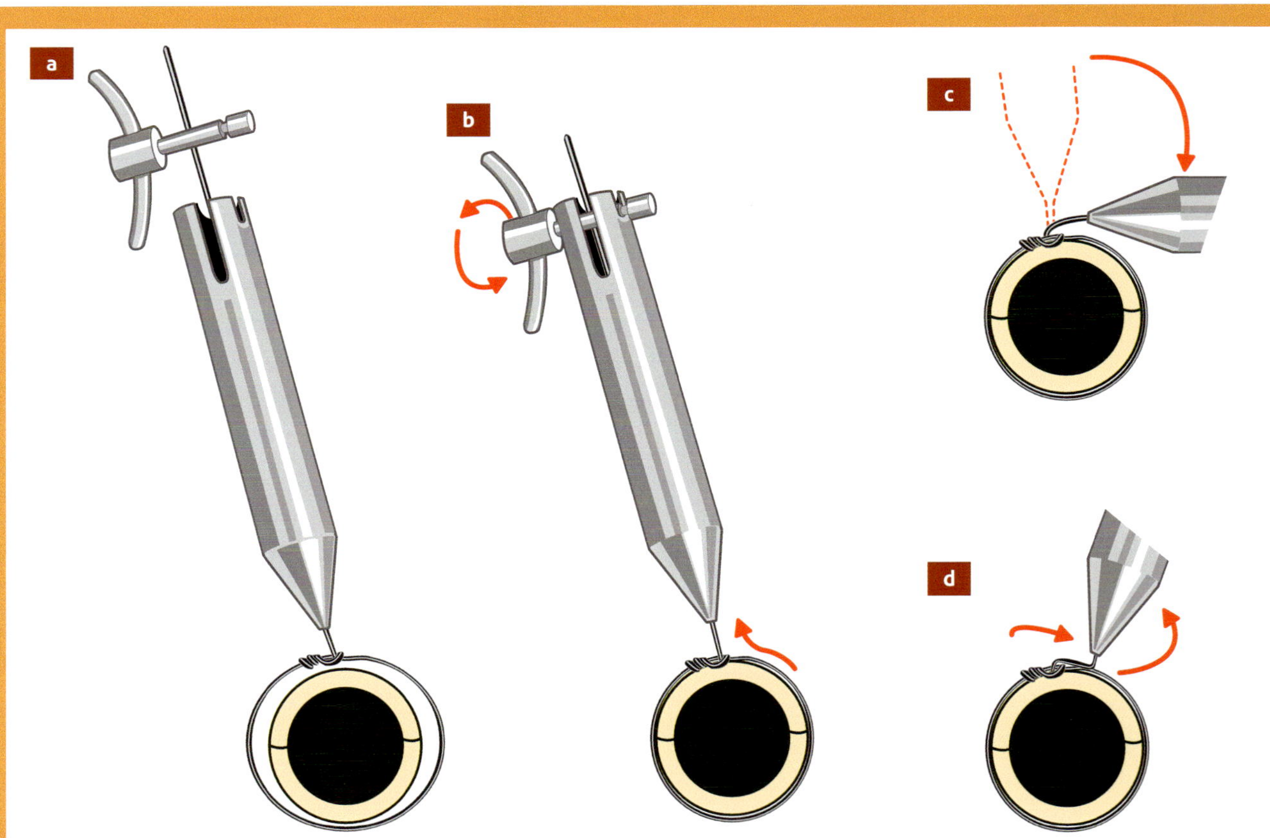

FIGURE 35. Procedure to tighten a cerclage with the help of a cerclage tightener.

Common errors that can be made when inserting a cerclage and that can cause treatment to fail

Regardless of the tightening system used, when a cerclage wire is set in place, the following must be kept in mind:

- The cerclage must be placed around the bone, in the area with the smallest perimeter, given that on the contrary, it could move towards the narrowest area, losing its stabilising capacity (Fig. 36). One possibility to avoid displacement is to make notches in the cortical bone where the wire is to be placed.
- It should be placed perpendicularly to the longitudinal axis of the bone. If it is in a slight oblique position, a small displacement will give it enough extra space to impede the correct stabilisation of the fracture (Fig. 37).

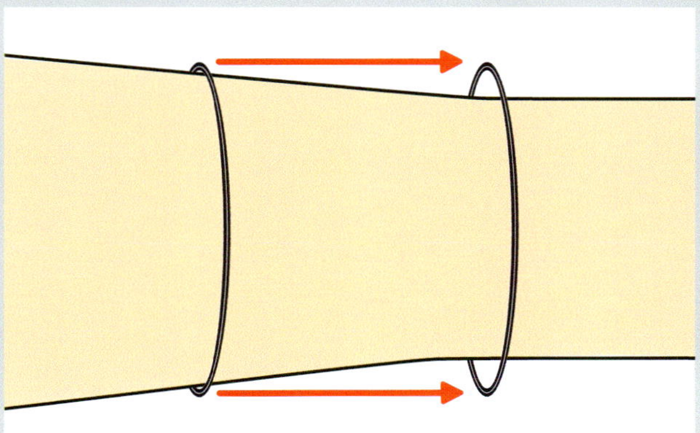

FIGURE 36. Diameter of the upper cerclage greater than the bone diameter as it has been tightened in a thicker area of the bone.

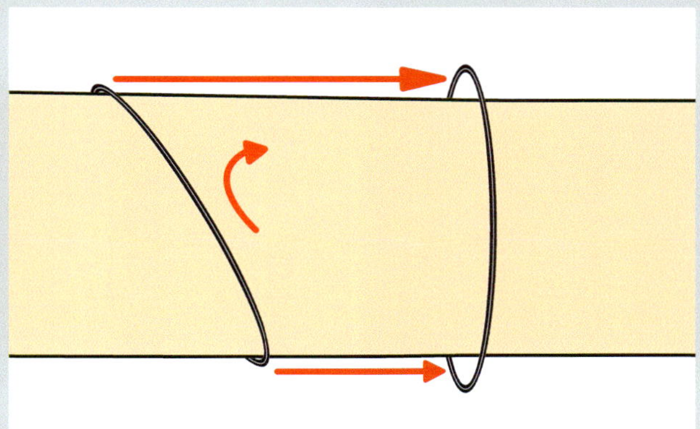

FIGURE 37. If the cerclage is placed diagonally, it can easily lose tension, as seen in the illustration.

If the fracture line is long enough, two separate cerclages should be used, with at least half a centimetre between them. This way, greater stability is achieved and movements parallel to the fracture plane are avoided.

Combination with other osteosynthesis systems

Intramedullary nails

As previously explained, cerclages alone are not capable of stabilising fractures. One of the most used combinations in veterinary bone surgery is the use of cerclages with intramedullary nails. This combination of systems avoids one of the significant problems of intramedullary fixation, as mentioned before: rotation of the fracture site. When the cerclage compresses the fracture lines, they fit together perfectly so that movements of rotation and displacement are avoided. The nail, resistant to forces of flexion, will stabilise the fracture, allowing for the bone to heal (Fig. 38). Of course, to select this treatment, the principals of the application of both cerclages as well as nails must be taken into account.

Osteosynthesis plates

The cerclages form a good combination with the osteosynthesis plates creating forces of compression, simultaneous with the neutralisation of the plates. Given that they must be perfectly adapted to the bone perimeter to carry out their function, they must always be placed under the plate and never above it (Fig. 39).

The exception constituted by certain specific plates such as those for double hip osteotomies should be mentioned, but in this case the cerclage does not act as a compression system, but simply as extra reinforcement so that the bone does not separate from the plate (Fig. 40).

Some surgeons use cerclages as a temporary stabilisation system until the plate has been moulded and inserted, at which point the wire is then removed.

Other applications

Cerclages or surgical wire can also be used for other purposes, although these applications are less frequent, with the exception of their combination with pins, which are

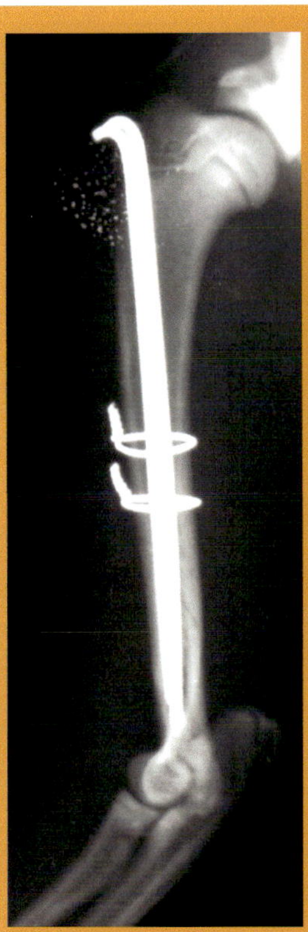

FIGURE 38. Femur fracture resolved with a combination of cerclage and intramedullary nails.

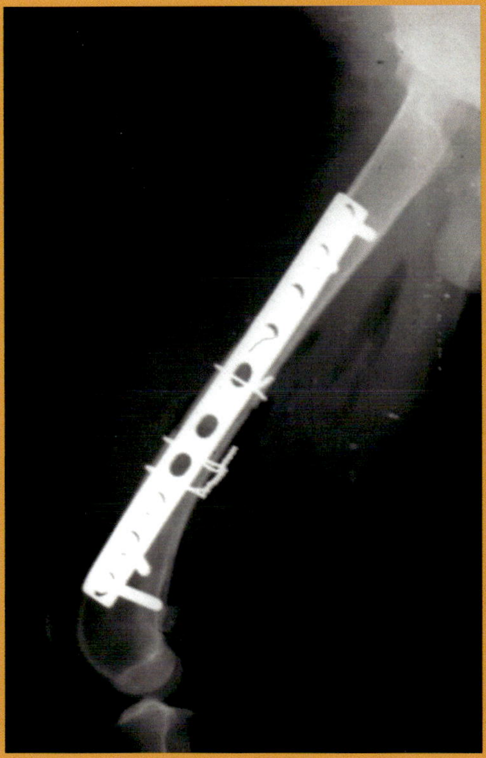

FIGURE 39. Oblique femur fracture treated with cerclages and a neutralisation plate. Take note of how the cerclages are placed underneath the plate.

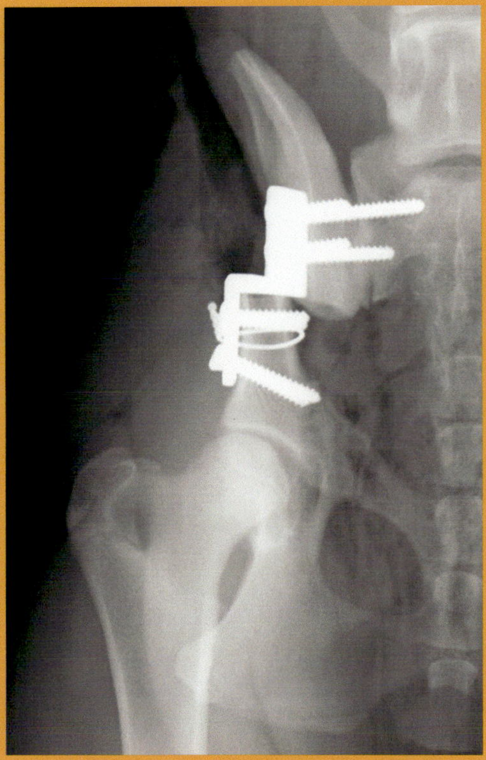

FIGURE 40. Double hip osteotomy. Note how the cerclage hugs the plate on top.

known as pins with tension bands, that will be discussed in another clinically-relevant section.

Other possible uses of surgical wire include the following:

Temporary substitution of tendons and ligaments

When an important tendon is injured, such as the patellar tendon, it must be temporarily substituted using a structure that resists strong forces of traction. It must be taken into account that when using a material such as wire, where there must be a flexible band, the metal will be subjected to cycles of flexion that will progressively cause strain to its structure causing it to break sooner or later. Depending on the diameter of the metal and the mobility of the joint, said breakage usually takes place in 4-5 weeks (Fig. 41). In order to delay breakage of the wire, another type of immobilisation system is usually used to temporarily limit joint movement, for example, external coaptation or temporary transarticular external fixation.

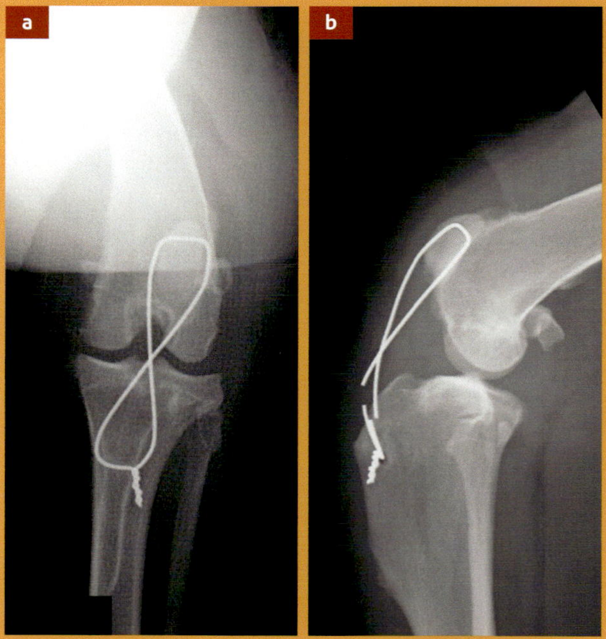

FIGURE 41. Patellar tendon tear stabilised with cerclage. Note how the wire has broken due to strain on the metal 5 weeks after the intervention.

The cerclage is anchored, in these cases, to the insertion points of the relevant tendon or ligament, through perforations in the bone or using screws or bone anchors.

While the cerclage resists the forces of tension, the lesion has time to heal.

There are currently flexible sutures available that resist strong forces of traction and thus have a longer half-life. They are progressively replacing the use of cerclages.

Creation of tension bands in certain orthopaedic techniques

Within this group of applications of wire cerclages, the most frequent are:

- Treatment of anterior cruciate ligament tears. For many years, and even today, certain surgeons have used wire cerclages to treat anterior cruciate ligament tears as an extracapsular stabilisation system. The cerclage is placed crossing the tibial crest until it reaches the area behind the lateral sesamoid bone, creating a band that impedes cranial displacement of the tibia (Fig. 42). The appearance of new techniques is reducing the frequency of application of this technique.
- This material has also been used in the treatment of coxofemoral luxations as material for iliofemoral sutures. The technique consists of creating a band that forces a medial rotation of the femur until reaching a relatively stable position against repeated luxations. The cerclage is thus placed from the trochanter major of the femur to a perforation in the body of the ilium, in the insertion point of the rectus femoris muscle (Fig. 43).

As in previous cases, flexible suture materials are now available with a longer service life than that of surgical wires, making use of the latter less and less frequent.

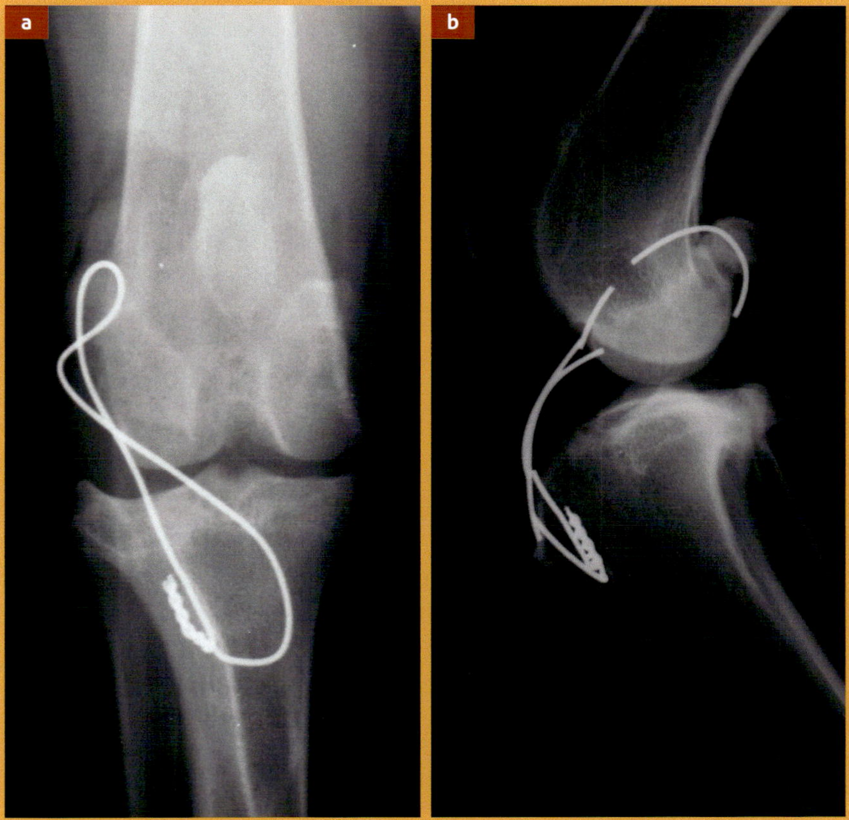

FIGURE 42. Extracapsular technique using cerclage wire to treat an anterior cruciate ligament tear (a). X-ray image four weeks later. Note how the cerclage has broken due to strain on the wire (b).

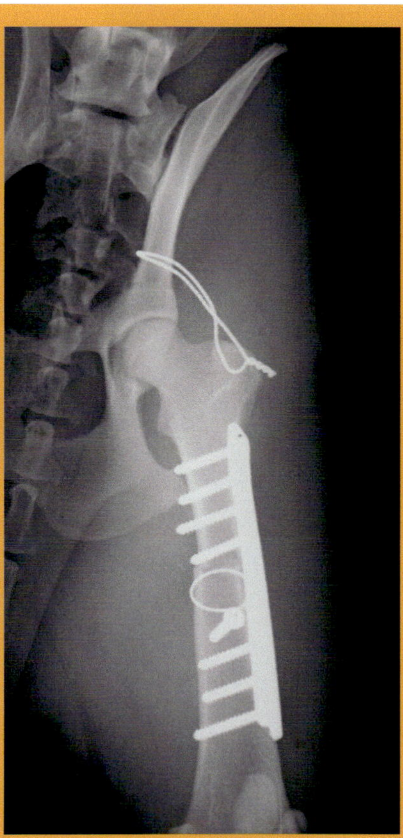

FIGURE 43. Iliofemoral sutures stabilised with cerclage that forces the femur to rotate in a medial direction until reaching a position that considerably reduces the possibilities of repeated luxations.

TENSION BAND PIN SYSTEM

This technique consists of the combination of several pins with a cerclage. The pins stabilise the movements of displacement and rotation and the cerclage counteracts the forces of traction.

Most implants function by impeding possible harmful movements that can be produced on the fracture site and by allowing for those that favour bone healing. Tension band pins, unlike other implants, are characterised by their capacity to reorient the forces that the fracture site is subjected to by transforming them into forces of compression. This effect is achieved thanks to the tension band principle, which is the same foundation by which cranes used in the construction of buildings have a weighted beam on the side contrary to that which bears the load to be lifted. When the crane lifts the load, the counterweight shifts the forces of gravity, which would tend to tip the crane over due to its lever beam, and transforms it into another that is transmitted through its structure towards the ground in a vertical direction (Fig. 44).

The tension band pins are used to stabilise avulsion fractures, that is, small bone fragments that tend to separate themselves from the bone when the patient uses the limb. Normally, these are insertion point areas for tendons or ligaments that transmit muscle contractions applying forces of traction on the bone fragment (Fig. 45).

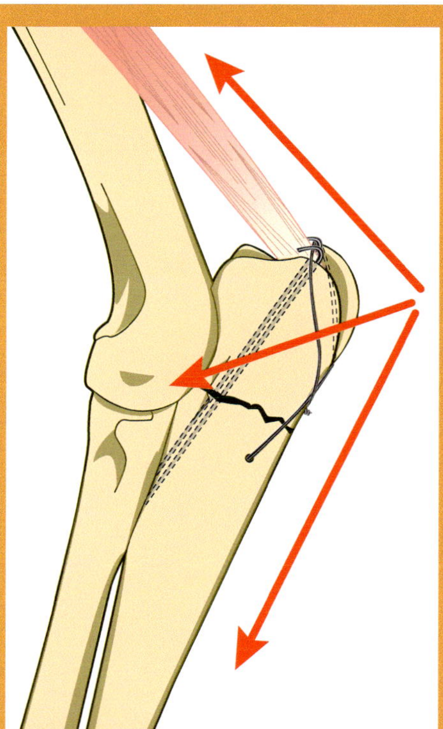

FIGURE 44. Diagram of the tension band principle. Note the reorientation of the forces in a fracture.

Avulsion fractures lead to the formation of small bone fragments that, frequently, cannot hold large osteosynthesis systems. For this reason, the only possibility to stabilise this type of fractures is by using pins.

That said, and as previously mentioned, pins used as an osteosynthesis system provide little resistance to bear forces of avulsion. On the other hand, pins with a small diameter must be used and they are not capable of resisting the angular forces that are produced in certain insertion points of tendons. This is especially the case when taking into account that tendons, almost always, are inserted on an angle.

Consequently, taking advantage of the mechanical resistance of the metals themselves against the forces of elongation, the forces exerted by the tendons on these fragments can be neutralised using a cerclage.

Placement procedure

The technique consists of reducing the fracture and stabilising the fragment using two pins. The insertion of two pins is ideal to stabilise movements of rotation of the fragment (Fig. 46).

The pins can be inserted in a normograde or retrograde manner (see page 38). In this case, no significant increase in the stability of the implant is achieved. Unlike the case with intramedullary nails, which are only anchored by the metal-bone coefficient of friction, in the specific case of tension band pins, the stability provided by the traction in a lateral direction from the cerclage must be added. The migration of the pins, if applicable, is a consequence of the side-to-side movements produced by the cyclical traction of the tendon. In the case of deficient contact between the fracture lines, either due to the existence of numerous fragments, or to inadequate surgical techniques, these movements will be greater.

Regarding the placement of the pins, one option is to insert one of them in a retrograde manner to later insert the second pin in a normograde manner, using the first as a guide (Figs. 47 and 48). It will thus be easier to correctly pull the tip of the pin through the fracture site without losing any stability from friction with the implant.

Subsequently, the tension band is put in place. The figure eight cerclage that is anchored on both sides of the fracture

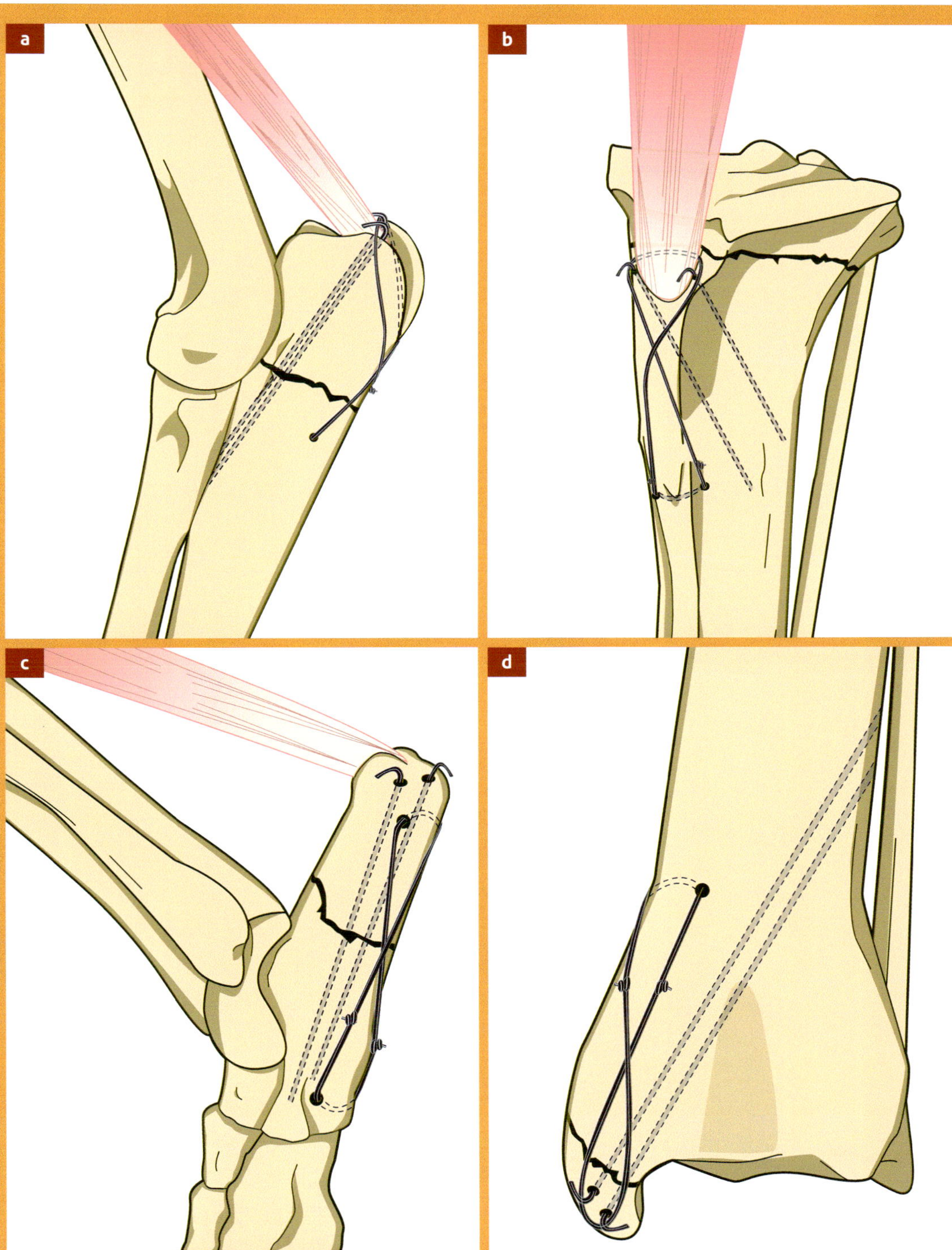

FIGURE 45. Different applications of the tension band pins in cases of avulsion fractures.

line performs this function. The first anchor point is formed by the portions of the pins that protrude and the second is a hole that must be made in the larger fragment, a certain distance away from the fracture line (Fig. 49).

The closer the perforation is to the edge of the bone, the more suitable the direction and effect of the traction will be. However, depending on the thickness of the wire, potency of the traction of the tendon, and hardness of the bone, certain minimal safety margins should be respected. In this sense, it must be taken into account that the forces of traction when the extremity bears weight are transmitted through the wire, producing halisteresis on the area of

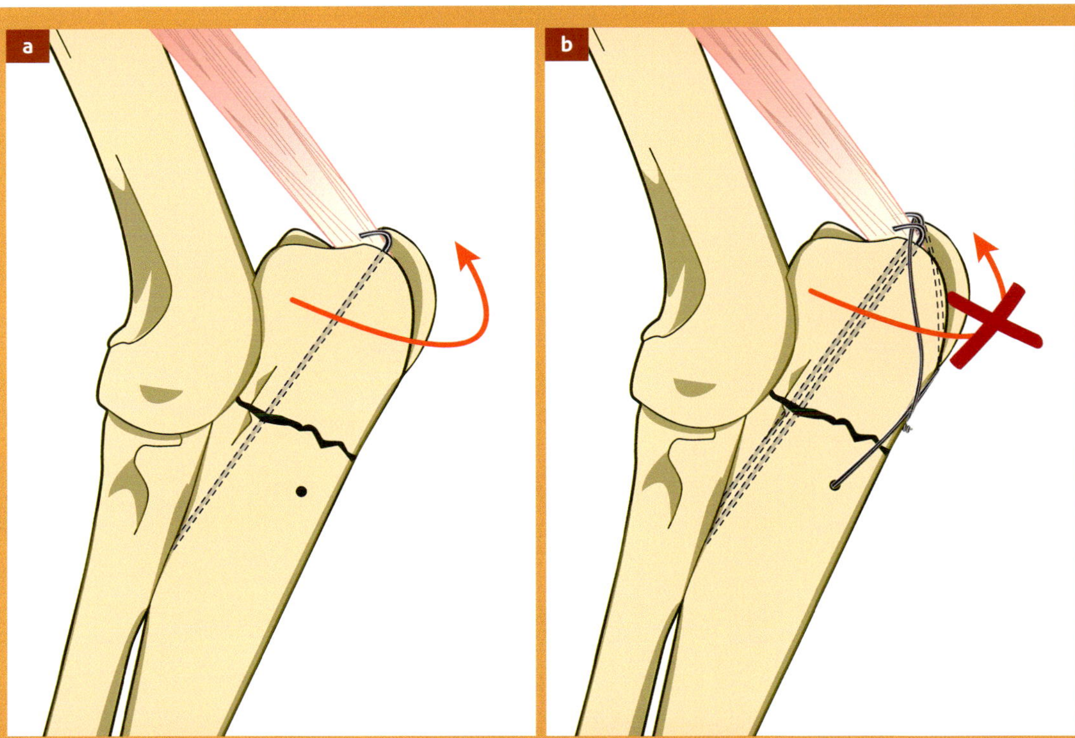

FIGURE 46. The placement of two pins impedes rotation of the fragment. As observed in the diagram, movements of rotation are possible with the placement of one single pin without any tension bands (a); this does not happen if a second pin and a cerclage are used as well (b).

the pin that is closest to the fracture line. If these safety margins are not respected, there is a risk that the cortical bone will break near the fracture site causing the tension band to lose its function. For this same reason, the bone should not be perforated close to the caudal cortical bone either.

The best option to achieve an ideal direction and traction effect is to perforate the bone as close as possible to the cortical bone located on the tension-bearing surface, however, a safety margin must be left.

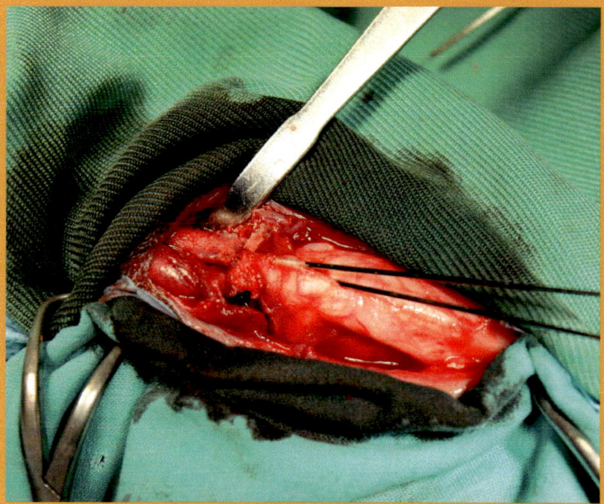

FIGURE 47. Placement of two pins following the normograde system in an avulsion fracture of the tibial crest.

The wire should rest over the tension-bearing surface of the bone. It must always be placed on this surface so that it can exert an opposing force to the forces of avulsion of the fracture site produced by muscle contractions (see Fig. 44).

Once the cerclage has been put in place, the ends should cross over each other on the tension-bearing surface to avoid displacement of the wire away from said surface (Fig. 50).

To achieve the proper tension of the band, the same method should be followed as that used to apply a cerclage, that is, twisting the ends to decrease their length. There are two possible procedures in the case of tension bands:

a. **Single loop**: This is the most frequent method to tighten a cerclage.

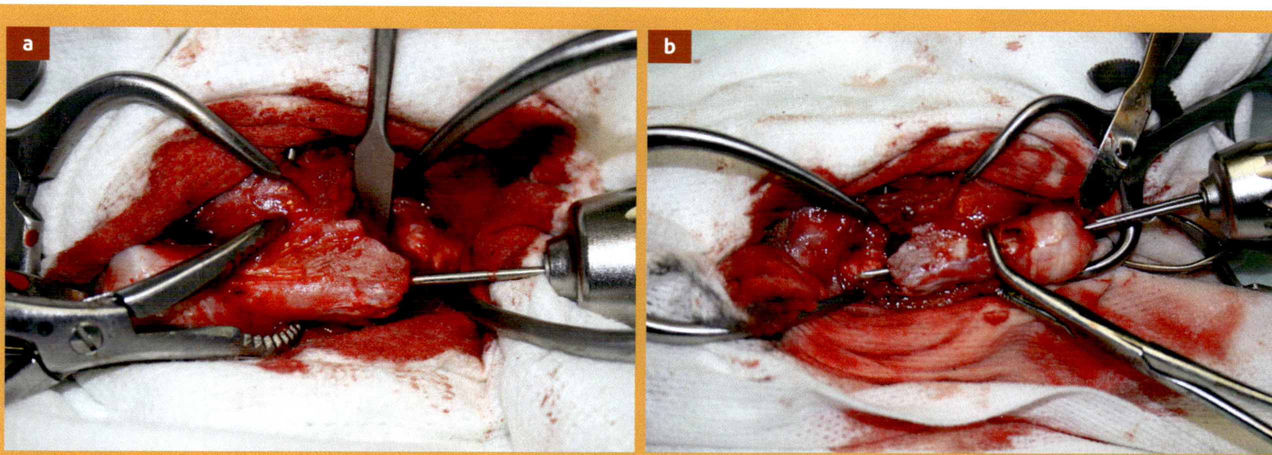

FIGURE 48. Insertion of pins in a fracture of the heel bone. The first is placed in a retrograde manner (a) and the second in a normograde manner (b).

It consists of twisting one end over the other while tractioning in the opposite direction to its point of insertion in the bone (Fig. 51). Once it has been sufficiently tightened, the "knot" will be located on side of the pins (it should be tied as close as possible to the end that comes out from the pins, Fig. 52). This way, if the implant needs to be removed, finding it will be easier and the incision needed for surgery will be smaller.

The disadvantage to this procedure is that the end of the wire where the "knot" is tied will always be tenser, as the other does not completely adapt to the bone. Consequently, as the tendon exerts forces of traction, the cerclage will adjust little by little, losing some of its initial tension.

To minimise this problem as much as possible, before tightening, the wire should be pressed against the bone on both sides of the hole where it will be inserted. This manoeuvre is easily done using reduction forceps or pliers, pushing one end of the wire against the other (Fig. 53).

b. **Double loop**: This procedure consists of tightening each wire at the same time, but independently.

Two "knots" must be tied, one on each side of the pins. This way, each knot is responsible for tensing its respective end of the cerclage, and the tension is distributed in a homogeneous manner, allowing the cerclage to properly adapt itself to the bone (Fig. 54). Once the cerclage is tightened, the ends of the wire are then cut and bent leaving at least three twists, to keep it from loosening, and we bend it towards the bone to avoid damaging the surrounding soft tissues (Fig. 55).

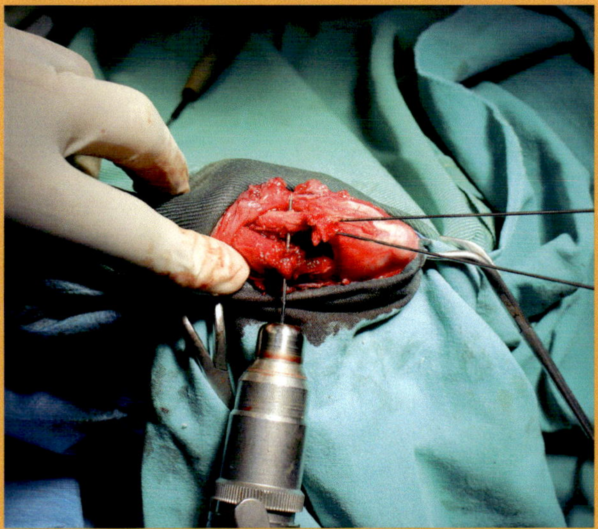

FIGURE 49. Perforation of the hole in the primary fragment. A minimum safety distance of 5 mm from the edge of the bone should be respected to avoid fracturing the cortical bone.

Next, the pins are cut and bent forming hooks that will ensure that the tension band does not loosen (Fig. 56). Logically, the hooks should be oriented towards the side opposite to where the cerclage is found (Fig. 57).

Before suturing the soft tissues, and to properly anchor the pins, gently tapping them with a hammer is recommended so that they are as closely placed to the bone as possible.

It is important to confirm the position of the cerclage regarding the tendon. If the pins are placed in the wrong position, when the wire is tightened, the tendon may be sectioned.

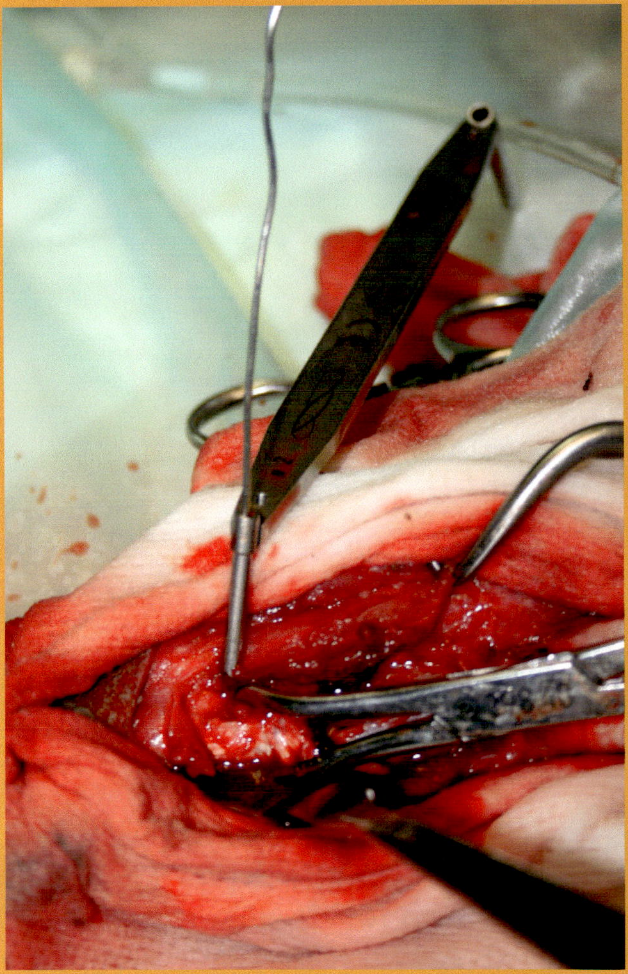

FIGURE 50. The perforation guide can be used to insert the cerclage to facilitate finding the insertion hole. However, care must be taken not to move it after making the holes.

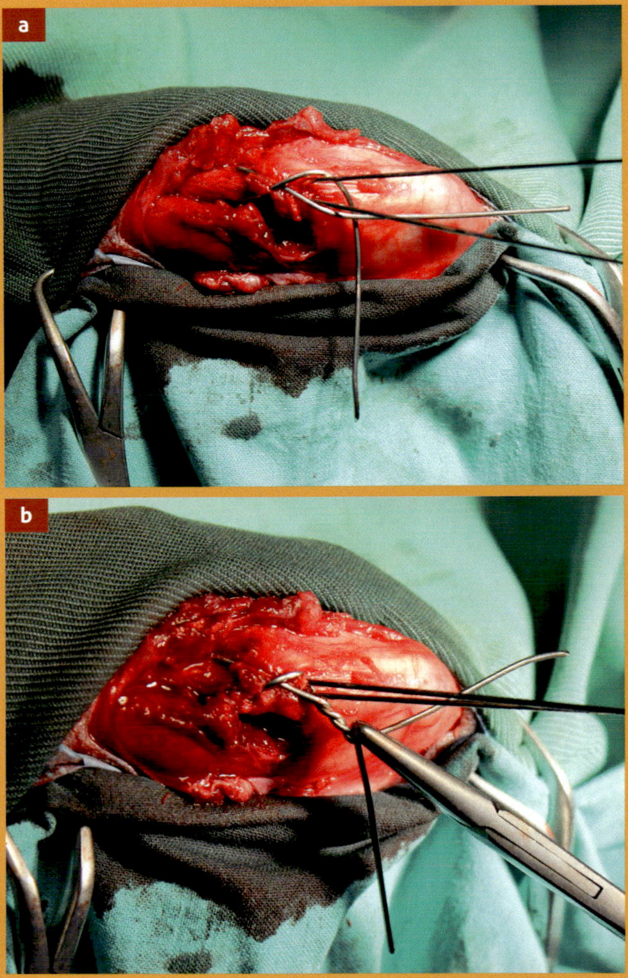

FIGURE 51. Tightening of cerclages using a single loop.

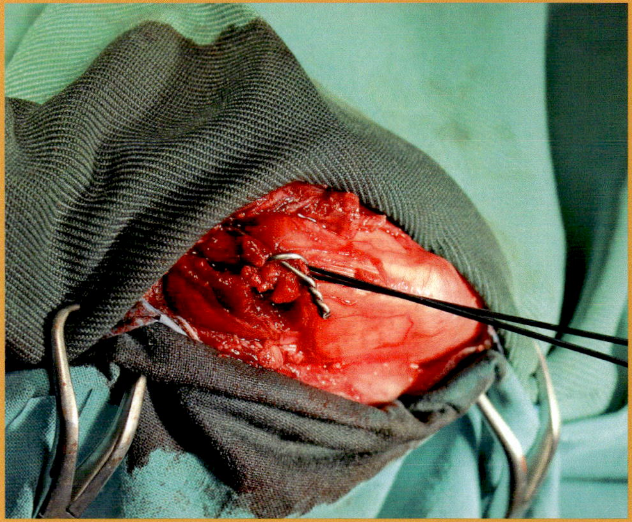

FIGURE 52. Note the location of the knot near the pins.

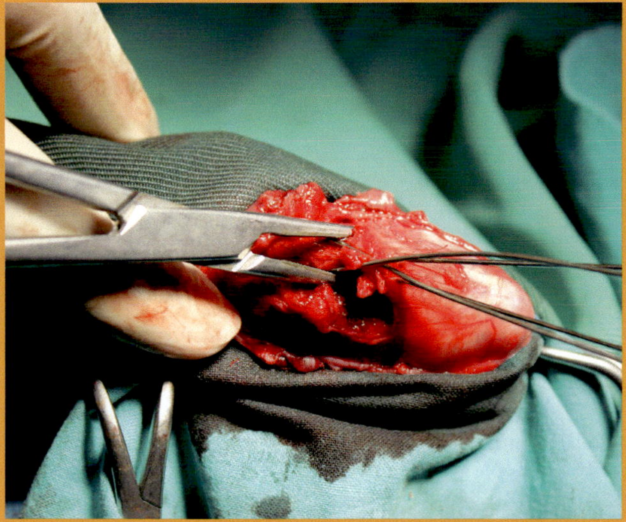

FIGURE 53. Procedure to adjust the cerclage before tightening it. The manoeuvre consists of pressing the wire against the bone with the help of reduction forceps or pliers.

In certain cases to avoid this problem, instead of fixing the wire to the ends of the pins, they can be fixed through another perforation made in the avulsed fragment. (Fig. 58).

It seems logical to think that the tension band pins only produce compression on the fracture area located underneath the cerclage. This idea is completely erroneous due to the tension band principle (see page 52). Every time the detached bone fragment is subjected to forces of traction produced by the tendon-ligament structure, they are voided by the resistance of the elongation of the surgical wire itself.

Also, these forces are partially redirected towards the cortical bone opposite of the bone in which the cerclage is placed (tension surface). That is, forces of compression are created on the cortical bone that is opposite from that where the implant is placed. This favours ossification (a displacement in the force vectors is originated). In this situation, the pins only suffer forces of flexion in the direction of the traction exerted by the tendon. For this reason, it is fundamental to perfectly set the opposing cortical bone where the cerclage is placed. On the contrary, the pins could bend or even break (Fig. 59).

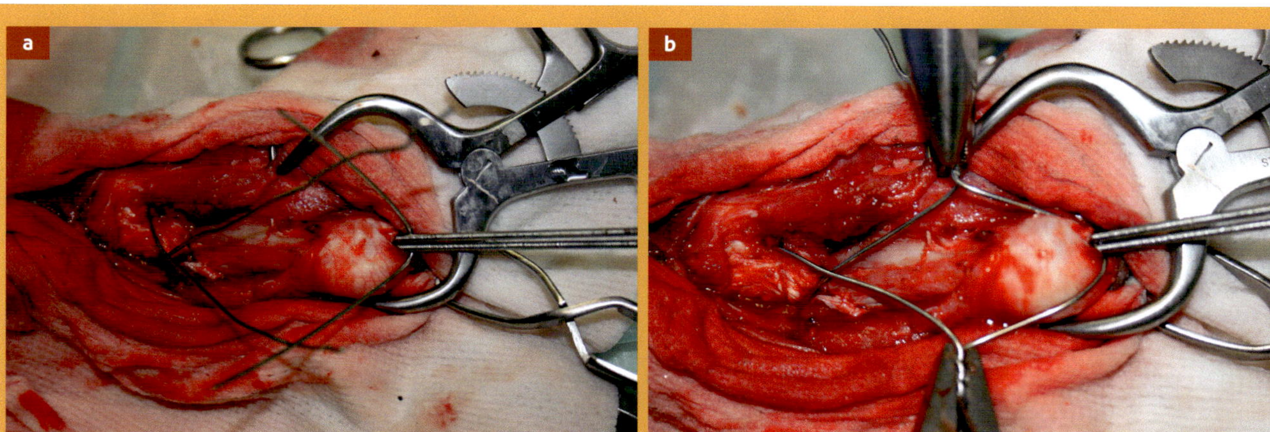

FIGURE 54. Tightening of the wire using a double loop. A knot is made on each side of the pins so that each one tenses their respective end of the cerclage.

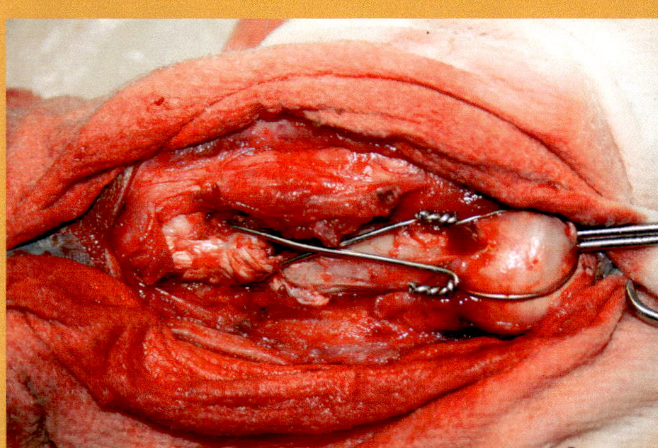

FIGURE 55. Once the cerclage has been tightened, the ends are cut and the knots are adapted to the cortical bone.

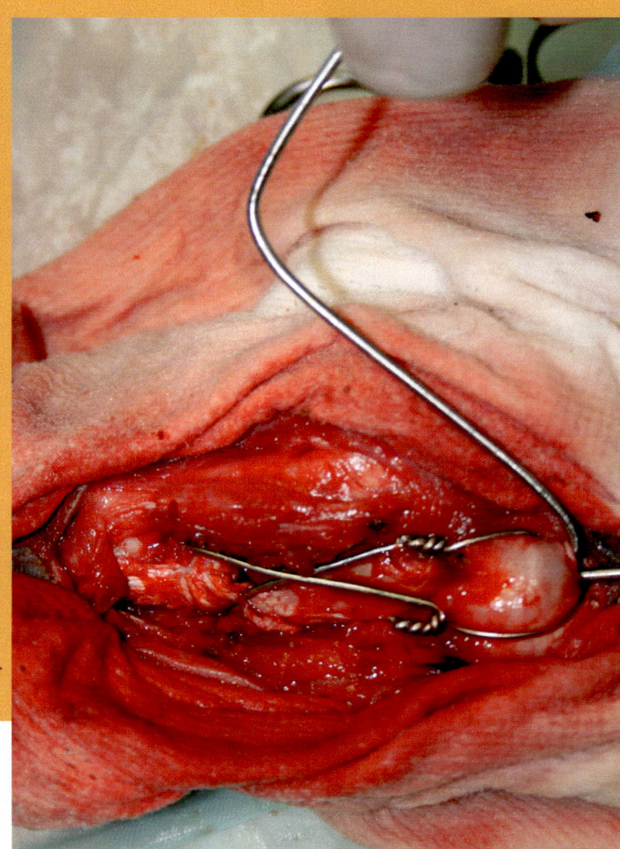

FIGURE 56. The ends of the pins are bent forming hooks that will impede the cerclage from loosening.

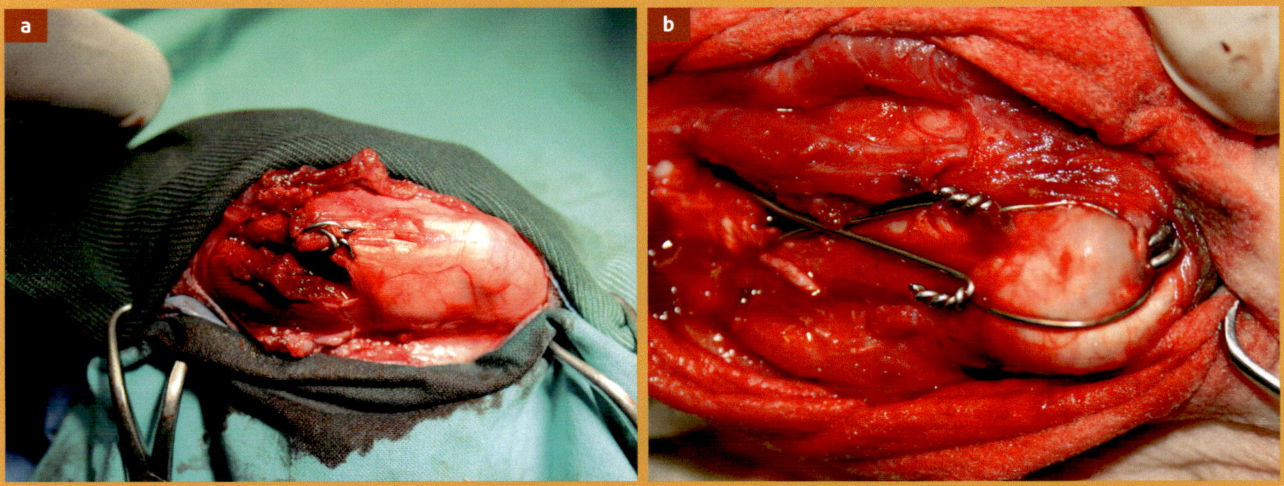

FIGURE 57. Detailed image of finished implants: single loop (a); double loop (b).

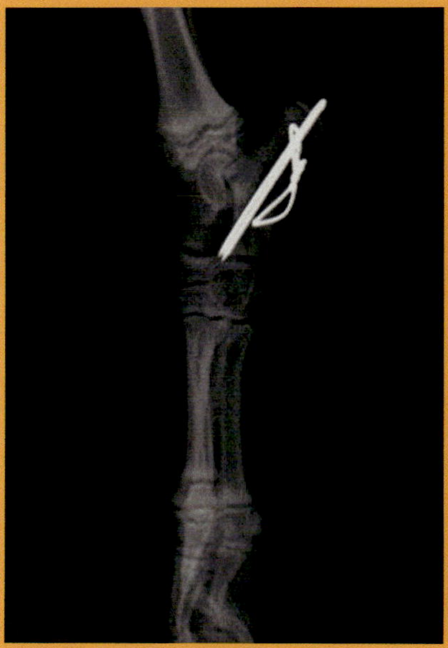

FIGURE 58. Latero-lateral X-ray of the tarsus where the placement of a tension band through two perforations can be observed.

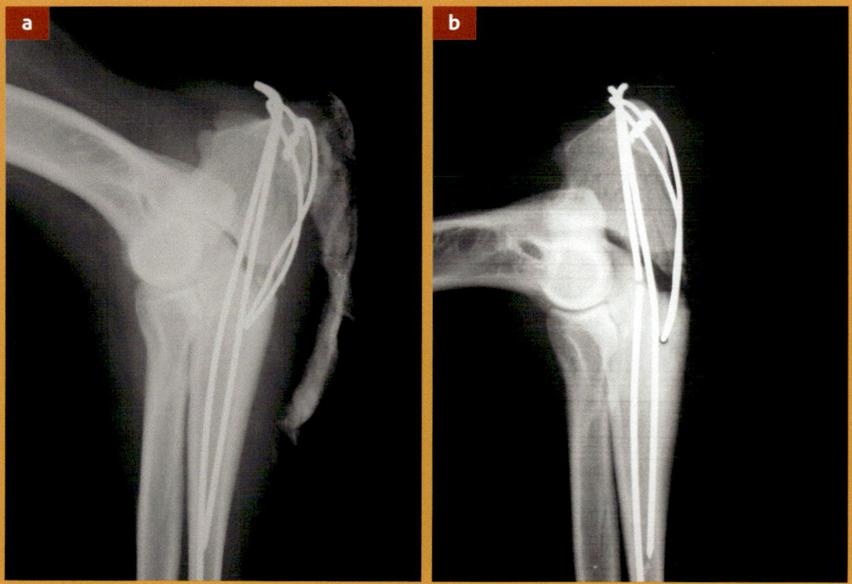

FIGURE 59. Latero-lateral X-rays of a patient that suffered an implant failure due to an insufficient reduction of the fracture site. X-ray after reduction of the fracture (a). Take note that one of the pins is broken and the other is bent (b).

EXTERNAL FIXATORS

External fixators include a series of osteosynthesis systems with a common characteristic that the system that provides stability to fractures is located externally.

This osteosynthesis system is based on a different philosophy than the rest of the previously studied systems, with the exception of the locking plates, which, as you will see in later sections, function like an external fixator.

The previously described implants basically serve to stabilise fragments in a rigid manner, impeding any movement of the fracture site. This system, however, attempts to minimise the undesirable movements of the fracture site, and when possible, allow for those that favour bone healing. That is, it impedes movements of rotation and shearing, allowing for those of approximation when bearing weight of the fracture site. Each time that the patient bears weight on the limb, both primary fragments move closer to the fracture site, causing the percutaneous pins to bend slightly, allowing for a margin to come together. When the load disappears, its normal elasticity returns both fragments to the starting point. This "accordion effect", carried out in the same direction as the longitudinal axis of the bone, favours healing.

Therefore, it is important to keep in mind that with this type of osteosynthesis system, healing depends, much more so than with other osteosynthesis systems, on the use and bearing of weight of the limb.

Components

Generally, an external fixation system has the following components:

- **Percutaneous pins**: nails or pins that cross through both cortical layers of a bone. Depending on the surgeon's needs, one or both ends stick out from the skin.

  To achieve optimal anchoring in the cortical bone, sometimes they have threads, preferably positive, either on the end, or on its central portion (Fig. 60). The use of positive threads, that is, that have a greater diameter than that of the rest of the body of the implant, reduces the concentration of forces, which in turn partially avoids causing strain to the metal and consequent risk of breaking it (Fig. 61).

  The nails are generally numbered from the most proximal to the most distal.
- **Connecting structures**: rods that are located outside of the skin holding the percutaneous pins in the correct position. These are the structures primarily responsible for bearing the loads of the fixator. They can be made of different materials, although they are usually steel or carbon fibre (Fig. 62).

  These structures, in some cases, are circular rings, known as Ilizarov fixators (Fig. 63), or more complex apparatuses that allow for the separation of the pins, lengtheners and catalysts (Fig. 64).
- **Clamps**: connections that connect the pins to the rods. They basically consist of two pieces of metal that when pressed against each other, they bring the rod and the percutaneous pin together until they are completely fixed. In veterinary medicine, the most used are the Maynard clamps due to their low cost (Fig. 65). There is another type that, at a much greater cost, offers

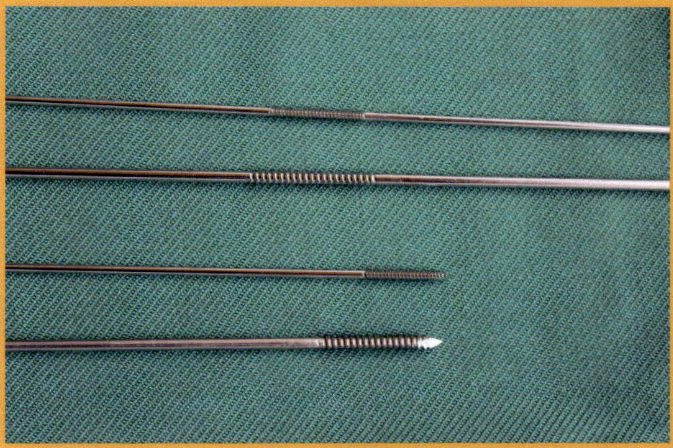

FIGURE 60. Pins with spade tips and threads on the end and centre.

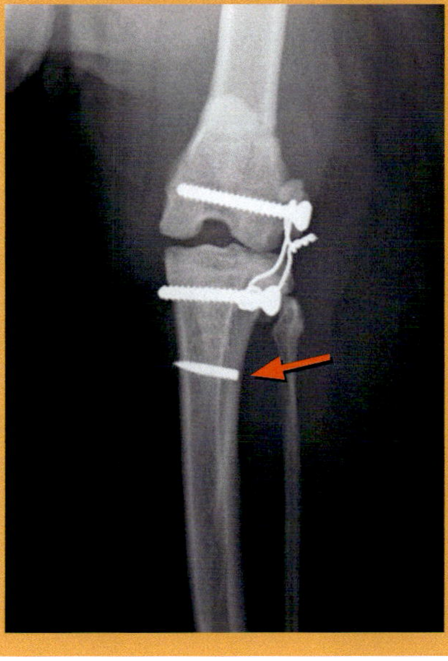

FIGURE 61. Pin with negative threading broken from strain on the bone-metal interface (arrow).

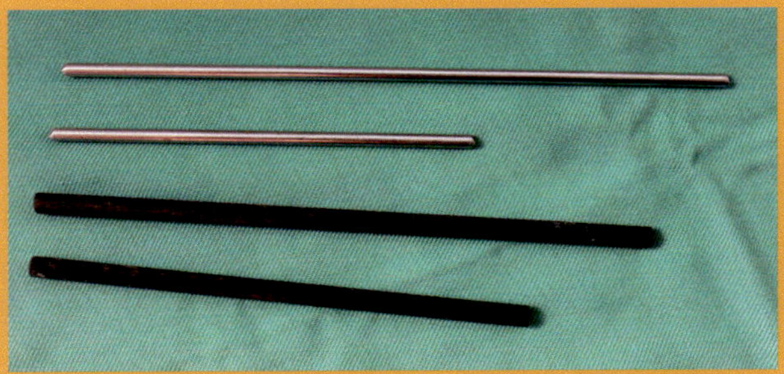

FIGURE 62. Carbon fibre (below) and steel (above) rods.

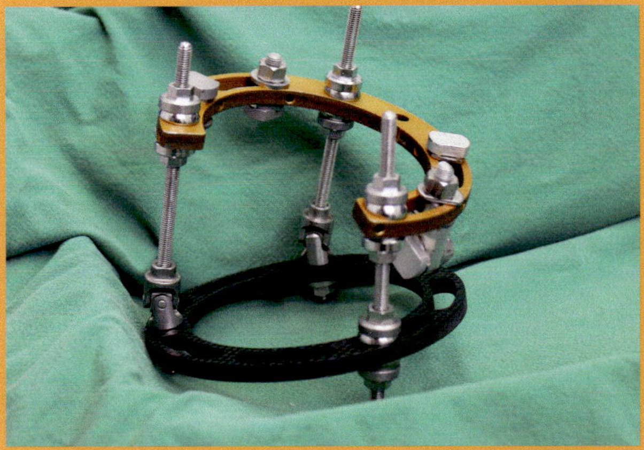

FIGURE 63. Ilizarov type fixators with rings of aluminium and carbon fibre.

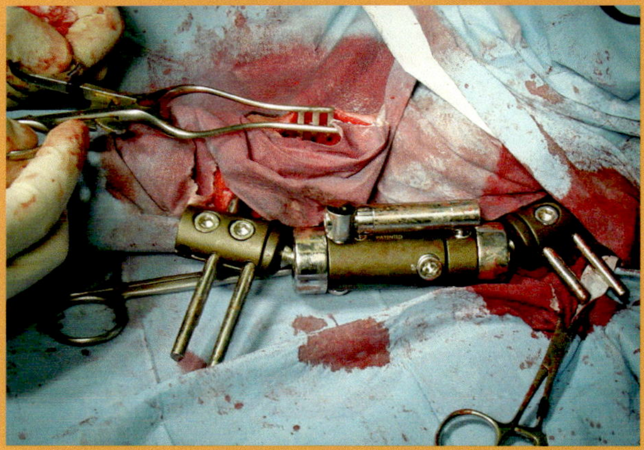

FIGURE 64. Unilateral elongators.

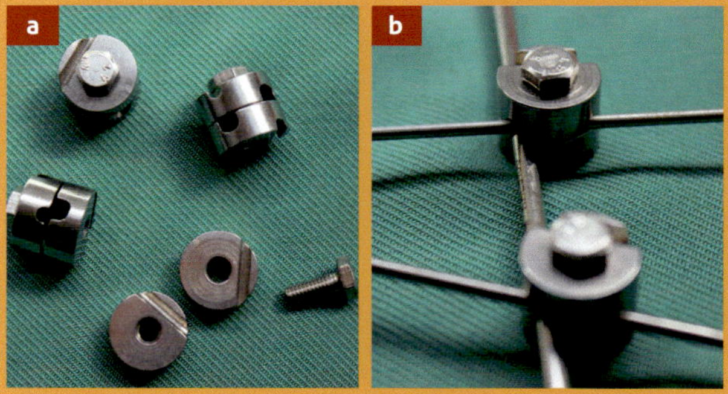

FIGURE 65. Maynard clamps.

more stability. They are generically known as Kirschner-Ehmer, although each manufacturer makes its own modifications (Fig. 66).

- **Articulations**: connections that join the rods together. There use is infrequent and their function is to provide rotational stability to three-dimensional or hybrid fixators.

Methyl methacrylate external fixators

Both the clamps as well as the connecting rods can be substituted by methyl methacrylates. These polymers adhere well to the percutaneous pins and, given their rigidity, they keep them perfectly stable (Fig. 67).

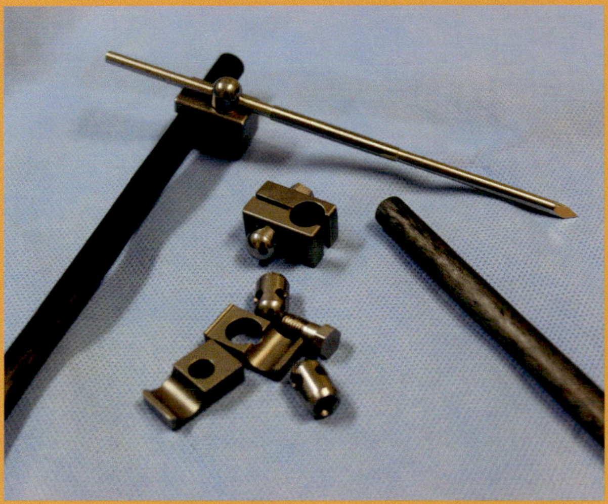

FIGURE 66. K-E type clamp for carbon fibre rods.

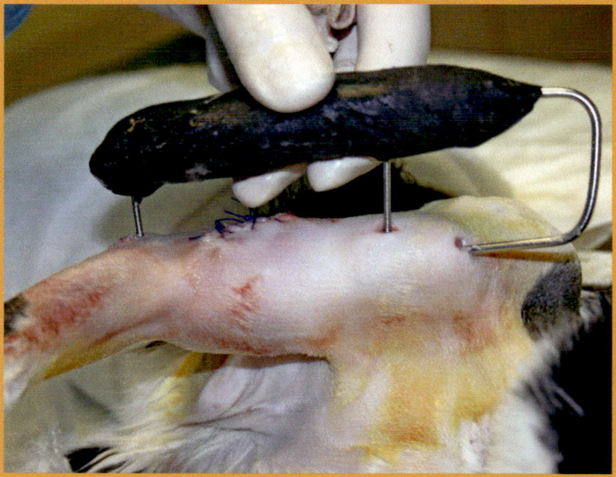

FIGURE 67. External tie-in fixator (hybrid fixation system that basically consists of the association of an intramedullary pin with an external fixator), done with methyl methacrylate.

This system possesses certain advantages that can be of great interest in certain cases. First, due to the absence of clamps and connecting rods, the total weight of the system decreases, which is useful when applied in small animals, primarily exotic species. In these cases, fixators with carbon fibre fixators are also useful.

The methyl methacrylate fixators, as they are made of malleable materials unlike classic fixators whose connecting rods are straight (rigid), allow for the creation of configurations with curves. This particular characteristic may be of use if the external fixation is applied to temporarily immobilise a joint or in the case of mandible fractures (Fig. 68). This configuration can also be achieved by bending the connecting rods if they are steel (Fig. 69). In the case of using carbon fibre rods, this alternative is not feasible; it is also not recommended when using titanium rods.

Another advantage of methyl methacrylate external fixators is that percutaneous pins with different diameters can be used. This is not feasible with clamps as they are designed for specific pin-rod combinations. In some Kirschner-Ehmer type clamp systems, this problem is less important as certain variations are acceptable regarding the diameter of the pins, however, this does not include the Maynard clamps.

Lastly, it is not mandatory that the percutaneous pins stick out forming one single plane with the use of methyl methacrylates; this is a necessary condition when fixating a rod. In that case, as this material is light, a sufficiently thick cylinder can be formed to entirely envelop the ends of the pins.

Types of fixators

There is a vast variety of fixators, depending on the number of pins, connecting rods or their configuration.

Single plane, unilateral external fixator (type I)

Also known as a unilateral fixator. The pins cross through the two compact bone surfaces of the bone, but only one skin surface. The connecting rod is placed on only one side of the bone (Fig. 70).

These are the best option for treating fractures in areas where, due to anatomical reasons, another rod cannot be placed on the other side of the limb (primarily, humerus and femur). Intramedullary pins are usually used for these types of bone. They are also useful to treat mandible or hip fractures.

Given the relative stability of this type of fixators, pins with the largest diameter possible should be used, and, if possible, with a positive threaded tip to increase the strength of the

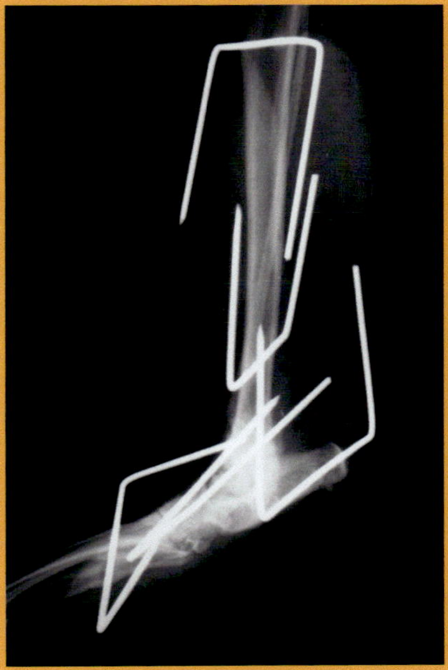

FIGURE 68. Temporary stabilisation of a tarsus in a functional position using external fixation with methyl methacrylate.

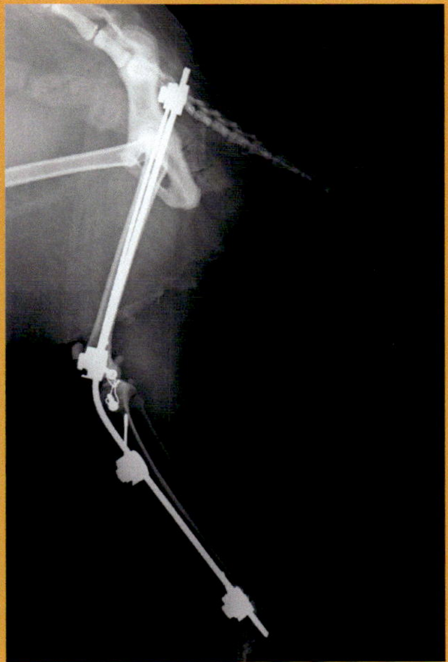

FIGURE 69. Temporary stabilisation of a stifle joint in a functional position through the bending of a connecting rod.

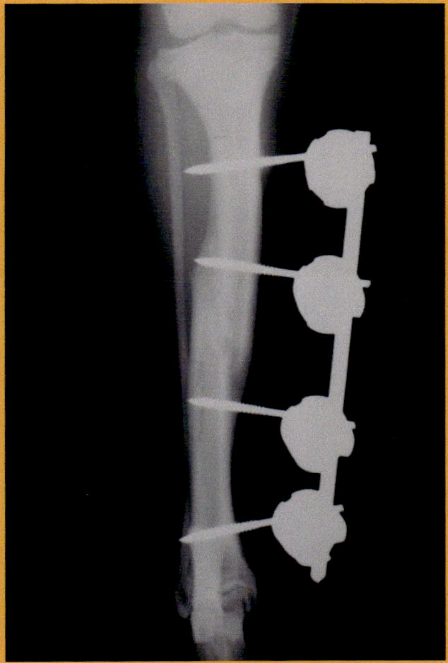

FIGURE 70. Unilateral, single-plane external fixator in the tibia.

anchoring to the bone. When using percutaneous pins without threads, they can be inserted in a convergent manner to avoid loosening, with an angle greater than 60º between them, although optimal anchoring will never be achieved (Fig. 71).

Single plane, bilateral external fixator (type II)

Also known as a double or bilateral fixator. The pins cross through both cortical bone surfaces as well as two skin surfaces. The connecting rods are placed on both sides of the limb (Fig. 72).

These fixators are the most used in radius and tibia fractures. They provide more stability than the type I fixators, given that the axial forces can only provoke slight flexion of the pins. The loads are distributed symmetrically between both rods, absorbed by the pins while bending like the leaf springs used for suspension in wheeled vehicles.

Three-dimensional external fixator (type III)

Also known as a "tent roof" fixator. It consists of a combination of the two previous types placed perpendicularly. The connecting rods are fixed together using others connected through the joints (Fig. 73).

This system provides great rigidity and is thus used frequently in unstable fractures or in those that will most likely take a long time to ossify. Its three-dimensional configuration impedes lateral displacement or "drawer-like" movements that are more probable when using the other types of fixators. Similarly, the "bending" movements that may be produced by type II fixators are stabilised.

Biplane-unilateral or biplane external fixator

This fixator consists of a combination of two type II external fixators placed more or less perpendicular to each other and connected using secondary rods and articulations. This configuration better compensates movements and decreases the structure's weight. When placing the connecting rods at a 90º angle, their size is reduced and they can thus be placed in bones in which type II and III fixators cannot be used (fractures in which a unilateral external fixator does not provide adequate stability).

Hybrid configurations

External fixation allows for numerous combinations, allowing for the structure to be adapted to the surgeon's needs. One of the most frequent configurations is the tie-in.

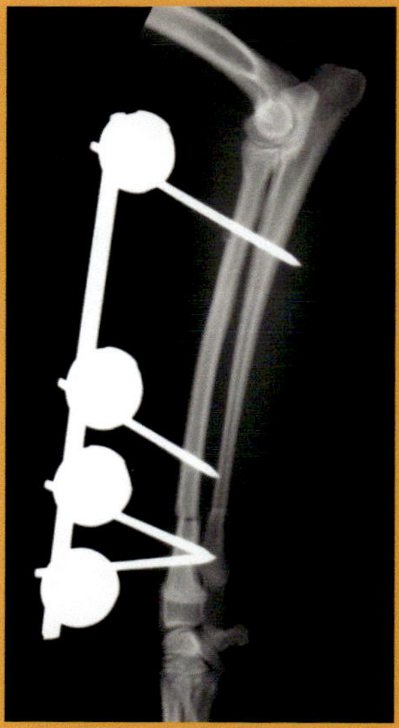

FIGURE 71. The un-threaded pins should not be placed parallel to each other to avoid premature loosening of the system.

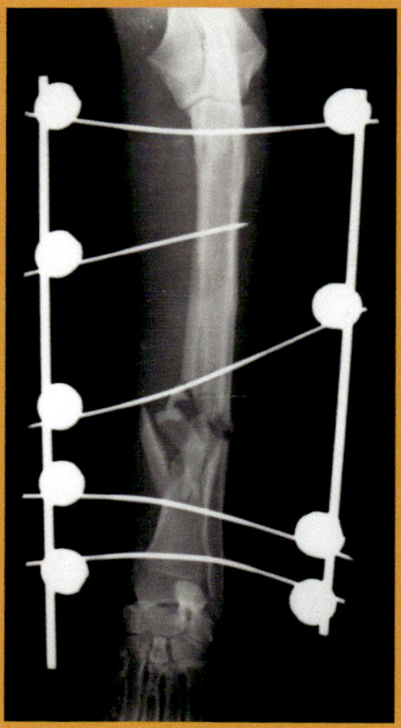

FIGURE 72. Bilateral, single-plane external fixator in the radius.

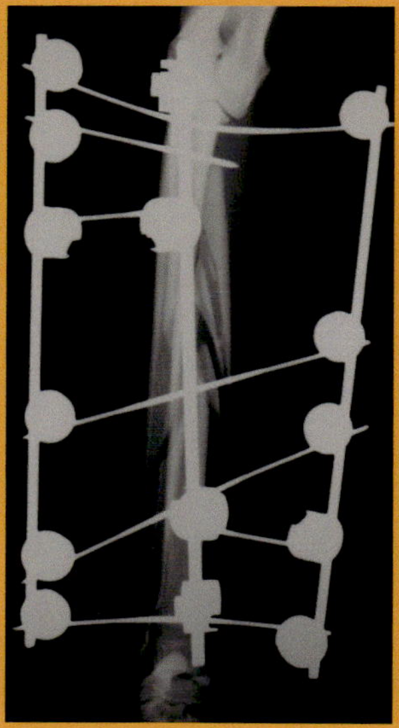

FIGURE 73. Three-dimensional external fixator in the radius.

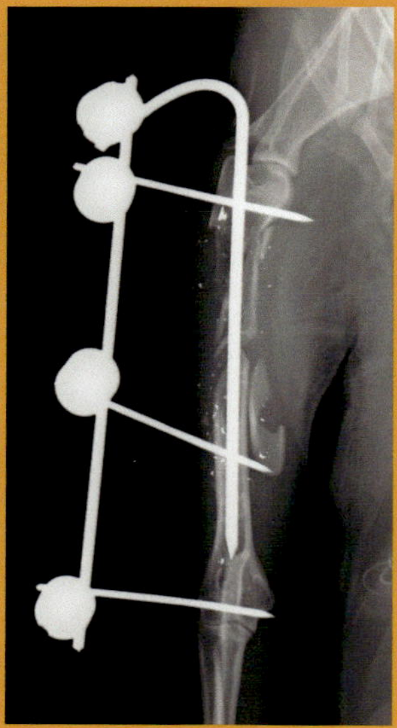

FIGURE 74. Tie-in type external fixator. Take note that the intramedullary pin and the connecting rod form one single element.

This system primarily consists of the association of an intramedullary pin with a single-plane, unilateral external fixator. Its peculiarity is based on the fact that the intramedullary pin and the connecting rod form one single element. Something similar to a bilateral, single-plane fixator is thus obtained in which one of the connecting rods is introduced into the medullary cavity. Given that the percutaneous pins cross through the cortical bone, migration of the intramedullary fixation system is avoided (Fig. 74).

In some cases, primarily when dealing with a humerus or a femur, due to the specific anatomical conditions of these bones, and depending on the fracture's stability, rods can be added to provide greater stability to the system. In this manner, hybrid fixations are obtained (Fig. 75).

Technique of application of external fixators

All external fixators must have at least two pins for each primary fragment. If only one pin is used, it would act as a hinge, allowing for the bone to rotate which would lead to a lack of stability. This issue is solved if the external fixation is associated with a complementary system that impedes said movement. The most typical example is the association of an intramedullary pin with a unilateral external fixator.

First of all, the pins are inserted in the positions farthest from the fracture site (proximal and distal), that is, number 1 and 4 of a fixator with four percutaneous pins (Fig. 76). To achieve optimal stability of the fixator, these pins should be placed as close as possible to the epiphysis, which means that the fixator must cover as much of the bone's length as possible.

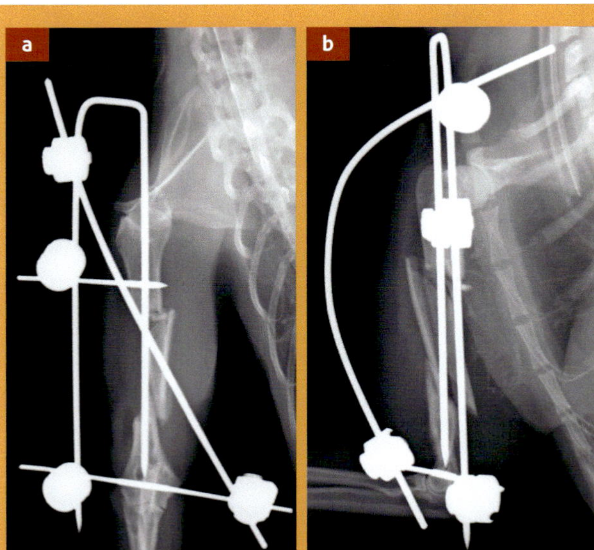

FIGURE 75. Tie-in hybrid external fixator. Take not of the different angles of the connecting rods.

When the percutaneous pin is being inserted, drilling it into place, care must be taken not to tug on the surrounding soft tissues. For this reason, before placement, a small incision should be made in the skin, reaching the bone, with the help of a scalpel.

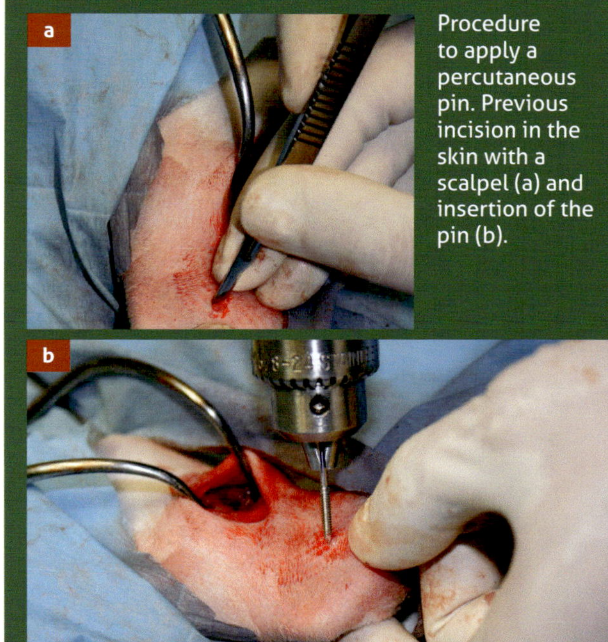

Procedure to apply a percutaneous pin. Previous incision in the skin with a scalpel (a) and insertion of the pin (b).

Once the pins are placed on the ends of the bone, they must be fixed to the connecting rods using clamps (Fig. 77). The placement of the clamps inside or outside of the connecting rods, that is, between the rod and the skin, or outside of the system, is not decisive to the correct functioning of the external fixator. However, placing Maynard clamps outside of the rods provides greater stability, while the Kirschner-Ehmer type clamps are placed inside.

Generally, a separation of 1 cm should be left between the clamps and the skin to avoid them becoming encrusted, especially taking into account that inflammation of the limb is frequent after surgery.

Once this first structure is assembled, which in the case of a type II fixator is like a frame, the position of the fragments can be slightly reduced, correctly reducing the fracture site. This is achieved by moving the primary fragments by tractioning the percutaneous pins.

To set the structure in its definitive position, there are two options:

a. Through direct observation, in the case of open reductions.
b. Using the position of the bone protrusions and the adequate direction of the joint movements as a reference, in the case of closed reductions.

Once the definitive position of the fixator has been decided, the rest of the percutaneous pins are then put into place (Fig. 78). To facilitate this process, a few clamps can be used on the connecting rods that will serve as a supporting point and guide to introduce the rest of the percutaneous pins.

When a pin is inserted, it must be taken into account that when perforating the cortical bone, friction is caused that produces heat, both at the tip of the implant and the bone. If the temperature rises past a certain point, it can cause bone tissue death around the area in question due to overheating. This phenomena is known as thermal necrosis (Fig. 79). When the osteocytes die, the bone is weakened or can even cause bone sequestrum around the implant, provoking the premature loosening of the osteosynthesis system, as well as pain when the affected limb bears weight.

Some fundamental aspects that must be taken into account when placing external fixations include:

- Generally, all percutaneous pins must be screwed into the bone, both if they stick out on both sides, in which case they would need to have central threading, as well as if they only pierce the skin on one side, in which case threading would only be necessary on the tip.
- Although the pin does not stick out on both sides, the implant must always cross through both cortical bone surfaces; if not, stability would be poor and allow for side-to-side movements. This is due to the fact that the grip of the pins or nails without threading depends on the coefficient of friction of the bone-metal interface. In these points of contact, between the cortical bone and the pin, the forces generated when the limb bears weight are absorbed. This produces a progressive loss of bone mass around the pin that will slowly enlarge the hole and eventually lead to the loosening of the pin.

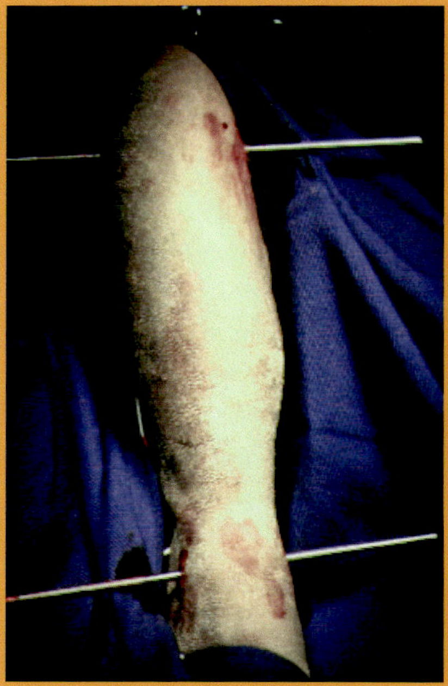

FIGURE 76. Insertion of the percutaneous pins 1 and 4 closest to the epiphysis.

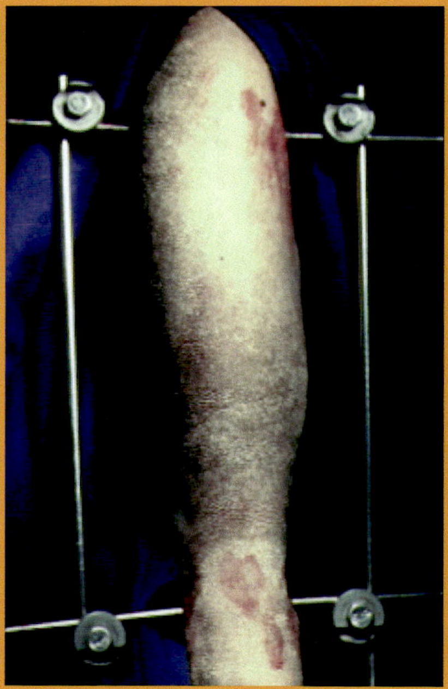

FIGURE 77. Fixation of pins 1 and 4 to the connecting rods.

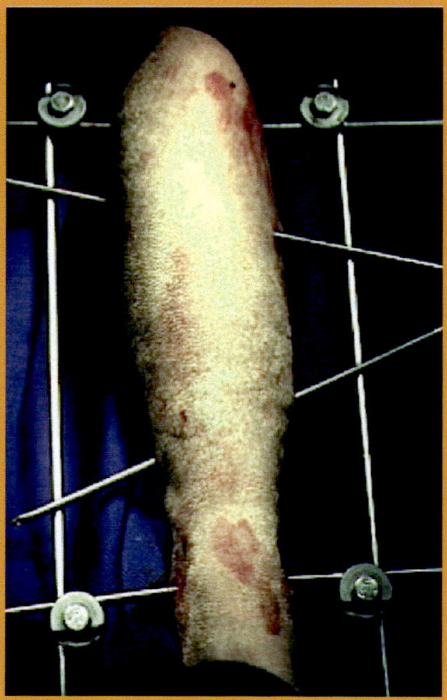

FIGURE 78. Placement of pins 2 and 3, supported by the connecting rods.

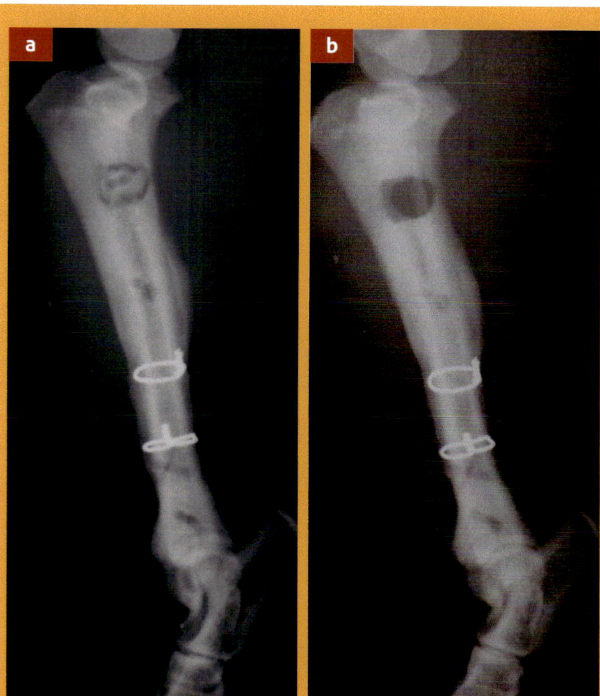

FIGURE 79. Thermal necrosis due to bone overheating. Take note of the radiolucency around the necrotised fragment (a). X-ray image after bone sequestrum has been eliminated (b).

If the pins loosen prematurely, the patient will experience pain when bearing weight on the limb, and consequently, the loads necessary to favour ossification will not be generated. On the other hand, when the percutaneous pins are loosened, the entire fixator may be displaced in a lateral direction which is known as "drawer-like" movement of an external fixator (Fig. 80).

- Although we have previously commented the advantages of using threaded pins, at least one for each primary fragment, if smooth pins are used, they should not be arranged in a parallel manner. That is, in the case of a type II fixator with four percutaneous pins, pins number 1 and 2 should maintain a certain angle between them, and the same goes for pins 3 and 4, to avoid lateral displacement. Pins 2 and 4, however, can be placed parallel, given that they would be anchored in different bone fragments.
- Another important aspect is the distribution of the pins along the length of the bone. As previously mentioned, the fixator should cover as much of the length of the bone as possible, that is, the pins on the ends should be placed on the bone epiphysis or metaphysis.

Overheating depends on various factors:

- **Diameter of the pin:** greater diameters lead to more friction. Before inserting the pin, it is recommended that the bone be perforated previously with a drill bit of a smaller diameter. This operation should primarily be done when pins with diameters greater than 1.5 mm will be used.
- **Perforation velocity:** greater velocity leads to greater friction. Perforations should not be made at more than 150 rpm. Drills designed for osteosynthesis do not usually surpass this number of revolutions. However, caution should be taken when using other types of adapted motors.
- **Friction time:** greater time leads to greater heating. Friction time is reduced when greater pressure is exerted with the tip of the implant on the bone leading to faster perforation.
- **Type of tip:** there are tips designed to minimise overheating.
- **Bone hardness:** harder bones cause more overheating. Precautions should be taken in surgeries with adult patients or when percutaneous pins are inserted in a diaphysis. The meta- and epiphyseal areas are formed by cancellous bone covered by a very thin layer of cortical bone, and thus these zones do not overheat as easily.

- For this same purpose, the pins closest to the fracture site should be placed close to the fracture line (as close as possible). Of course, a safety margin should be kept between the percutaneous pins and the edge of the fracture (minimum 3-5 mm) so that when perforating the cortical bone, no new fracture lines are caused.
- If the surgeon chooses to perform an open reduction, care should be taken to not place the pins in the surgical incision area as this would cause a delay in healing.

Once all of the pins have been set in place, they are then fixed to the rods with the corresponding clamps, tightening them as much as possible.

If considered necessary at this time, an X-ray can be taken to assess the result of the surgery. If satisfactory, the

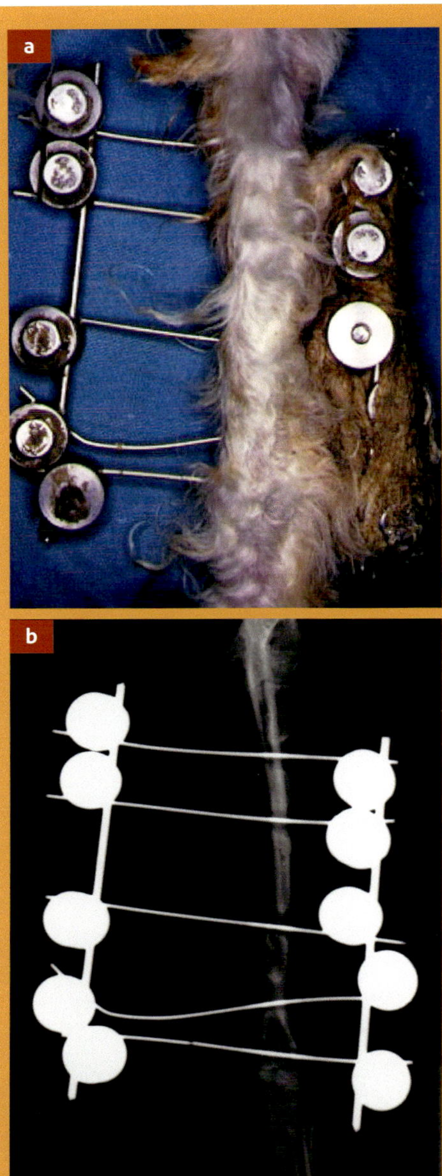
FIGURE 80. Lateral displacement or "drawer-like" movement of an external fixator.

ends of the percutaneous pins can be cut to level them with the clamps to avoid causing any damage to the patient or to elements near the patient.

It is important that the surgeon possesses in-depth knowledge of the anatomical structures when the pins are inserted to avoid the areas where important structures reside, primarily blood vessels and nerves. Similarly, crossing through important muscle masses should also be avoided. This would cause discomfort to the patient, an increase in the production of exudate around the pin, as well as the premature loosening of the implant as a result of constant movement. The ideal areas for insertion are called safe corridors.

***Safe corridors:** trajectories of anatomical regions where the probability that the insertion of percutaneous pins may damage important structures such as nerves or blood vessels is lower.*

Advantages of the application of external fixators

One of the primary advantages of external fixators is their low cost as many of their components can be reused. Also, no large investment in specific instruments or storage of material is needed.

On the other hand, it must be taken into account that although the price of the implants is lower, a patient treated with external fixation must be monitored more closely during the postoperative period and a second surgical intervention is mandatory to remove the implants. The cost of this system compared to osteosynthesis plates is practically the same.

This technique, like all surgical techniques, must be performed in a rigorously aseptic manner. In this sense, its primary advantage is that is preserves the blood supply and integrity of the surrounding soft tissues, in such a way that the possible problems of iatrogenic infection are minimised and bone healing times are shortened.

Another advantage of this osteosynthesis system is the possibility to stabilise the fracture without opening it up and exposing the fracture site. However, if an open reduction is necessary, a narrower approach can be performed than that used when a fixation system is placed using other osteosynthesis methods, primarily plates. This is due to the fact that only the space needed to associate some other system or confirm the correct reduction of the fracture site must be exposed.

When dealing with open fractures, external fixation also offers interesting benefits that are explained below in the section Type of fracture.

Selection of the type of external fixator

When selecting the proper osteosynthesis system, obtaining the greatest stability with the minimum amount of osteosynthesis material should prevail. There are no fixed rules as everything depends on the stability of the fracture, the patient's age, the bone affected, the manufacturer of the fixator, etc. Consequently, when a fixator is selected, different aspects must be taken into account.

Physical limitation

The anatomy of the limb to be treated must be considered. From an anatomical point of view, a bilateral, single-plane fixator cannot be used in a femur fracture given that a connecting rod cannot be placed on the medial face. For this type of bone, the possibility to apply biplane fixators should also be rejected as there are potent muscular masses on both the cranial surface as well as the caudal surface that should not be crossed through. Therefore, the use of type II fixators is limited to stabilisations that are performed in distal areas of the elbow and stifle.

The distal portions of the femur and humerus may tolerate connecting rods on their medial surface in some cases (Fig. 81). This possibility can be exploited to use hybrid configurations (combining different types of fixators).

Diameter and number of pins

Mechanically, the greater the diameter of the percutaneous pins, the greater the stability that can be achieved at the fracture site. However, as previously mentioned, external fixation does not achieve absolute rigidity.

The thickness of the pins presents certain physical limitations. Sections that surpass one third of the bone's diameters should not be used. If so, the hole would weaken the mechanical resistance of the cortical bone with its consequent risk of fracture.

Regarding the number of pins per fragment, it has been experimentally confirmed that a higher number of pins leads to more stability. This is due to a better distribution of forces, which decreases the stress on the bone-pin interface. The pins are therefore able to remain stable for more time. Another advantage of inserting a greater number of pins is that the movements of cranio-caudal angulation are better compensated.

Connecting rods

The connecting rods are what truly confer stability to the structure. When an external fixator has more rods, its resistance to deformation will be greater. The problem is that bones do not always tolerate all structures. One possibility to partially compensate this problem is to add another temporary connecting rod parallel to one that is already in place (Fig. 82). This configuration also presents the advantage that once a few weeks have passed, the temporary connecting rod can be removed, allowing for the bone to bear more weight which will in turn favour

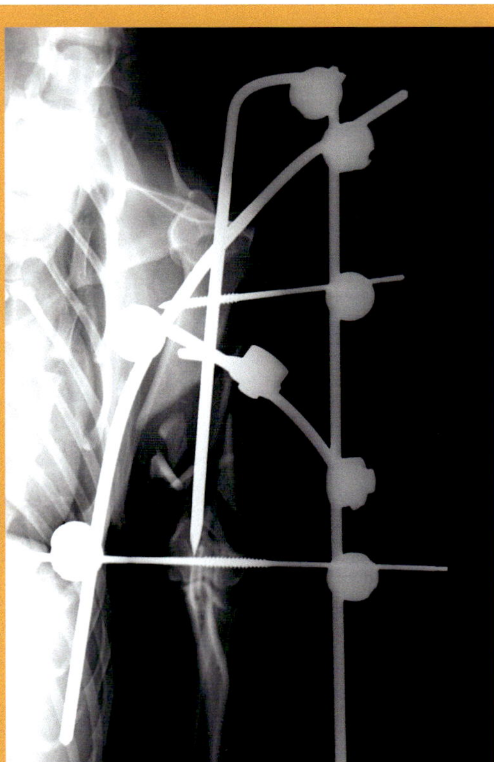

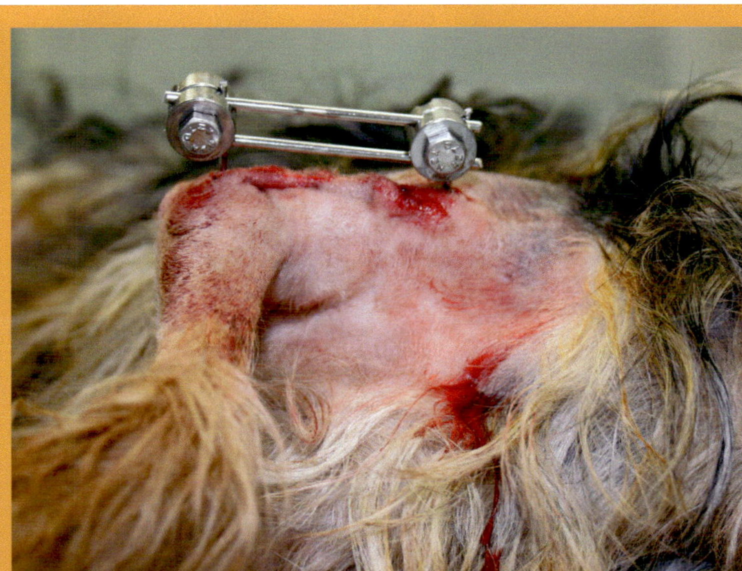

FIGURE 82. Unilateral external fixator with a double connecting rod. The double connecting rod provides resistance to the fixation structure.

FIGURE 81. Connecting rod placed on the medial surface of the distal epiphysis of the humerus in a tie-in hybrid.

ossification. This is referred to as the dynamisation of an external fixator.

Another important point is the type of rods used. Generally, metal is more elastic (steel, more than titanium which is lighter, is more rigid). Carbon fibre rods are extremely light and thus greater diameters can be used. Diameters of 2 to 4 mm are used with steel whereas diameters from 4 up to 10 mm can be used with carbon fibre.

If carbon fibre rods are used, which only accept Kirschner-Ehmer clamps (much more stable than Maynard clamps), complex structures should not be used as the rigidity of the system may thus be excessive.

Dynamisation of an external fixator: *consists in the progressive elimination of temporary rods connected to the fixator, so that the weight supported by the bone increases and, consequently, bone healing is favoured.*

Age of patient

Generally, fractures in younger patients heal faster, which means that the fixator must perform its function for less time; therefore:

- If non-threaded percutaneous pins are chosen, there will be no time for the bone-pin interface to produce the loosening of the implants.
- On the other hand, as the healing potential in young patients is much greater, less rigid structures can be used; the relative instability of the fracture site is perfectly compensated.

Consequently, the age-healing speed must be taken into account, applying more rigid structures in accordance with the patient's age.

Type of fracture

The most important point to be kept in mind regarding the type of fracture is its stability after reduction.

Considering the external fixator and the bone as an interrelated biomechanical system is important. The stability of this system not only depends on the configuration of the external fixator, but also on the contact between the bone fragments, as well as the stability achieved in the fracture site as the healing process takes place.

In cases of comminuted fractures or in those where an external fixator is used to elongate bones, all stability will depend on the fixator. In these situations, the fixator bears all of the axial loads that the limb is subjected to. These forces will produce areas of stress on the bone-pin interface, that, consequently, will cause halisteresis with loosening of the pin. For this reason, in this type of fractures, it is always recommended that three-dimensional fixators are used, as well as threaded percutaneous pins.

If there is contact between the bone fragments, the axial forces will be partially transferred to the cortical bone. In this case, the fixator must only compensate part of the forces of the load, as well as those of rotation, avulsion and shearing.

When dealing with transversal or short oblique fractures that can be reduced, the axial loads may almost be entirely transferred from one primary fragment to another. Consequently, the external fixator has to compensate primarily forces of flexion and rotation in this type of fractures.

However, as previously mentioned, it must be taken into account that the short oblique or transversal fractures with only one small fracture plane do not tolerate instability well. Any movement of the fragments is transformed into great displacement between the fracture lines (high index of movement per linear fracture unit). That is, although transversal and short oblique fractures are very stable and easy to correctly reduce, they are not ideal for stabilisation using dynamic systems; rigid osteosynthesis systems are preferable.

There are certain cases where external fixators are the treatment of choice, although not the only choice. This system is more advantageous than others for certain types of fractures for the following reasons:

Open fractures

One of the primary advantages of this type of fixation is that it does not introduce any type of osteosynthesis material in the fracture site (introducing foreign material in the infection site makes both the elimination of necrotic material as well as the rest of healing processes more difficult). Also, better revascularisation is achieved of the fracture site by enabling the new formation of blood vessels through the medullary cavity and in the soft tissues surrounding the bone (disadvantage of osteosynthesis with plates). Quick revascularisation favours the activation of the cells responsible for acting against infection, as well as the antibiotics that should be administered to the patient.

Another advantage of the external fixators in this type of fractures, especially grade III open fractures, is that they allow for direct treatment of the infected area (Fig. 83).

The last advantage is the possibility to carry out temporary stabilisations until other treatments can be applied if necessary.

Highly comminuted fractures

At least one of the primary fragments is very short which impedes stabilisation using osteosynthesis plates.

Generally, external fixation produces good results in fractures that apparently cannot be reduced. These are fractures in which the movement index per linear fracture unit is very low, that is, the displacement between the primary fragments is divided between the multiple fractures, causing a very slight displacement between them.

In this type of fractures, closed techniques are usually used, giving priority to the length and alignment of the bone and preserving the surrounding soft tissues. On the other hand, as previously mentioned, more rigid fixation structures are needed.

Fractures of the mandible

External fixation can be of great use in the treatment of mandible fractures due to a series of factors including the following:

- Limitation of space, due to dental roots.
- Weakness of the cortical bone, in the caudal portion of the mandibular ramus.
- Frequent existence of multiple fragments, that are frequently of a small size.
- Suspicions of contamination due to the opening of the oral mucosa.
- Need for perfect occlusion between teeth.

For all of these reasons, one of the most used systems in this type of fractures is stabilisation by means of external fixation with methyl methacrylates.

The advantage of these materials over rigid rods, as previously mentioned, is that they allow for the placement of all necessary percutaneous pins without the need to keep them in one single plane (Fig. 84).

Once in place, the mouth is closed to obtain the perfect occlusion of the teeth. Intubation is recommended through

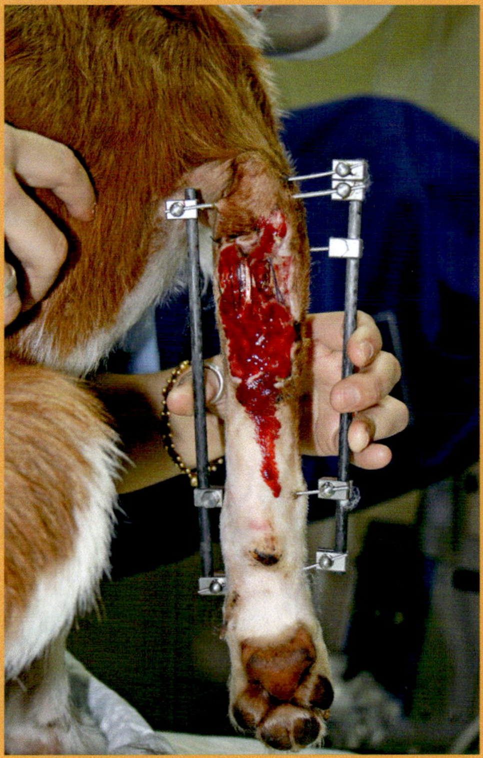

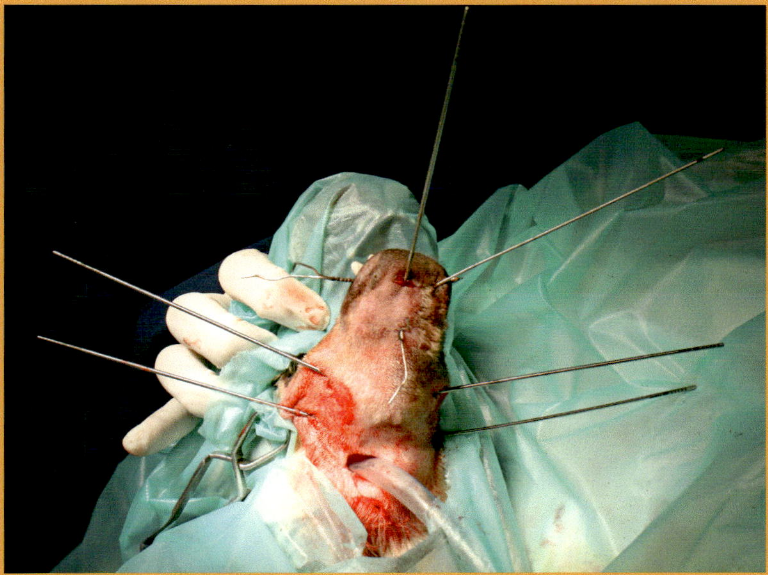

FIGURE 84. Placement of two percutaneous pins per fragment in a mandible fracture.

FIGURE 83. External fixator in an open fracture from an animal bite where a great loss of soft tissues is observed. Note that the arrangement of the rods allows for the injury to be treated.

a pharyngostomy to avoid the endotracheal tube from impeding correct assessment. After, and while keeping the patient's mouth shut, stabilisation is performed using methyl methacrylates. There are two ways to apply acrylic cements:

a. Bending the ends of the pins and manually applying the product around them in a semi-solid phase (Fig. 85).

b. Placing a silicone tube that crosses the percutaneous pins and injecting the cement in its liquid phase into the tube (Fig. 86).

The external fixation with methacrylates is the best system to stabilise mandible fractures due to the possibility of placing the pins of different diameters in different planes.

You can find more in-depth information regarding fractures of de jaw in the chapter titled Head Fractures (page 118).

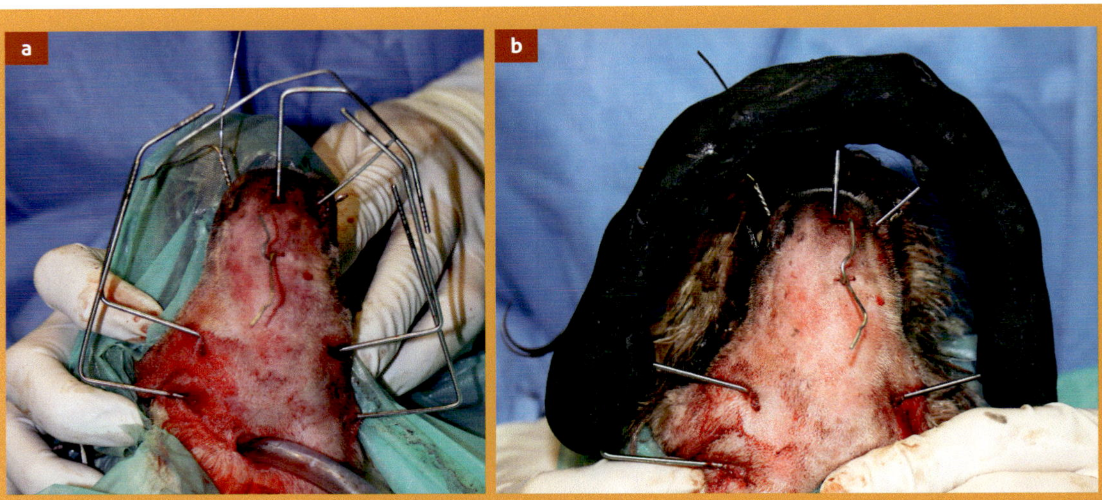

FIGURE 85. Bending of the pins in occlusion (a). Stabilisation with semi-solid methyl methacrylate (b).

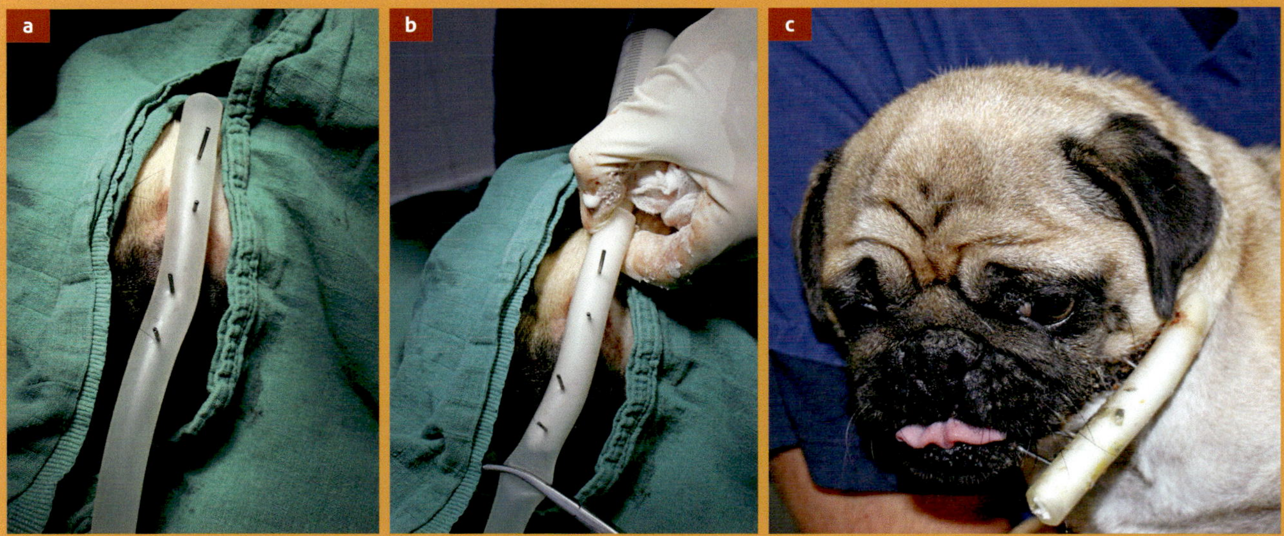

FIGURE 86. Sequence of injection of the cement through a tube. Placement of the tube in the pins (a); filling of the tube with the cement (b), and final result (c).

SCREWS

Types of screws

The principal application of screws in bone surgery is to fasten plates to bones. However, we will discuss this osteosynthesis system in another section in order to properly clarify certain concepts that should be taken into account.

First, we must be familiar with the different types of screws that are currently available on the market. Depending on the type of threading, there are two large groups:

Cortical bone screws

Cortical bone screws (Fig. 87) are designed to fasten tightly to the cortical bone found in the diaphyses of long bones. This tissue is compact and its thickness, depending on its location and the patient's age, allows for a resistant anchoring. The screws inserted in the diaphysis of a bone, which resembles a tube (hollow inside), are only fastened to the cortical bone (Fig. 88). If the screw crossed through the entire bone, it would be screwed into the proximal cortical bone (the head of the screw), and in the distal cortical bone (the tip). That is, it is fixed in two points, one close to the head and the other close to the tip.

Cancellous bone screws

Cancellous bone screws (Fig. 89) are designed to be applied to metaphyseal and epiphyseal areas where there is more cancellous bone. This bone is much more labile compared to the previous type. There is no cortical bone in these areas as the entire bone cylinder is solid, that is, it is nearly entirely filled with bone tissue (Fig. 90). Practically the entire length of the screw is anchored, achieving optimal fastening.

They are easily distinguished due to their different design. The cortical bone screws have a thread pitch (the number of spirals per unit of length) greater than that of the cancellous bone screws (Fig. 91). Second, given that the cancellous bone is less resistant, achieving correct fastening requires that more material be fastened between each spiral. For this purpose, the difference between the diameter of the thread and the nucleus is greater in the cancellous bone screws. This way, more bone is covered between the spirals in this type of screw.

Understanding the concept of both diameters is of great importance. The diameter of the nucleus should be equal to the diameter of the solid portion of the screw (Fig. 92). The diameter of the thread is the distance between the most protuberant areas of the spirals (Fig. 93), that is, where the screw presents its greatest diameter. The screw is identified by the diameter of its thread expressed in millimetres. A 3.5 screw thus presents a distance of 3.5 mm between the most protuberant portions of the spirals.

In veterinary bone surgery, there is a great variety regarding the thickness of the screws as there is a great diversity in the size of patients. These go from 1.5 mm thick, to systems of 5.5 mm, used in equine bone surgery. The largest diameter is 6.0 mm, corresponding with cancellous bone screws of the 4.5 system (Fig. 94).

The diameter of the nucleus indicates the diameter of the drill bit that should be used to perforate the bone for the screw to fasten properly to the bone tissue. Each system, logically, uses a drill bit according to the size of the nucleus of the screw (Table 1).

In order to reach an equilibrium between the resistance of the nucleus of the screw and its capacity to fasten to the bone, the difference between both diameters has been studied thoroughly. Almost all companies respect these difference in diameters, as well as the thread pitches of all screw systems. However, when changing from one brand of material to another, it should be confirmed that the standard sizes are respected.

Confirming that reference sizes are respected is important when changing the brand of material used.

After having discussed both basic types of screws available on the market, their function should be taken into account. With one single screw, depending on the steps followed for its placement, two different functions can be achieved. This way, depending on the function produced by a screw, it is classified as a position screw or a compression screw.

Position screws

This is the most frequent function of screws. They are used to fasten plates in the treatment of fractures. When a plate is placed, its attachment to the bone must be firm and solid, for which the screws used must be anchored to both cortical bone surfaces. The position screw is thus a screw

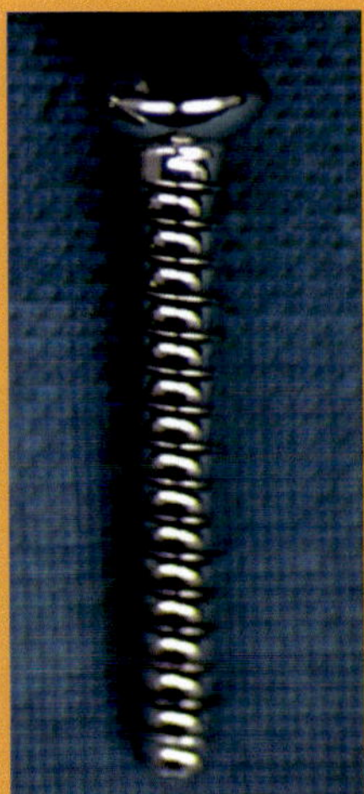
FIGURE 87. Image of a cortical screw.

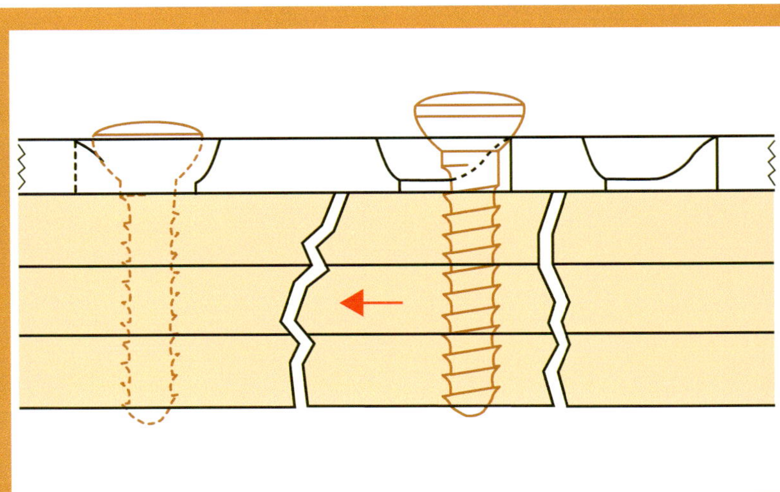
FIGURE 88. Diagram showing how the screw is anchored to both cortical surfaces.

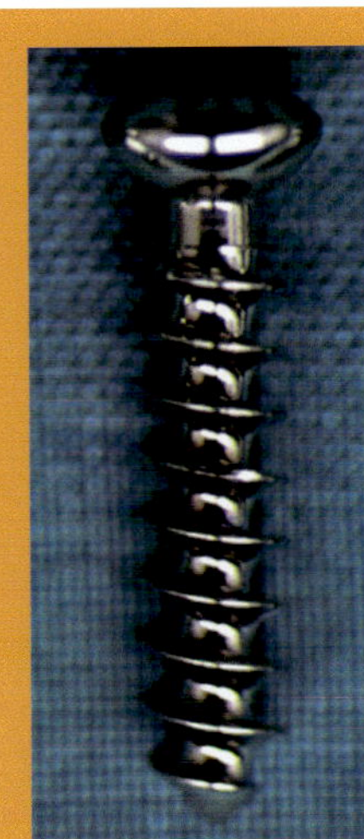
FIGURE 89. Image of a cancellous screw.

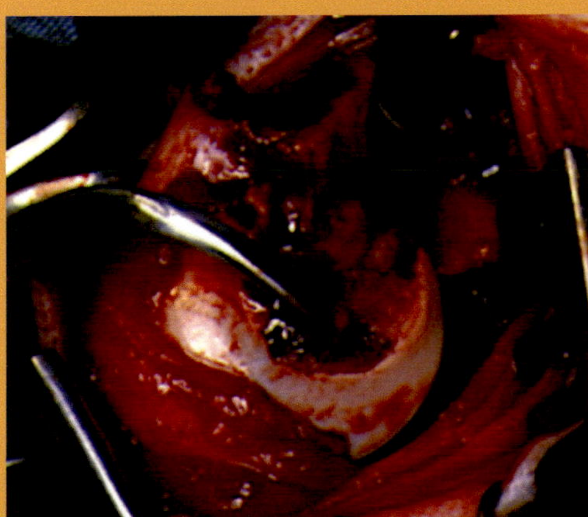
FIGURE 90. Epiphyseal cancellous tissue in a Salter-IV fracture in the lateral condyle of the humerus.

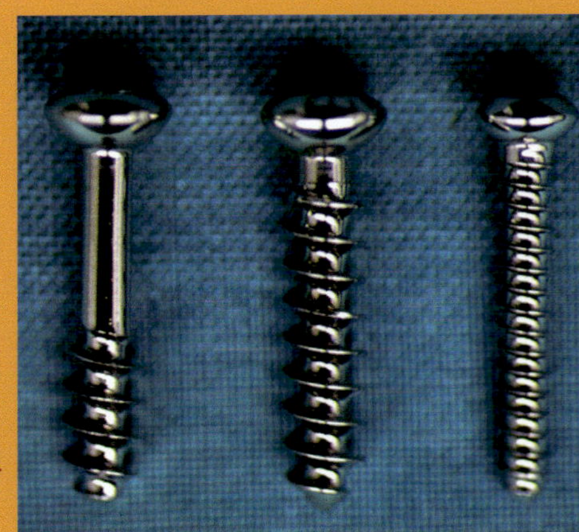
FIGURE 91. Comparative image of the threading of both kinds of screws.

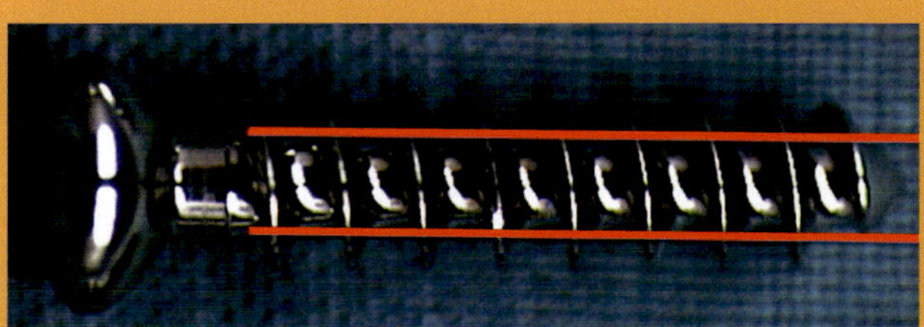
FIGURE 92. Representation of the diameter of the nucleus.

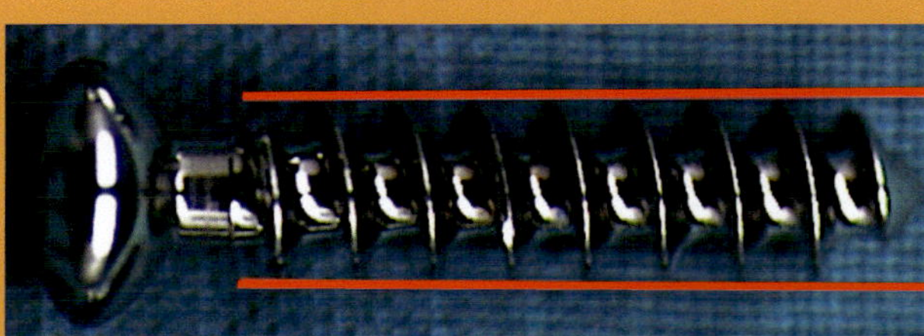
FIGURE 93. Representation of the diameter of the threading.

that is almost always fastened to both cortical bone surfaces of a bone.

Procedure to place position screws

To ensure that a screw is properly anchored, a series of steps must be carefully followed. First of all, a hole must be made that allows for the entry of the screw in the bone. To do this, a drill bit corresponding with the diameter of the nucleus of the screw is used. As previously mentioned, each system is assigned its proper drill bit (Table 1).

It is important that the perforation is made using a guide of the same diameter as the drill bit. These guides have small teeth on their tip that avoid the displacement of the drill on the surface of the cortical bone surface of the bone (Figs. 95 and 96). Once set in the desired position and direction, the drill is inserted in the interior to start the process

TABLE 1. Table of diameters.

Screw	Type	Cortical					Semi-cancellous	Cortical	Cortical	Cancellous
	Diameter (mm)	1.5	2.0	2.4	2.7	3.5	4.0	4.5	5.5	6.5
Diameter of the drill bit for the gliding hole		1.5	2.0	2.4	2.7	3.5	4.0	4.5	5.5	4.5
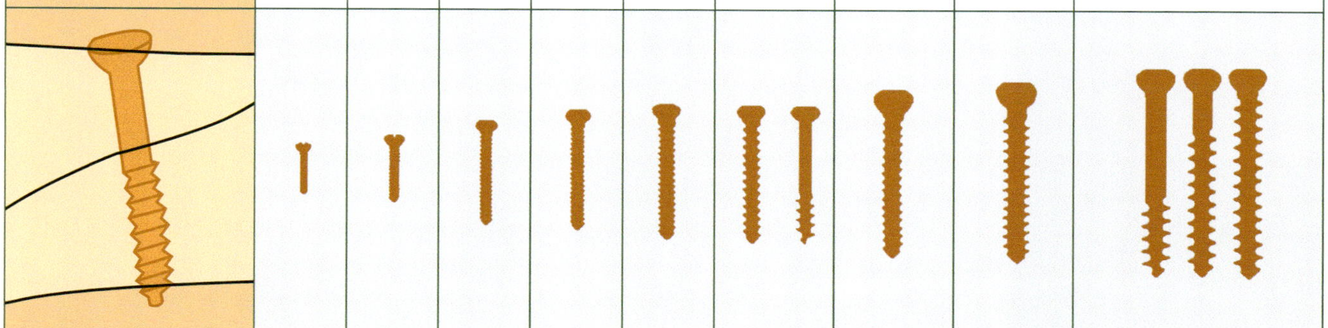										
Diameter of the drill bit for the hole with threading		1.1	1.5	1.8	2.0	2.5	2.5	3.2	4.0	3.2
Thread insert to carve threading		1.5	2.0	2.4	2.7	3.5	4.0	4.5	5.5	6.5

(Fig. 97). This way the tip of the drill bit does not slip when beginning the perforation.

As always when perforating, the friction of the drill bit on the bone produces an increase in temperature that should be avoided. This overheating varies depending on different factors.

- **Age of patient**: older patients usually have harder bones. Also, the layer of cortical bone is usually thinner in young patients.
- **Type of bone to be perforated**: the cortical bone, as it is more compact, is harder. Overheating does not usually take place in the metaphyseal or epiphyseal areas as they are made of cancellous bone.
- **Other factors**: diameter of the drill bit, its sharpness, and the velocity of perforation.

The problem of the drill bit overheating resides in the possibility that thermal necrosis could be produced (cellular death due to excessively high temperatures), which would lead to the premature loosening of the screw when the material in which the spirals of the screws are anchored dies and is reabsorbed.

Overheating of the drill bit can cause thermal necrosis of the bone and, consequently, loosening of the screw due to reabsorption of the bone layer to which the screw is anchored.

To avoid this issue, drill bits in good condition should always be used to perforate, and said perforation should be done at low revolutions. The bone overheats less if the pressure is increased when perforating instead of the number of revolutions of the drill. The perforation tip should be kept cool during the entire process. The use of a flow system of saline solution is sufficient through which isotonic solution is flushed over the bone while perforating.

Once the hole is made, the length of the screw to be used must be chosen. Logically, each system has screws of different lengths. Generally, the increment of length of each screw regarding the previous is 2 mm in the most common size and diameters. Only those of 1.5 mm present an increment of 1 mm due to the small diameter of the bones in which they are applied. For certain lengths and in

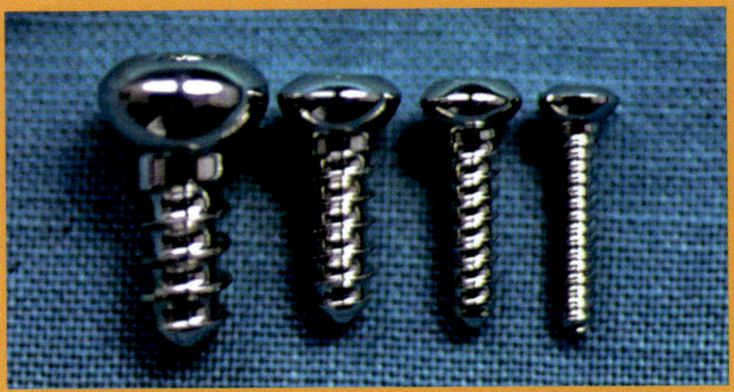

FIGURE 94. Different systems of screws.

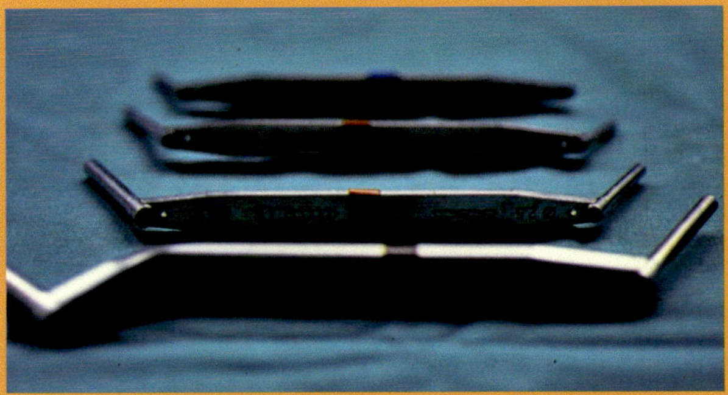

FIGURE 95. Different perforation guides are shown in the image.

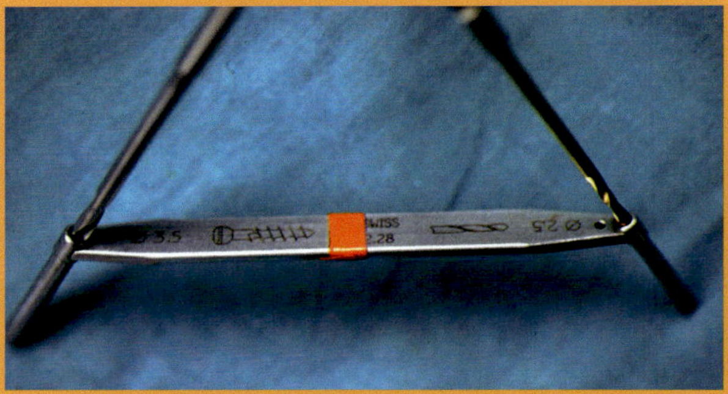

FIGURE 96. Note how the drill bit is introduced into the interior of the guide. This impedes the drill bit from slipping on the bone surface.

screws with large diameters, the difference of the length of one and the next is 5 mm.

To determine the length of the screw, a depth gauge is used (Fig. 98). This instrument is basically a hollow tube that slides over a measuring stick which extends along a rod with a bent tip (Fig. 99). To measure the length, that is, the diameter of the bone where the perforation has been made, said rod is inserted in the hole until the tip sticks out through the distal cortical surface. Slightly inclining the gauge, it is slowly pulled out until the bent tip is "hooked" on the cortical bone surface that we cannot see (Fig. 100).

To avoid overheating:

- Use drill bits in good condition.
- Drill at low revolutions.
- Increase the pressure instead of the speed.
- Cool the process using saline solution.

Once its in place, the tube that envelops the rod is slid until it comes into contact with the proximal cortical bone surface, showing the length of the perforation (Fig. 101). Generally, we should always select a screw with a length that is one size greater than the depth measured. The selection of a longer size is important to ensure that the screw sticks out at least one thread pitch from the distal cortical bone surface. This way we ensure proper anchoring on both cortical surfaces.

Once the screw is selected, the thread must be carved. This process consists of creating a spiral with the same thread pitch as the screw on the walls of the perforated

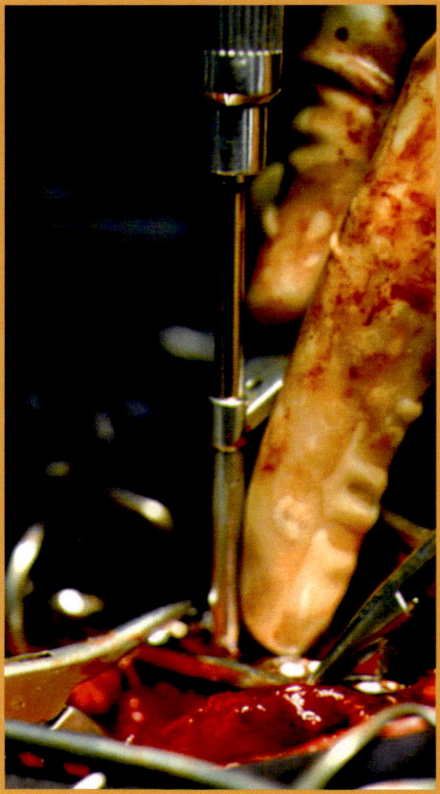

FIGURE 97. Detailed image of a thread insert introduced in the guide to carve the threading.

hole, as if it were a nut. To do this, a thread insert or a tap and die tool, which is nothing more than a long screw with the same diameter and threading as the screw selected, are used. The end of this thread insert has longitudinal fluting that allows for the shavings of bone material from drilling to come out (Fig. 102). Obviously, each system possesses its own specific thread insert.

There are currently self-tapping screws on the market, that is, screws that, due to their design, can be introduced in the hole made in the bone without having to insert the thread insert previously. This is achieved thanks to the design of the tip, which is capable of creating its own threading in the bone as the screw is introduced (Fig. 103).

The primary advantage of this system is not that the placement process is faster, but that, while carving the threading, the screw itself is better anchored to the bone. This phenomena is more important when the bone in which the screw will be inserted is softer.

Once all of the steps are completed, the screw is inserted and tightened. The force to be used to tighten a screw depends fundamentally on the resistance of the bone and the difference between the diameter of the threading and the nucleus of the screw. That is, the difference between diameters will logically be smaller for smaller screws. The depth of the spiral of a 1.5 mm screw is 0.2 mm, while that of a 4.5 screw has a depth of 0.65 mm.

In adult individuals, both the thickness of the cortical bone as well as the bone density are greater than in growing patients.

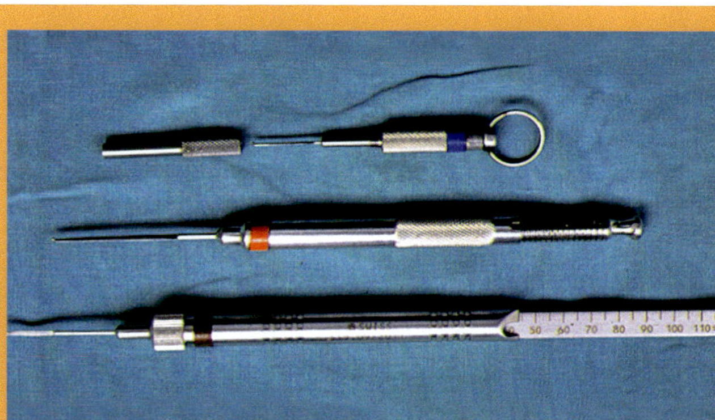

FIGURE 98. Different depth gauges are shown in the image.

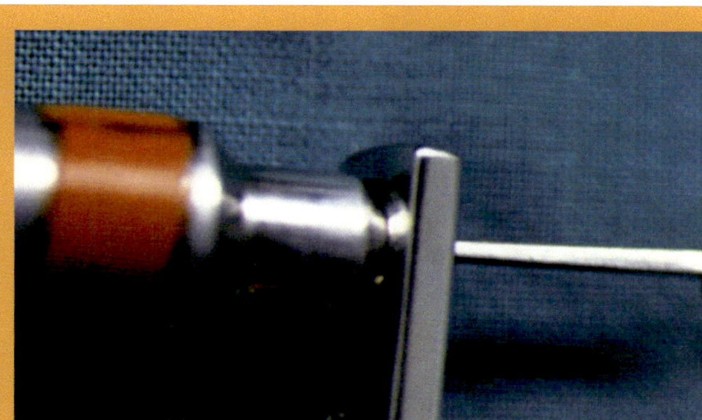

FIGURE 99. Detailed image of the gauge that is introduced in the bones to determine the depth of the hole made. Take note of the bent tip of the rod.

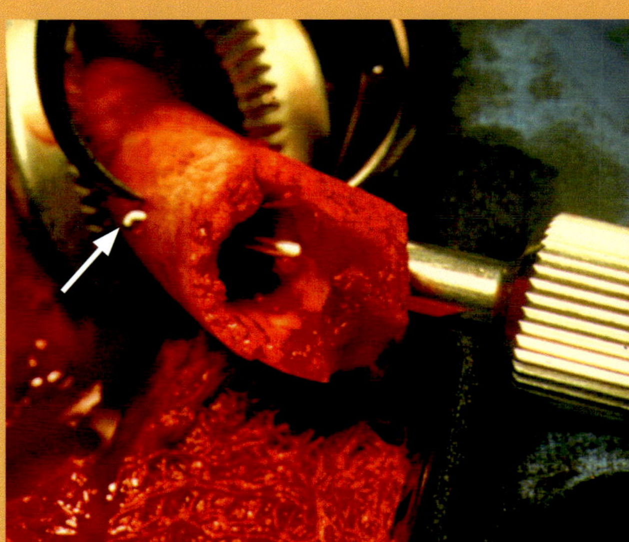

◀ FIGURE 100. Detailed image of the rod introduced in the bone and hooked onto it by its bent tip (arrow).

▼ FIGURE 101. Detailed image of the ruler of the gauge.

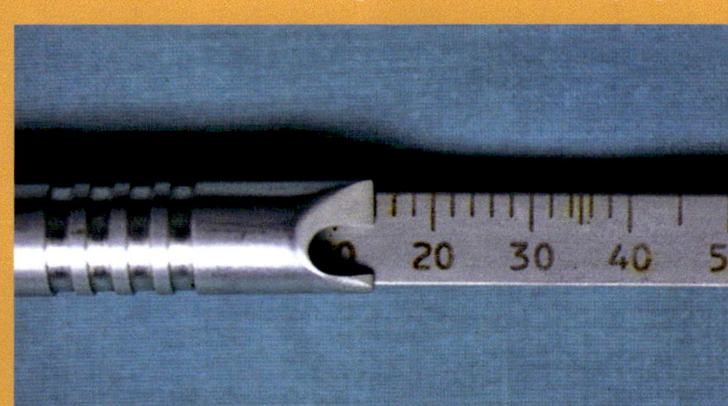

Compression screws

Unlike position screws, the primary function of compression screws is to apply a force that compresses the fracture line. Proper stability is thus achieved and the healing process is faster, as postulated by the Roux Law.

Procedure to place compression screws

A screw compresses a fracture if it is made to function like a nut and bolt. When being screwed into place, the nut and the head of the screw move towards each other, applying pressure to the cortical bone surfaces so that the fracture line located between both fragments is compressed.

In bone surgery, there are nuts that can be used with traditional screws (Fig. 104), however, this is not usually the case. This is done by substituting the nut with the distal cortical bone surface, which is perforated using a drill bit with the same diameter as the nucleus, and later the corresponding threading is carved. Nonetheless, the hole in the proximal cortical surface is perforated with the diameter of the threading. When the screw is introduced, it slides without resistance in the proximal cortical surface and penetrates in the perforation performed on the distal cortical surface (Fig. 105). When turning it, it screws into the distal cortical surface and penetrates until its head comes into contact with the proximal cortical surface in which, as previously mentioned, it does not screw into. From this moment on, as the screw is tightened, the head exerts pressure on the cortical bone surface, pushing it towards the other cortical bone surface, and thus achieves the desired compression.

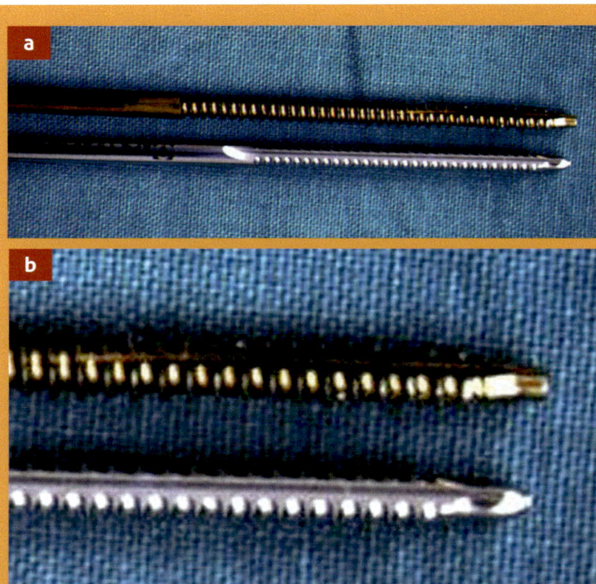

FIGURE 102. Sample of two thread inserts (a) and detailed image of the thread inserts (b).

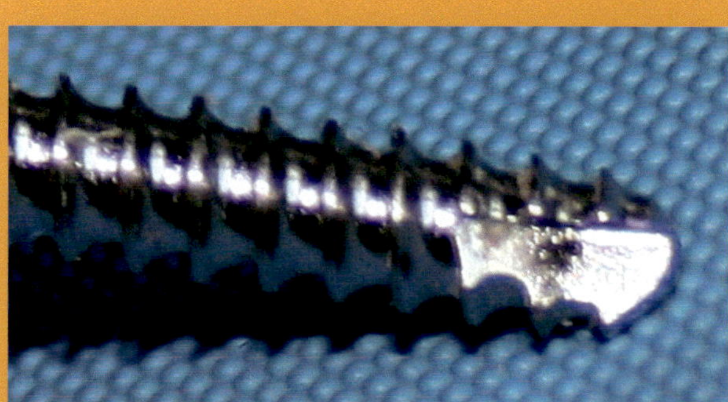

FIGURE 103. Detailed image of the tip of a self-tapping screw. Note its similarity with the tip of a thread insert.

To stabilise a fracture using a screw of this type, proper reduction of the fragments must first be achieved as, if not, when applying pressure on the fracture line, the desired effect would not be achieved.

Once the fracture line is reduced, the fragments must be kept firmly stabilised throughout the entire process of placing the screw. Two-point reduction forceps are especially useful to do this (Fig. 106).

In order to take advantage of the tractioning effect of the screw, it should be placed in the most proximal direction possible to an imaginary line that perpendicularly crosses the fracture plane (Fig. 107). Second, certain safety margins should be respected between the edges of the fragments and the holes to be perforated. If they are made too proximal, when tightening the screw, there is a risk of causing another fracture. The safety margin depends on the diameter of the screw and the hardness of the bone.

Once the diameter of the screw, its position and its direction have been chosen, the perforation of the holes can be performed.

First, as previously mentioned, only the proximal cortical surface will be perforated with the diameter of the threading of the screw in the predetermined direction using the corresponding perforation guide (Fig. 108). This hole is called the "gliding hole". Next, the distal cortical surface is perforated using the drill bit with the same diameter as the nucleus ("traction hole"). To maintain the direction selected, the guide is inserted through the first hole until it comes into contact with the endostium of the distal cortical surface (Fig. 109). These guides, or centring sleeves, are specifically designed for each system of screws.

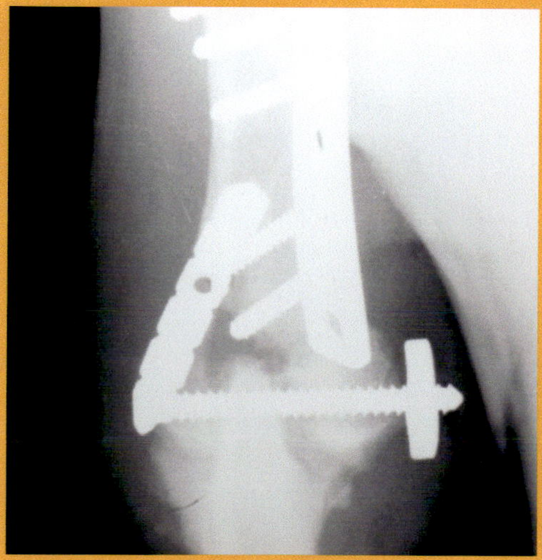

FIGURE 104. X-ray that shows the placement of a nut.

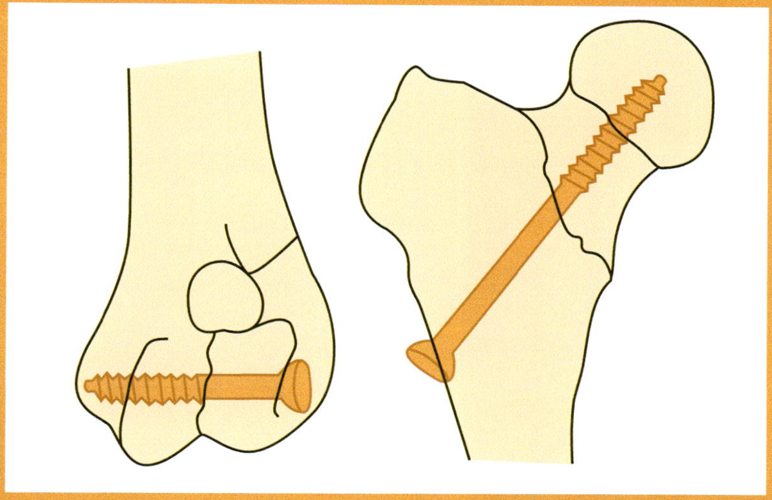

FIGURE 105. Diagrams that show the placement of compression screws anchored to the distal cortical surface with no need for nuts.

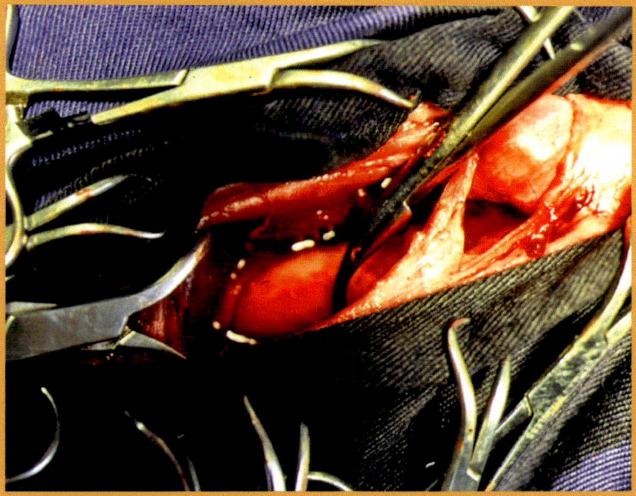

FIGURE 106. Two-point reduction forceps used to hold the fragments of the fracture firmly while it heals.

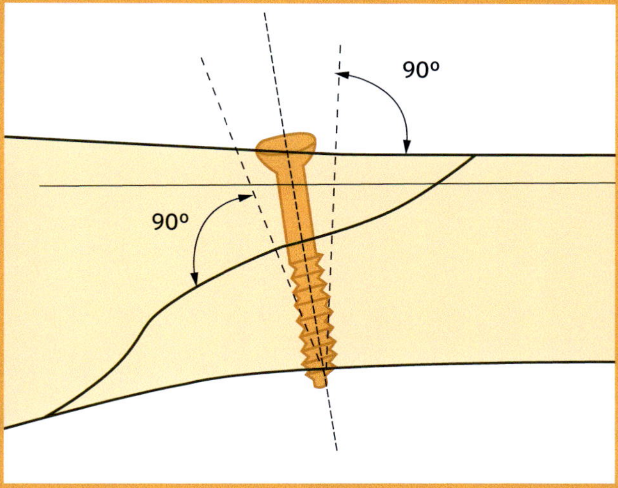

FIGURE 107. Diagram showing how a screw should be oriented to achieve maximum traction.

The external diameter coincides with the diameter of the threading, while the internal diameter coincides with that of the nucleus. This way the distal cortical surface can be perforated while maintaining the direction and keeping the drill bit from slipping.

When compression screws are placed in cortical bone, the area where the head of the screw will be should be countersunk. Countersinking consists of carving a wedge for the screw head so that its pressure is distributed over a greater bone surface (Fig. 110). Osteolysis, which is produced in the areas of metal-bone contact, is delayed and the function of the compression screw is prolonged by avoiding its premature loosening.

When this type of screw is applied in epiphyseal areas or in soft bones, as these areas are formed primarily by cancellous bone, countersinking is contraindicated. Due to the weakness of the bone, if we eliminate the cortical layer, the head of the screw will break the bone structure and penetrate into the bone (Fig. 111). To achieve proper distribution of the pressure over these areas, washers are used between the screw head and the bone (Fig. 112).

In epiphyseal areas or soft bones, countersinking is contraindicated as it weakens the area where the screw head exerts pressure.

To finalise the process, the other steps are followed as usual. The length of the screw is measured using a depth gauge. The threading is carved if self-tapping screws are not used, and the screw is introduced, tightening it until the desired tightness is achieved (Fig. 113). In the case that the threading must be carved, if the bone is soft enough, the thread insert can be turned only a few times to start the creation of threading and then leave the screw, although it is not self-tapping, to continue introducing itself. Optimal anchoring is achieved this way.

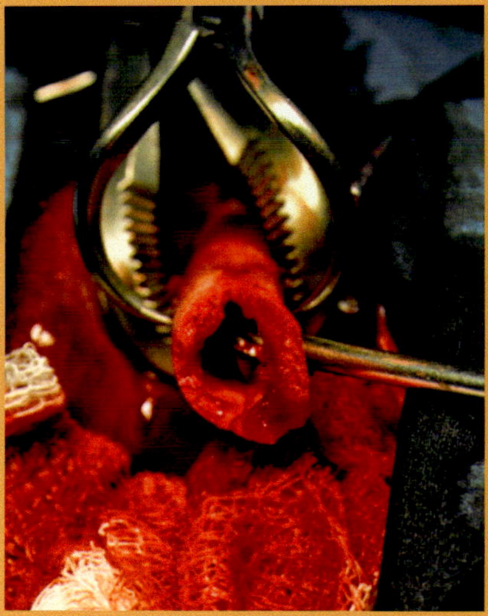

FIGURE 108. Perforation of the cortical surface of the bone with the diameter of the threading of the screw. The gliding hole is obtained.

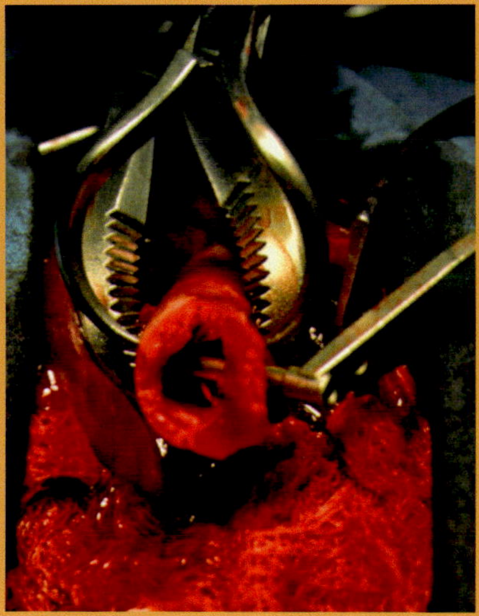

FIGURE 109. Insertion of the screw to the distal cortical surface. The guide is used to maintain the screw in the correct direction.

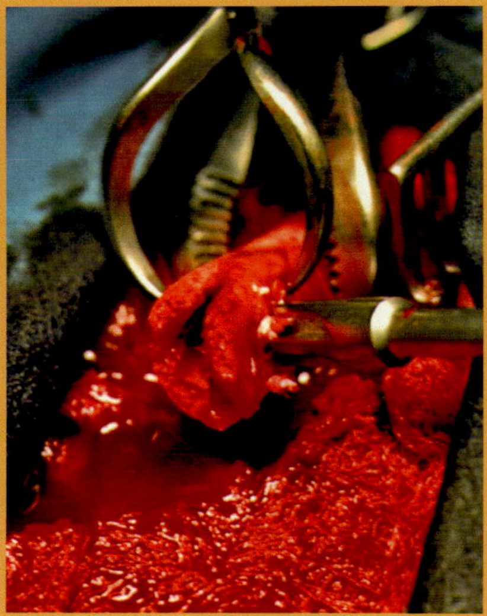

FIGURE 110. Detailed image of the countersinking of the bone in which the screw will be inserted.

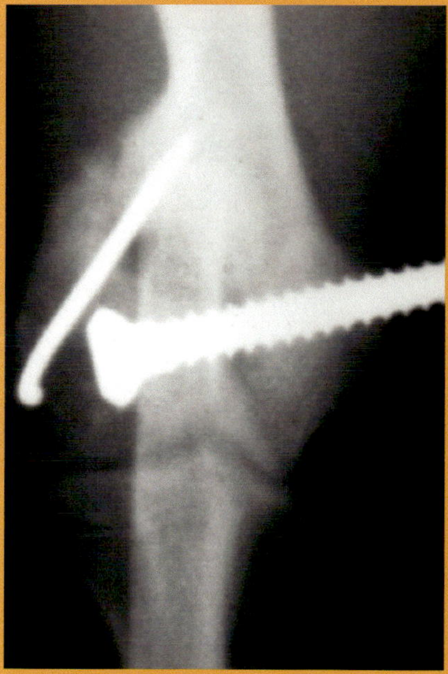

FIGURE 111. This X-ray shows how the screw has been inserted into the bone as the bone structure was broken.

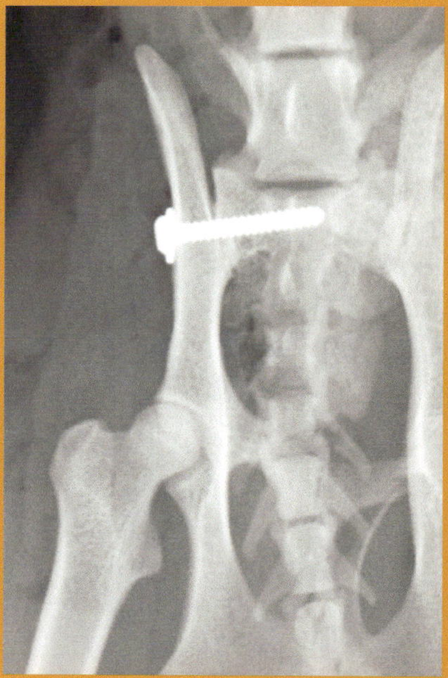

FIGURE 112. X-ray showing the washer used to distribute the forces exerted by the screw and prevent the bone from breaking.

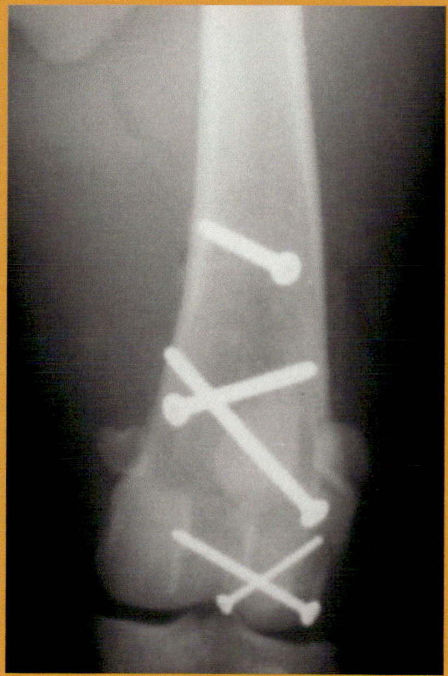

FIGURE 113. X-ray image that shows the different placement of screws.

PLATES

The use of plates as an osteosynthesis system dates back to 1886. However, it was not until the sixties when, thanks to the formation of two study groups on internal fixation, the Association for the Study of Osteosynthesis (AO, from its German name *Arbeitsgemanschaft für Osteosintesefragen*) and the Association for the Study of Internal Fixation (ASIF), its use became popular.

An osteosynthesis plate is basically a surgical disk made of metal, steel or titanium, whose function is to stabilise a fracture by being tightly attached to the bone using screws. When the heads of said screws come into contact with the plate, they push the implant against the cortical bone surface, achieving the desired stability.

Another type of plates came onto the market a few years ago, called locking plates, which will be discussed at the end of this chapter. In this system, unlike the previous one, the head of the screw is also screwed into the plate. Consequently, the implant does not exert pressure on the cortical surface which can be advantageous in several aspects.

Regarding the identification of the different plates available, it must first be taken into account that the plates are named depending on the type of screws they use. That is, there are plates that go from 1.5 (because they use screws with that diameter), to plates of 4.5, which are fixated using 4.5 mm screws, and greater (5.5 and 6.5) (Fig. 114).

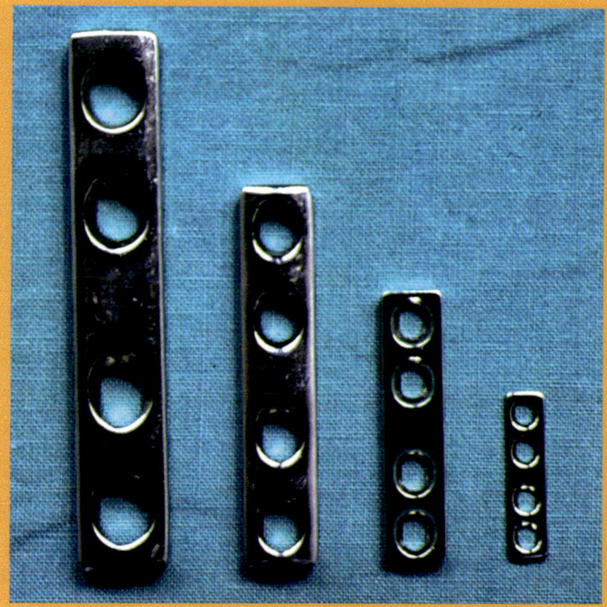

FIGURE 114. Different plate sizes.

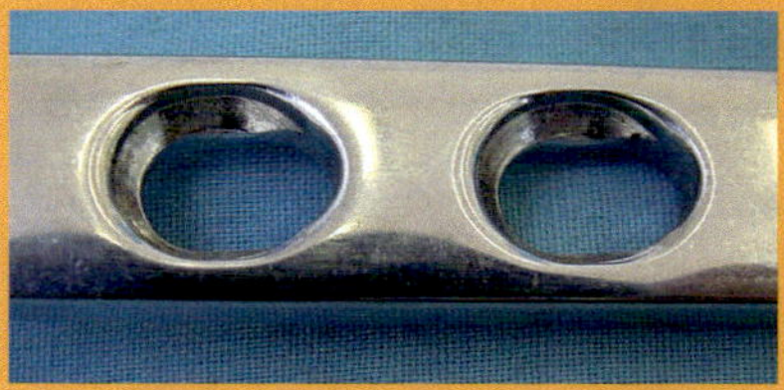

FIGURE 115. Plates with oval holes.

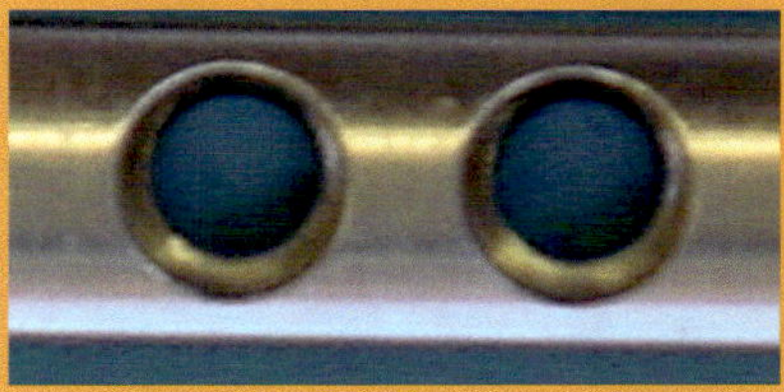

FIGURE 116. Plates with round holes.

Classification of plates according to their design

There is a great variety of plate types on the market. From a manufacturing perspective, they can be divided into two large groups depending on the shape of their orifices.

The following classification can be made according to the design of the plates' orifices: dynamic compression plates (DCP), with oval orifices (Fig. 115), through which axial compression can be applied to the fracture site, and neutralisation plates, with round orifices (this type of compression is not achieved with this latter type of plate) (Fig. 116). Meanwhile, depending on the resistance of these plates against forces of flexion, they are sub-divided into proper neutralisation plates, and plates for lengthening or support.

The appearance of DCP was a breakthrough in the bone surgery field by discovering how to apply axial compression on a fracture site in a simple manner. Another breakthrough recently took place with the introduction of locking plates.

Dynamic compression plates

According to the Roux studies, and as discussed in the chapter on Bone Growth and Healing, fracture lines must be subjected to forces of compression for proper healing (see page 12). These forces can be achieved through axial loads, that is, the limb bearing weight, or through the effect of implants.

At the beginning of the use of internal fixation systems, attempts were made to achieve axial compression through the placement of plates in transversal and short oblique fractures. For this purpose, a complicated apparatus was developed that was screwed into one of the bone fragments, immediately proximal or distal to the plate, after it had been fixed to the other bone fragment. Once the fracture was reduced, this device was anchored using a hook at the end of the implant. In this position, one of the fragments was pressed against the other by turning a screw which in turn pulled on the plate and compressed the fracture line (Fig. 117). When the desired inter-fragmentary compression was achieved, the plate was fixated using the corresponding screws and the tensioning apparatus was removed.

This system required a broader approach that included the creation of an additional hole in the bone that, occasionally, caused secondary fractures. For this reason, DCP plates were developed.

If a longitudinal cut is made to a DCP plate (oval holes), you can see that it is not symmetrical. The edge of each hole that is closest to the fracture site has a small ledge, so that the holes have a smaller diameter on the side of the plate that is in contact with the bone than that which is in contact with the heads of the screws. However, the edge of the hole that is farthest from the fracture site is straight, that is, the hole has the same shape on both sides (Figs. 115 and 118).

Meanwhile, the head of the osteosynthesis screw is slightly spindle-shaped, similar to the body of a spinning top (Fig. 119).

The unique shape of the head of the screw and the special design of the holes in the plate cause the partial displacement of each primary bone fragment towards the fracture site (this effect is slightly greater in the holes located on each side of the fracture line).

For a plate to be firmly fastened, it must be placed using screws that are anchored on both cortical surfaces of the bone, that is, using position screws. It must be taken into account that whether the plate is a compression plate or not, all of the screws, except in very rare occasions, are position screws.

As covered in the section on screws (see page 71), to insert a position screw, a hole must first be perforated on both cortical surfaces with a drill bit that corresponds with the diameter of the screw nucleus. When the screw is going to be used with a plate, the perforation must be made with a special guide designed so that the tip fits perfectly in the holes made in the bone (Fig. 120). This helps to impede the screw from lateral displacement or excessive inclination. If this occurred, when tightening the screw, the bone

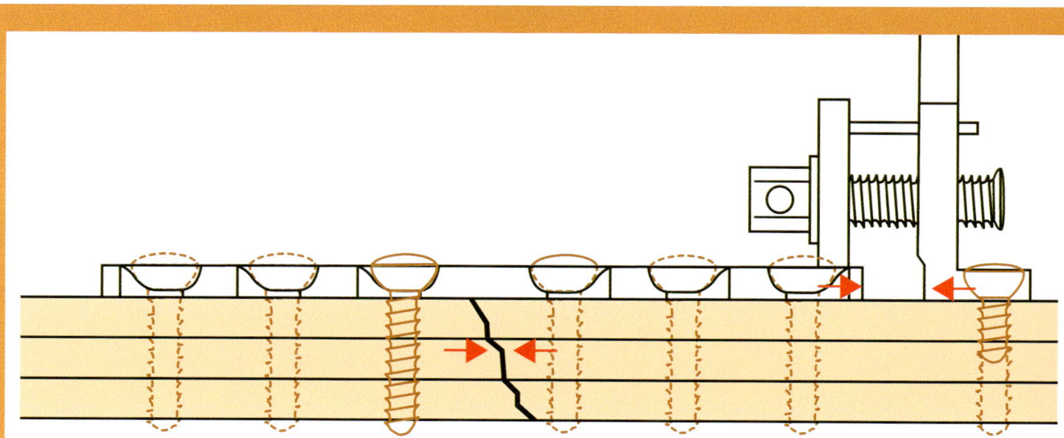

FIGURE 117. A tensioning apparatus used to bring the fracture edges together.

FIGURE 118. Longitudinal cut of the plate. Note the inverse symmetrical orientation of the holes from the centre of the plate.

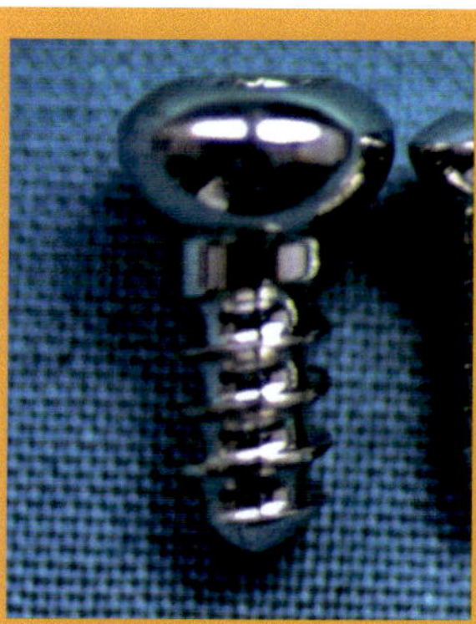

FIGURE 119. Image of a screw. Note the conical form of the "head", which is similar to the body of a spinning top.

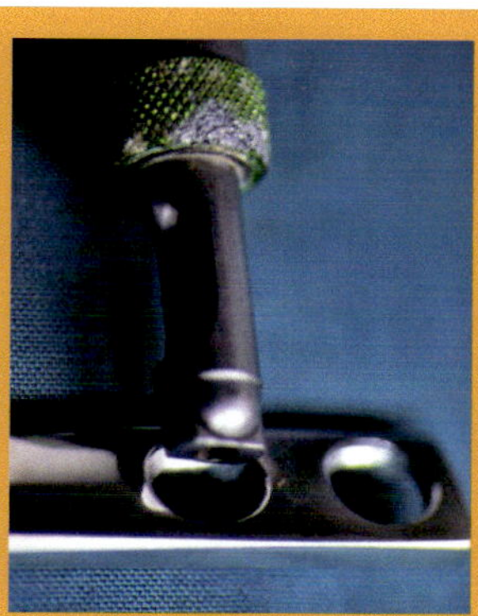

FIGURE 120. End of the guide designed to fit into the holes of DCP plates.

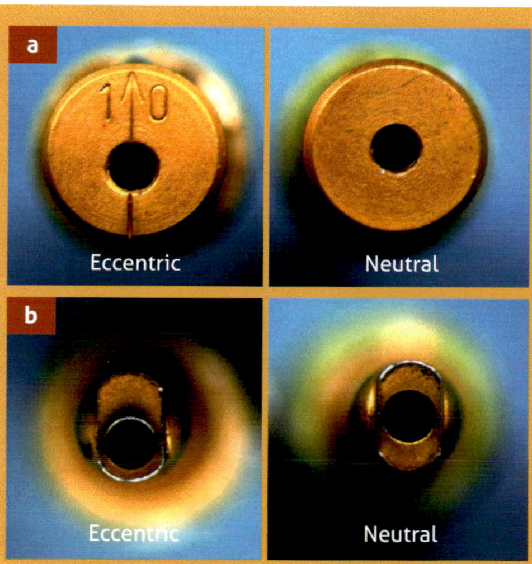

FIGURE 121. Differences between neutral and eccentric guides, seen from both sides.

fragments could be displaced, with the respective loss of reduction of the fracture. Logically, each plate system has its own guide that corresponds with the diameter of the screw that is uses (page 73). Each guide is double, with two slightly different sides (two guides) that are used depending on whether compression is needed or only to fasten the plate to the bone. If you look at both guides, you can see that the tips are different regarding the position of the hole where the drill bit will be inserted. On one of the sides, the hole is perfectly centred, serving as a guide for neutral perforation, while on the other side, the hole is slightly displaced to one side, serving as a guide for eccentric perforation (Fig. 121).

DCP plates compress the fracture site in an axial manner due to the relative position in which the hole is perforated when the screws are placed closer to the fracture site. If the neutral guide is used for drilling, the perforation will be located in the centre of the plate's hole. This way, when the screw is tightened, its head will come into contact with the plate and held in the centre of the hole, pushing the implant against the bone without displacing it (Fig. 122).

If the eccentric guide is used for perforation, the hole can be drilled slightly away from the fracture site or even in the other direction (Fig. 123).

To displace the fragments towards the fracture site through compression, an eccentric perforation should be made, in the opposite direction than the fracture site. To do so, once the two cortical surfaces are drilled, the screw is then inserted. The body of the screw is placed so that it is practically in contact with the edge of the hole found farthest from the fracture site.

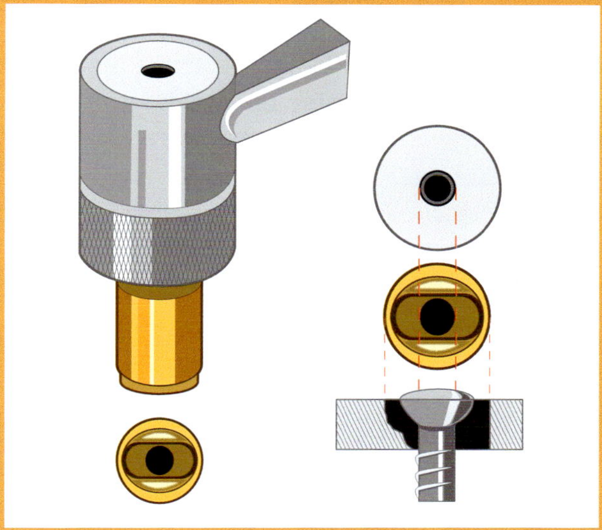

FIGURE 122. Neutral guide and effect that it produces on the position of the screw and, therefore, on the fracture site.

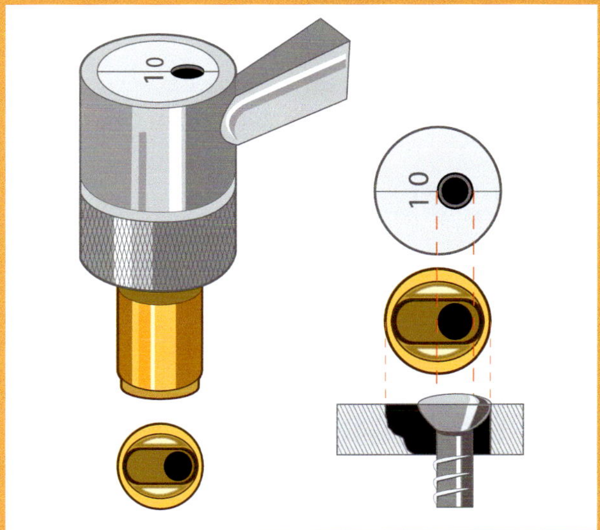

FIGURE 123. Eccentric guide and the effect it produces.

When the head of the screw comes in contact with the edge of the hole of the plate that has no recess in its upper portion, its cone shape forces the bone to progressively displace itself towards the fracture site, achieving the desired axial compression (Fig. 124).

If, by error, the perforation is made towards the fracture site, which should always be avoided, the implant's design would impede the undesired effect: when tightening the screw, its head would get stuck on the "ledge" or recess that each hole of the DCP plates has on the side opposite to the fracture site, and thus the effect would be the same as if the perforation would have been done with the neutral guide.

As previously mentioned in the Classification of Fractures chapter, the only ones that can tolerate an axial compression force without losing their reduction are the transversal and short oblique fractures. No other types of fractures benefit from the application of eccentric screws; on the contrary, a detrimental effect would be obtained, given that if applied in an oblique fracture, for example, a displacement of the fracture site would be produced.

To optimise the effect of the displacement of the primary fragments, the eccentric screws should be placed as close as possible to the fracture site.

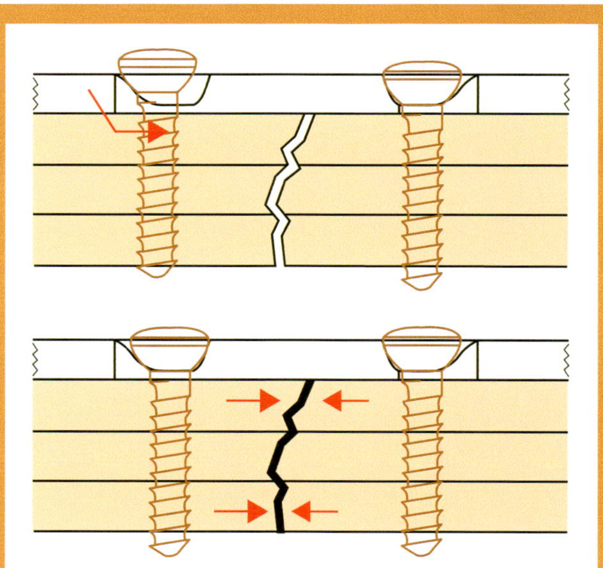

FIGURE 124. When a second eccentric screw is inserted, it forces the bone to displace itself towards the fracture site.

The DCP plates also present another particularity: to avoid any holes being left without screws, there is a greater separation between the two central holes; the fracture is set in this place and is thus equidistant from both holes.

Respecting a minimal distance between the perforation and the edge of the fracture is important to avoid the formation of any fissures from the hole made. The safety distance depends on various factors, primarily the diameter of the screw, and the thickness and resistance of the bone. The maximum limit that should never be reached is that of the diameter of the threading of the screw to be used.

Respecting a minimal distance between the perforation and the edge of the fracture is important to avoid the formation of fissures.

On these occasions, it must be taken into account that the risk of secondary fractures is much greater when using eccentric screws than with neutral screws.

Once the fracture has been properly reduced, the two eccentric screws are then placed and tightened until achieving compression of the bone fragments. The holes closest to the fracture site should be used or this purpose, and never those on the ends of the plate. If the latter were used, when the fragments move against each other, pushed from their ends, a separation of the plate or lateral displacement could be caused, losing the reduction of the fracture and, therefore, the effect of the compression. The rest of the screws that attach the implant to the bone should be placed neutrally.

A frequent error is to think that a greater number of eccentric screws used would lead to greater compression of the fracture site. This is false, given that as the plate is firmly fixed to the bone by the eccentric screws, it is impossible that the plate and the bone move one over the other (a displacement that would be necessary to increase compression).

More than two eccentric screws in one plate should only be used in the case of two fracture lines, which is quite frequent (Fig. 125).

Neutralisation plates

Characteristically, all of the orifices in these places are round and they have identical diameters on both sides. To make them more polyvalent and avoid the need to have a great amount of material on hand, these plates have holes all along their entire length. For this reason, when they are used in oblique, multiple and comminuted fractures, a few holes should be left unused because, as previously mentioned, a screw should never be inserted into a fracture line as it would complicate the healing process.

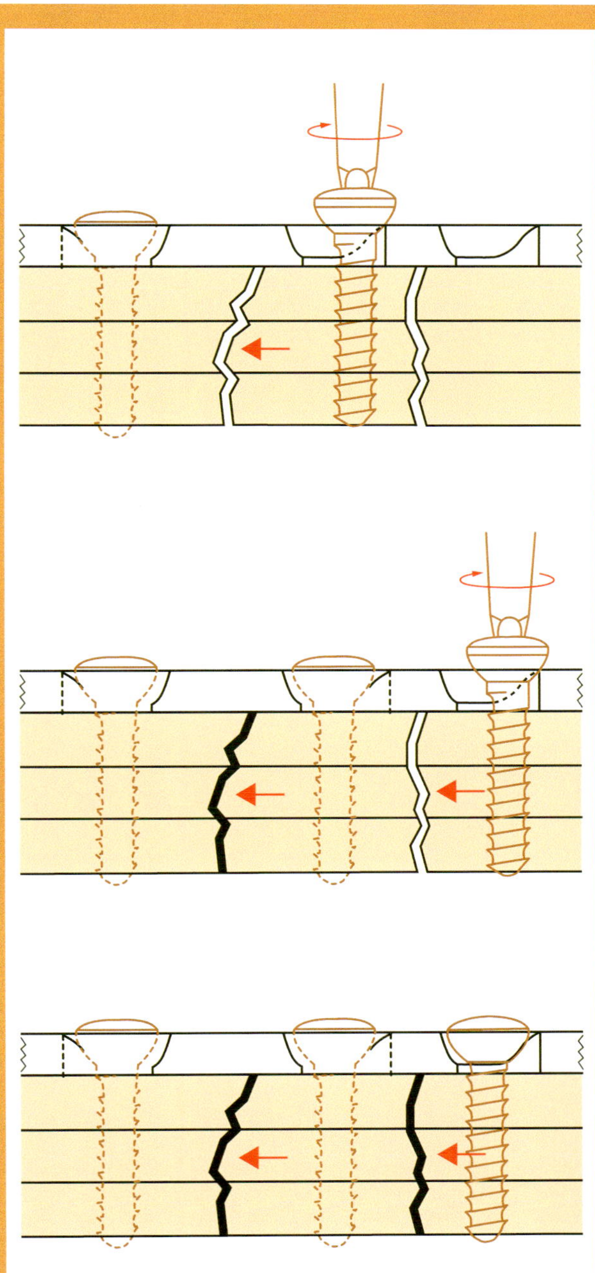

FIGURE 125. The insertion of two eccentric screws is a manoeuvre that is only performed in cases with two consecutive fracture lines.

Screws should never be inserted into fracture sites as this would complicate the healing process.

To place a neutralisation plate, the same process is followed as that used for DCP plates. The only difference is that the neutral guide should be used to perforate all of the holes.

One aspect that may seem erroneously irrelevant is the position of the implant in regard to the area of contact between the cortical surfaces of a fracture site.

When a fracture is properly reduced, that is, when most of the fracture perimeter of both fragments is in contact, the axial loads can be transmitted throughout the bone without creating excessive forces of flexion. On the contrary, when dealing with a bone in which there is no contact at any point of its perimeter near the fracture site (comminuted or poorly reduced fractures), there is a strong tendency to flexion. The problem arises when part of the perimeter is in contact and another part is not. In these cases, the tendency to flexion is greater on the side where the edges are not in contact. When the implant is put in place, the possibility of movement is much greater if the plate is set over the area of contact than if it is set over the area with no contact (Figs. 126 and 127). One of the situations where partial contact can cause problems is in transversal fractures, in

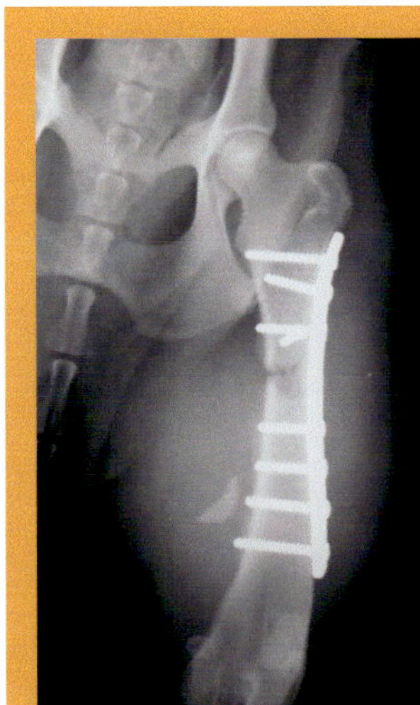

FIGURE 126. Femur fracture with a small separation in the cortical surface opposite from the plate.

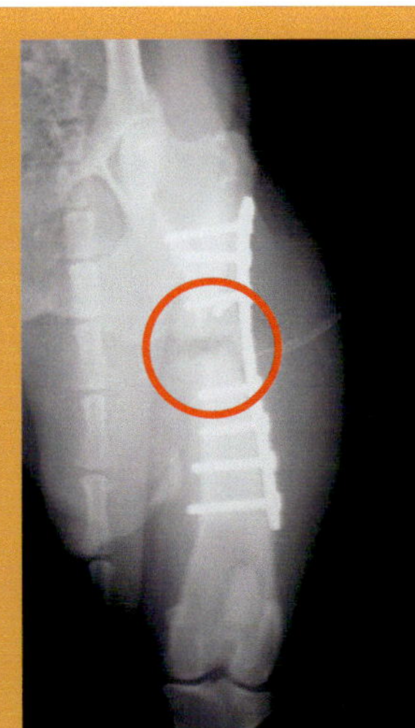

FIGURE 127. Delay in the healing process as a result of the lack of contact.

which when evaluating the reduction from the visible side, the separation cannot be seen on the opposing cortical surface. For this reason, and to avoid problems with this type of fractures, the plate can be bent slightly towards the bone, right where it will be placed over the fracture line. This way, close contact is ensured with the cortical surface on the opposite side of the implant.

In the previously mentioned fractures, and primarily in comminuted fractures, until the fracture callus acquires adequate resistance, the plate has to bear all loads. The problem arises when said loads surpass the resistance threshold of the metal, which could lead to the deformation of the implant.

For these cases, there are basically two possibilities: the plastic deformation of the metal, and the structure breaking from strain on the implant. The deformation is produced as a consequence of a lateral load that surpasses the resistance to flexion of the metal. This primarily occurs when a plate is selected of a thickness that is inferior to that needed by the patient, or when the metal is excessively soft. For this reason, which implant to use must be analysed.

The choice depends on the size of the patient and the bone to be stabilised. However, other factors such as the type of fracture, activity, habitat and age of the patient, as well as its weight, should be taken into account (Table 2).

TABLE 2. Illustrative table on size of the implants according to the weight of the patients. Adaptation of W.O. Brinker, D.L. Piermattei, G.L. Flo. *Handbook of Small Animal Orthopedics and Fracture Repair*. Saunders, 1997.

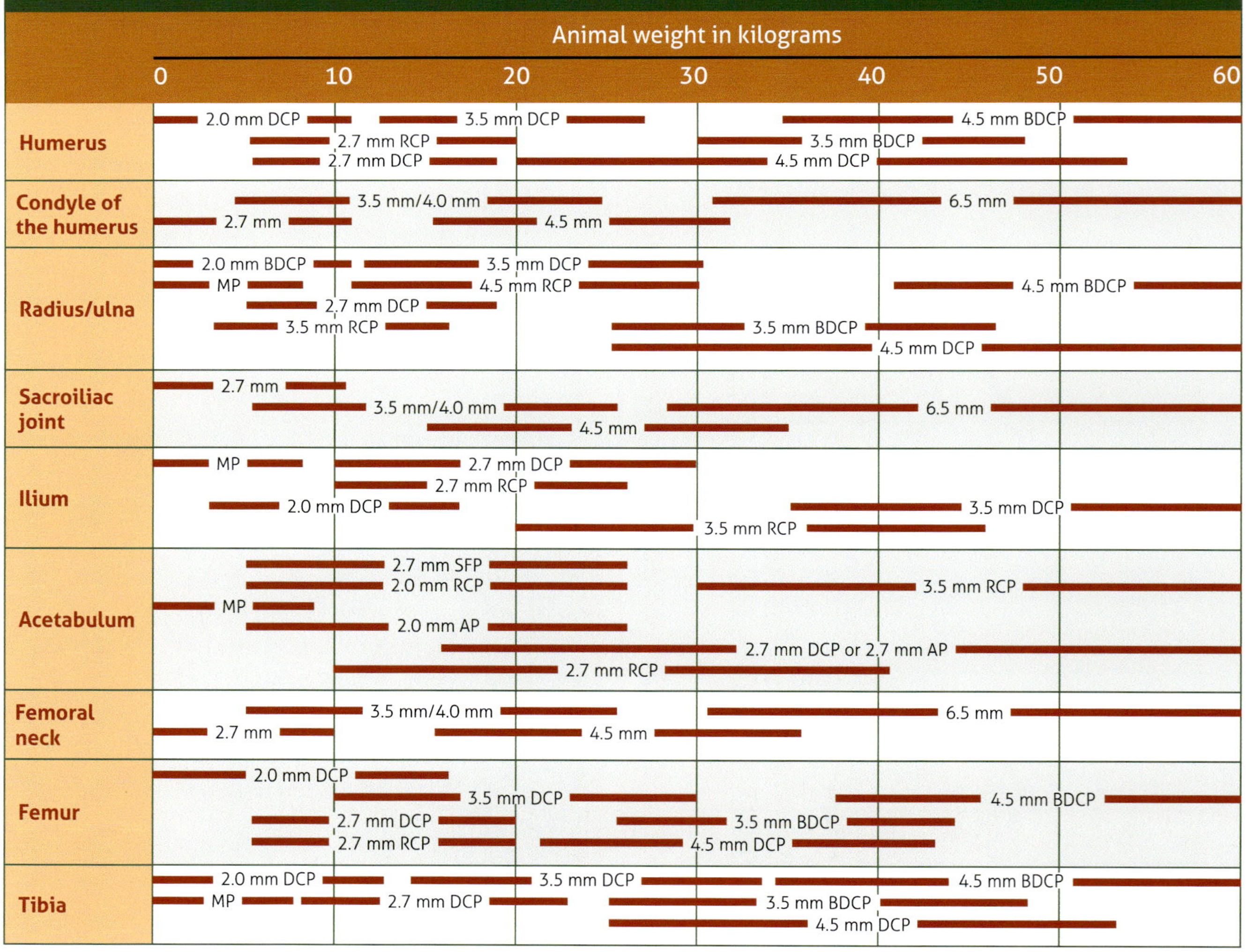

DCP: Dynamic compression plate
BDCP: Broad dynamic compression plate
AP: Acetabular plate for veterinary use
SFP: Small fragment plate
RCP: Reconstruction plate
MP: Miniplate

One example of the importance of the size of the implant is found in the appearance of the 2.4 system. The use of these implants in veterinary medicine began to cover a spectrum of fractures that primarily affect the radius in small dogs and cannot be covered with 2.0 or 2.7 plates. Currently, it is most likely the most used in feline bone surgery.

If the selection of a fixation system is incorrect, implant failure is generally produced during the first two weeks after surgery. The patient will normally bear less weight on the affected extremity and a modification of the longitudinal bone axis can be observed.

Another cause that leads to this problem is the use of plates, that although of the right size, are excessively soft (Fig. 128).

These plates are manufactured with "soft" surgical steel. In these cases, the implant is subjected to a process of annealing, heating at high temperatures and slowly cooling which gives it greater plasticity. This procedure is carried out in adjustable and reconstruction plates. For the latter, it is done to make the intraoperative cutting process easier given that the sterilisable shears, due to the fact that they are made of surgical steel, have a duller cutting edge than those made of hardened steel. Regarding the reconstruction plates, they are made of this material to facilitate moulding to sharper angles, as well as to be able to bend them in the direction of the wide plane of the implant. These soft plates that can be easily bent should not be used in fractures that will be subjected to heavy loads (Fig. 129).

In cases where this type of implants must be used, their resistance should be increased by associating them with other osteosynthesis systems such as intramedullary pins or external fixation.

In the specific case of adjustable plates, as they are thinner than normal plates, two plates, one on top of the other, can be used in what is known as the "sandwich" system (Fig. 130).

However, implants break as a consequence of loading cycles, that is, by a phenomena known as metal fatigue. Each time the bone is subjected to an axial load in a fracture whose edges are not connected, the plate suffers microdeformation that is absorbed by the metal. If these flexions continue for a long period of time without the fracture healing, the metal's own structure weakens progressively, until, in some cases, it breaks (Fig. 131).

Implant failure can be the consequence of the inadequate position of a plate, the wrong size or the wrong choice of material.

Breakage occurs in plates made of rigid metals, whereas plates made of soft metals tend to bend. Titanium, as it has a Young's modulus (measurement of the elasticity of

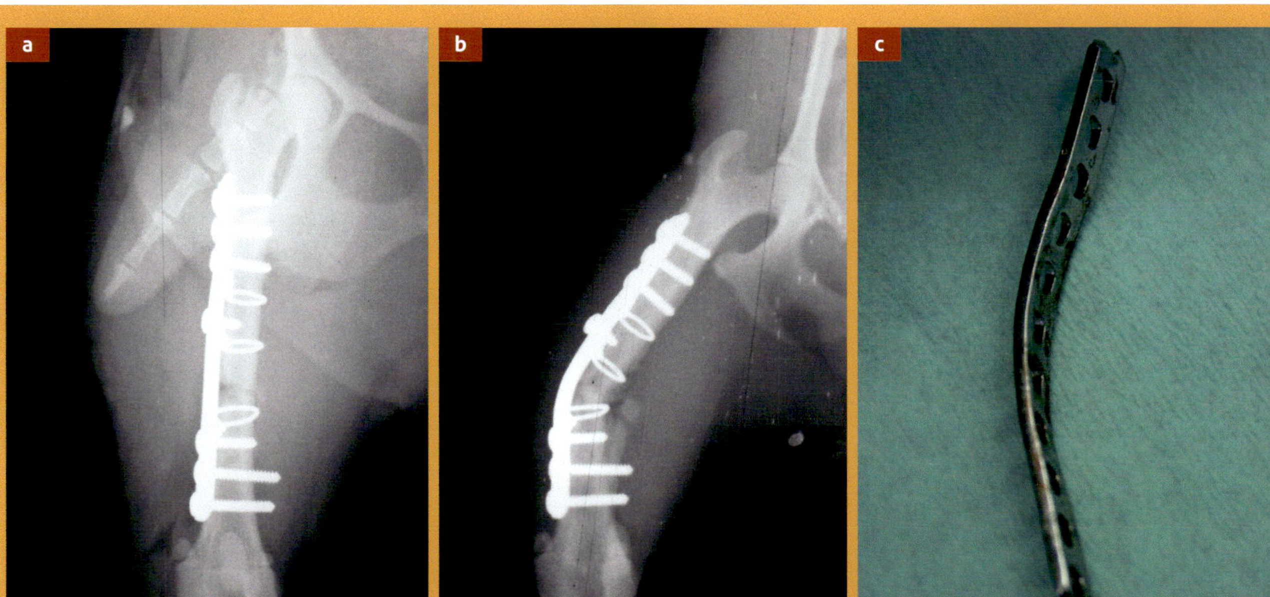

FIGURE 128. Adjustable plate (a). X-ray showing how the plate has been bent due to the effect of the loads (b). Detailed image of the plate (c).

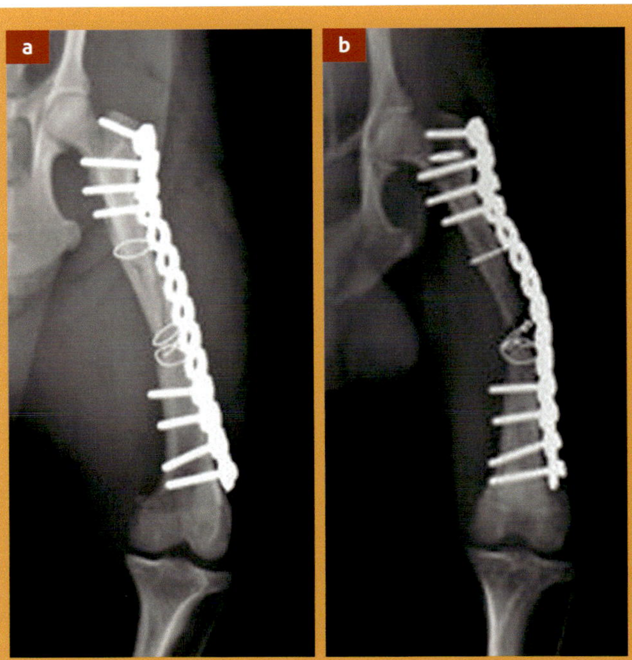

FIGURE 129. Bent reconstruction plate (a). Its "soft" structure has given way to the effect of the loading forces (b).

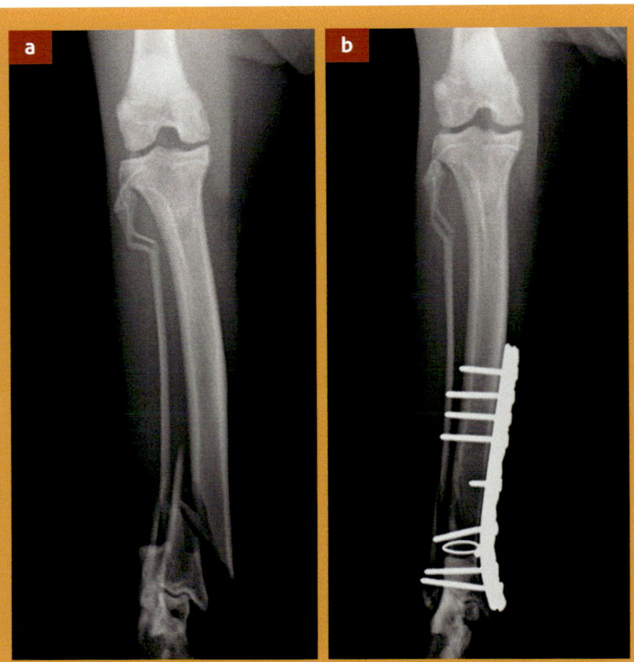

FIGURE 130. X-ray image showing the placement of two plates, one over the other ("sandwich" system) in an unstable distal fracture of the tibia. X-ray showing a fracture (a) and placement of a "sandwich" plate (b).

a metal) lower than that of steel, is much more rigid, and consequently, titanium plates rarely bend, but it can break.

The forces of flexion are concentrated on the portion located between the screws that are closest to the fracture site as the rest of the implant is anchored to the bone forming a single block. The weak point of the plates are their holes as their capacity of absorption is decreased due to the smaller amount of metal. It has previously been mentioned that screws cannot be placed into all holes in oblique, multiple and comminuted fractures, which increases the possibilities of the implant breaking. If one single hole is left open in the fracture site, all of the forces are concentrated in the portion of metal found on both sides of the hole, that is, on only two points. However, if two or more holes are left open, the forces are distributed to four or more weak points, which releases the intensity of the load of each point and decreases the fatigue of the metal.

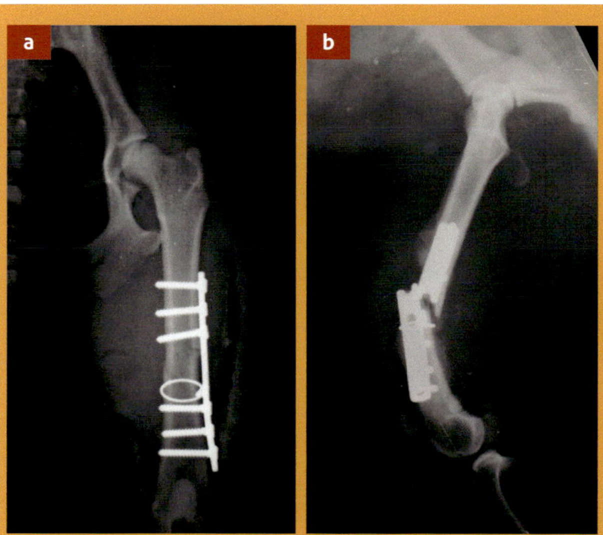

FIGURE 131. Broken plate in a femur due to metal fatigue. Immediately after surgery (a) and a few days later (b).

By leaving more than one hole free over a fracture site, the intensity of the load on the plate is released and metal fatigue is reduced.

In cases where it is necessary to leave holes of a plate unoccupied, at least two should remain free. In the specific case of implants made of titanium, as this metal is less elastic, more free holes are needed to avoid the implant from breaking (Fig. 132).

Plates for lengthening

To avoid the breakage of implants, plates for lengthening or support have been developed. These plates can be distinguished from normal plates by the distribution of their holes, which are grouped on both ends leaving the central portion of solid metal (Fig. 133). This configuration eliminates the weak points.

In plates for lengthening, the holes do not need to be prepared to hold eccentric screws, and due to their round, and not oval, shape, they are located closer together. This characteristic allows for them to correctly fasten the plate even in cases where there is less bone length available on the ends, which is frequently the case with comminuted fractures (Fig. 134).

Given that in veterinary medicine the incidence of multiple or comminuted fractures is relatively high, and that these patients, unlike humans, show little cooperation during the postoperative period, plates for lengthening have been developed over the last few years for almost all sizes.

After having explained the different types of osteosynthesis plates available on the market, it should be mentioned that their classification according to their function is more important.

Classification of plates according to their function

Compression plates

The plate exerts axial compression on the fracture site. This compression is mechanical and depends exclusively on how the screws are placed in the plate.

Static compression plates

The principal indication for this type of plates are transversal or short oblique fractures of the diaphyses of long bones (Fig. 135). This function of compression can only be achieved using DCP plates.

Dynamic compression plates

Dynamic compression is produced by the effect of bearing weight on the extremity, that is, without bearing weight, the effect would not be produced. This is based on the tension band principle, whose mechanical justification is explained in the Tension Band Pin System section (page 52). The effect is achieved by placing the plate over the tension bearing surface of the bone. When the patient bears weight on the limb, the cortical surface that is right under the plate will attempt to separate itself. This attempt is neutralised by the plate and reconverted in forces of compression on the opposing cortical surface.

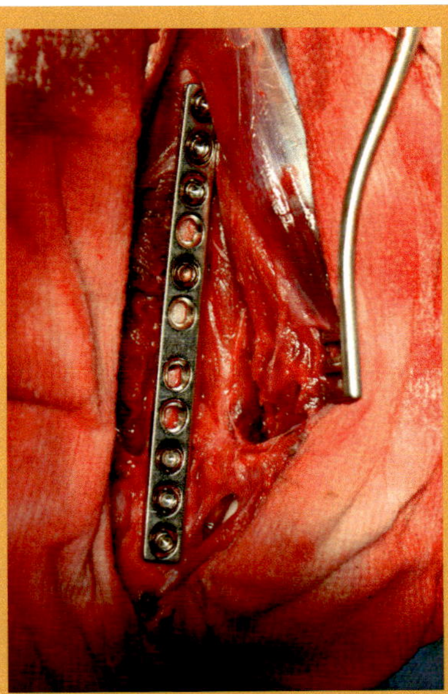

FIGURE 132. Surgery to place a titanium plate. The hardness of this material requires that various holes be left free around the fracture site to avoid the concentration of the forces of flexion.

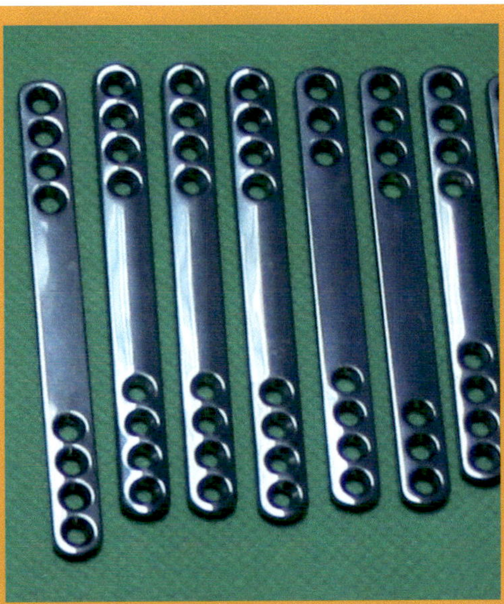

FIGURE 133. Image showing the different sizes of plates for lengthening.

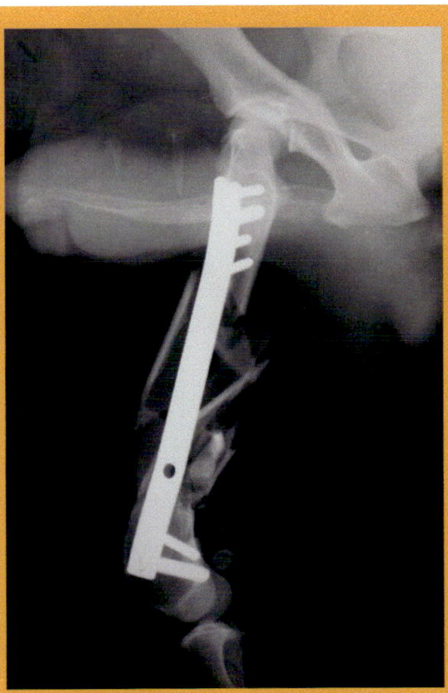

FIGURE 134. X-ray showing the anchoring of a plate for lengthening in the metaphysis and epiphysis of a femur that presents a comminuted fracture.

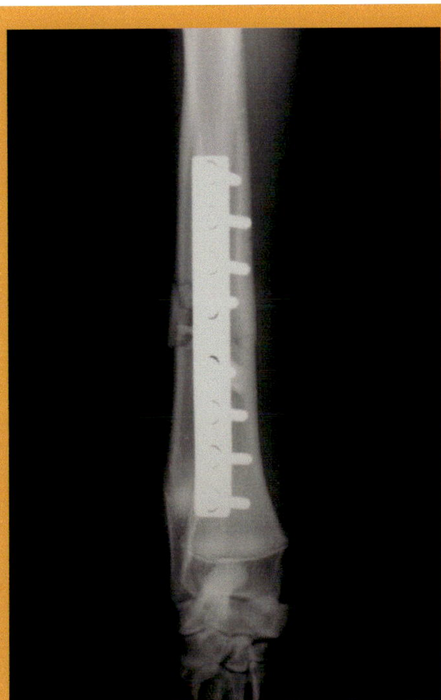

FIGURE 135. Compression plate in a transversal radius fracture.

The plates with a strictly dynamic compression function are rarely used given that when compression is needed, DCPs are the most frequent choice. The implant should always be placed on the tension-bearing surface when possible to add the dynamic effect to the static effect.

The clearest example of a dynamic compression plate is the treatment of a fracture of the acetabulum, in which the implant is applied to the implant in the dorsal acetabular rim (Fig. 137).

This can be done with all types of plates as it only depends on the bone's position.

Neutralisation plates

The function of the plate is only to protect the fracture site from forces of flexion, torsion and shearing, as in this case the compression around the fracture lines is achieved by the application of other fixation systems such as compression screws or cerclages.

This system is primarily used in long oblique fractures, and spiral or multiple fractures with a small number of large fragments (Fig. 138).

The neutralisation function can be achieved with all types of plates.

Supporting plates

The function of this type of plate consists of keeping the primary fragments aligned, protecting the fracture site from all movement and to serve as the base of the biological osteosynthesis, which is mostly applied to comminuted fractures.

What is the tension-bearing surface of a bone?

Basically, the cortical bone surface that is subjected to forces of avulsion (in the opposite direction) during physiological weight-bearing at a structural level. Transferring this concept to the case of a specific fracture, it would be the surface that when a patient uses its limb, the edges tend to separate.

Normally all plates should be placed on the tension-bearing surface, as if they were placed on the opposite side, the plate would bend. This is due to the scarce resistance of the metal to the forces of flexion, compared to those of avulsion (Fig. 136).

A plate placed on the tension-bearing surface of a bone absorbs all avulsion forces and transforms them into forces of compression at the level of the fracture site. This is the tension band principle exerted by the plates.

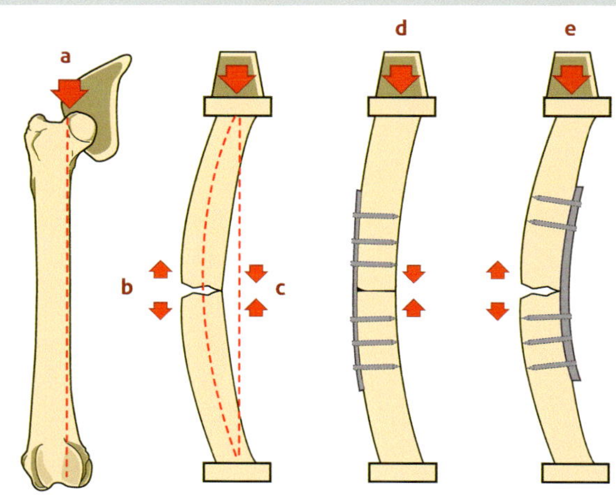

a. Physiological load: axial compression.
b. Tension-bearing surface: forces of tension or avulsion.
c. Compression surface: forces of compression.
d. Correct placement of the plate.
e. Incorrect placement.

FIGURE 136. Representation of the effect of the loading forces on the tension-bearing face of a bone.

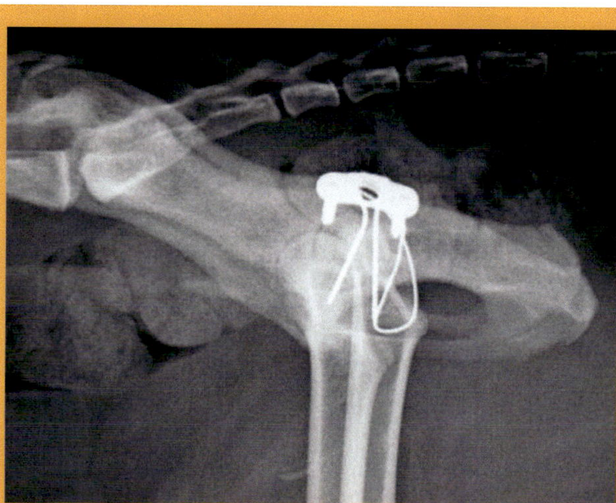

FIGURE 137. Plate in the dorsal acetabular rim. This type of plate is an example of dynamic compression plates.

This can be done with all types of plates, however, plates with greater resistance than those discussed in the previous cases should be used, or the previously described plates for lengthening (Fig. 139).

Plate application technique

Traditionally, the AO postulated that perfect reduction of all fragments with inter-fragmentary compression of the greatest number possible of fracture lines was necessary to achieve bone consolidation. Currently, however, fractures are generally treated with biological osteosynthesis, which consists of fixating only the primary fragments to maintain alignment and the functional length of the bone without taking into account the intermediate fragments.

There are two possible biological osteosynthesis techniques to reduce fracture sites:

- **OBDT** (Open But Don't Touch). This technique consists of accessing the fracture site and inserting the implant without manipulating the free fragments (Fig. 140).
- **MIPO** (Minimally Invasive Plate Osteosynthesis). This technique is similar to the previous one, but the bone is only accessed through two incisions, just large enough to allow for the insertion of the plate underneath the soft tissues and any necessary screws (Fig. 141).

Each fracture reduction technique has its benefits and disadvantages, and thus the surgeon must evaluate the best option depending on his/her experience and the particular characteristics of each fracture. In this sense, the following principal should be taken into account: the simpler and easier to reduce a fracture, the greater the reason to apply rigid osteosynthesis techniques with inter-fragmentary compression. On the contrary, the more fragments the fracture has, the greater the reason to select biological osteosynthesis.

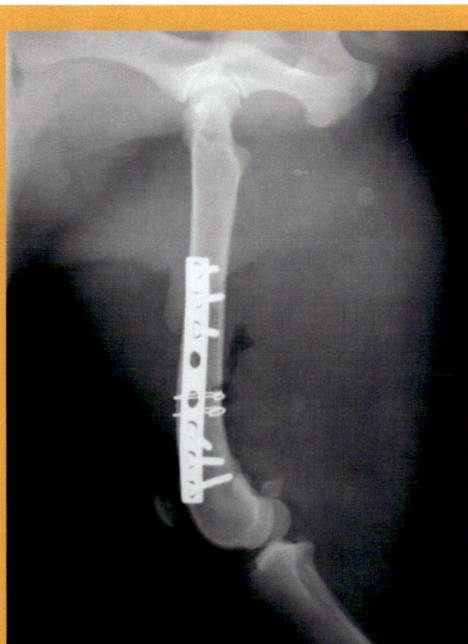

FIGURE 138. Neutralisation plate associated with cerclages in a femur fracture.

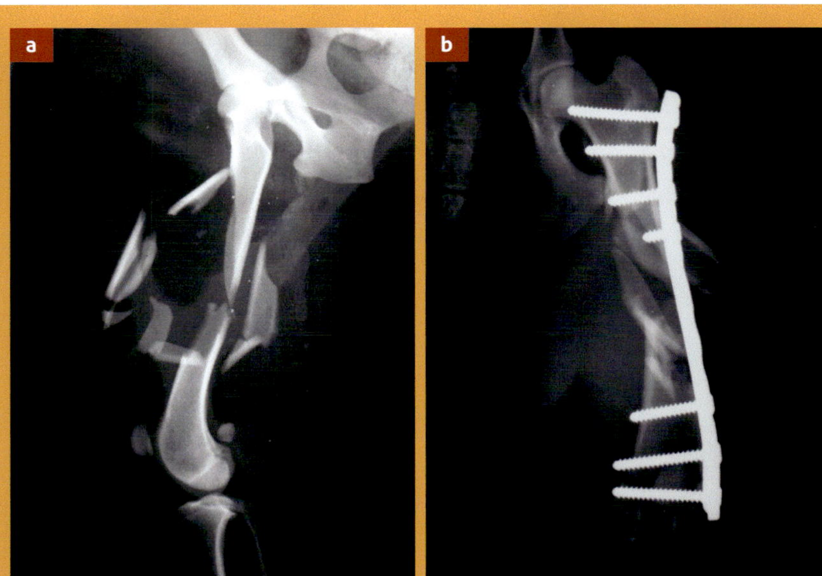

FIGURE 139. X-ray image of a comminuted fracture (a), resolved with a supporting plate, using a standard plate (b).

The perfect reduction of the fracture site, a rigid technique, facilitates the moulding of the plate and avoids the creation of poor unions, that is, preventing the surgeon from making mistakes in the alignment of the axis of the bone; this is much easier to perform for those surgeons with less experience in the application of osteosynthesis plates. Biological osteosynthesis, however, is less harmful to the surrounding soft tissues and therefore the healing process is faster. It is the best technique for comminuted fractures, although the surgeon must be more skilled in the surgical technique. Lack of experience could lead to making mistakes.

The rigid techniques are more indicated in cases of simple fractures, which can easily be reduced, while biological osteosynthesis is recommended for comminuted fractures.

If a rigid technique is chosen, the fracture should be transformed into a simple fracture, that is, with two primary fragments and one single fracture plane. To do so, if possible, compression screws or cerclages are used that reduce and keep the fragments stabilised, while they simultaneously exert forces of compression on the fracture lines. It must be taken into account where the plate will be placed so that the heads of the compression screws or the knot of the cerclages do not impede its insertion. This technique to reduce fractures can only be performed in multiple fractures in which the bone fragments can be reduced (Fig. 142).

Once the fracture is converted into a simple fracture, or in the case of oblique and transversal fractures, the primary fracture plane is then reduced to achieve complete alignment of the bone.

For oblique fractures, temporary stabilisation of the fracture site can be performed using two-point reduction forceps or by applying compression with screws or cerclages. For transversal fractures, the assistant must temporarily hold the reduced fragments using reduction forceps until the surgeon moulds and stabilises the plate with its corresponding screws.

Next, once the fracture is reduced, the plate size must be chosen depending on the size of the bone, the patient's age, weight and character, and the type of fracture. Regarding its length, it must be long enough for at least three screws

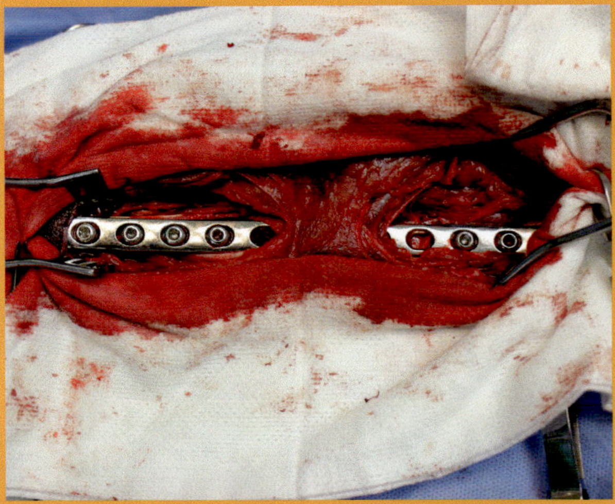

FIGURE 140. Comminuted tibia fracture treated with an OBDT system.

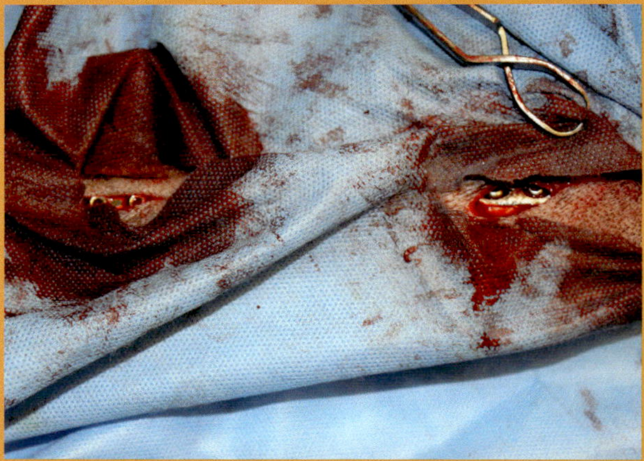

FIGURE 141. Tibia fracture treated using a MIPO system with opening of the skin.

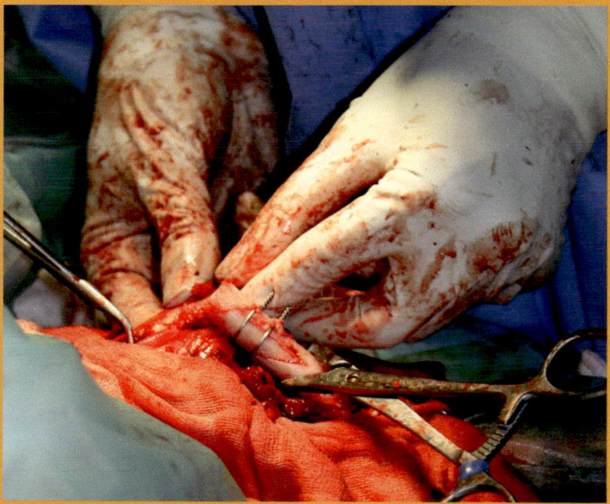

FIGURE 142. Placement of cerclages to convert a multiple fracture into a simple fracture (two primary fragments and one single fracture plane) and application of a rigid technique.

to fit for each primary fragment, that is, the plate must have at least six screws to achieve adequate stability.

In this sense, it must be kept in mind that a normal fracture should be anchored by at least five cortical surfaces in each primary fragment, taking into account that each screw screws into two cortical surfaces. The sequence of the neutralisation of forces depending on the number of screws used is described below:

- Movements of rotation over the longitudinal axis of the bone, and movements of separation-approximation of the fracture site are neutralised with one screw per fragment (Fig. 143b).
- With the screws, the movements of rotation that are produced when the screws serve as an axis, that is, the side-to-side movements, are also stabilised with two screws (Fig. 143c).
- The stability needed to impede the screws from being ripped out of the cortical surfaces is achieved with the third screw (Fig. 143d).

Regarding locking plates, the minimum number of screws per fragment is reduced to two as the screw is also anchored to the plate and acts as a second "cortical surface".

The following step is to adapt the plate to the anatomical shape of the bone. Each bone has its own curves to which the plate must be perfectly adapted. This is the most critical point of the placement of rigid osteosynthesis systems using traditional plates. If after perfectly reducing the fracture site the plate does not adapt to the bone correctly, the reduction will be lost when the screws are tightened due to the fact that the screws traction the bone fragments towards the bone.

If the moulding of a traditional plate does not adapt to the shape of the bone, the reduction will be lost when the screws are tightened.

In the case of locking plates, as the fixation is produced by anchoring the screw to both the plate and the bone, this displacement is not produced. This is one of the principal advantages of these plates.

One option to facilitate the moulding of the plates is to use aluminium templates. These are made of fine sheets of metal that, once the fracture is reduced, are situated in the position where the plate will be placed. As they are

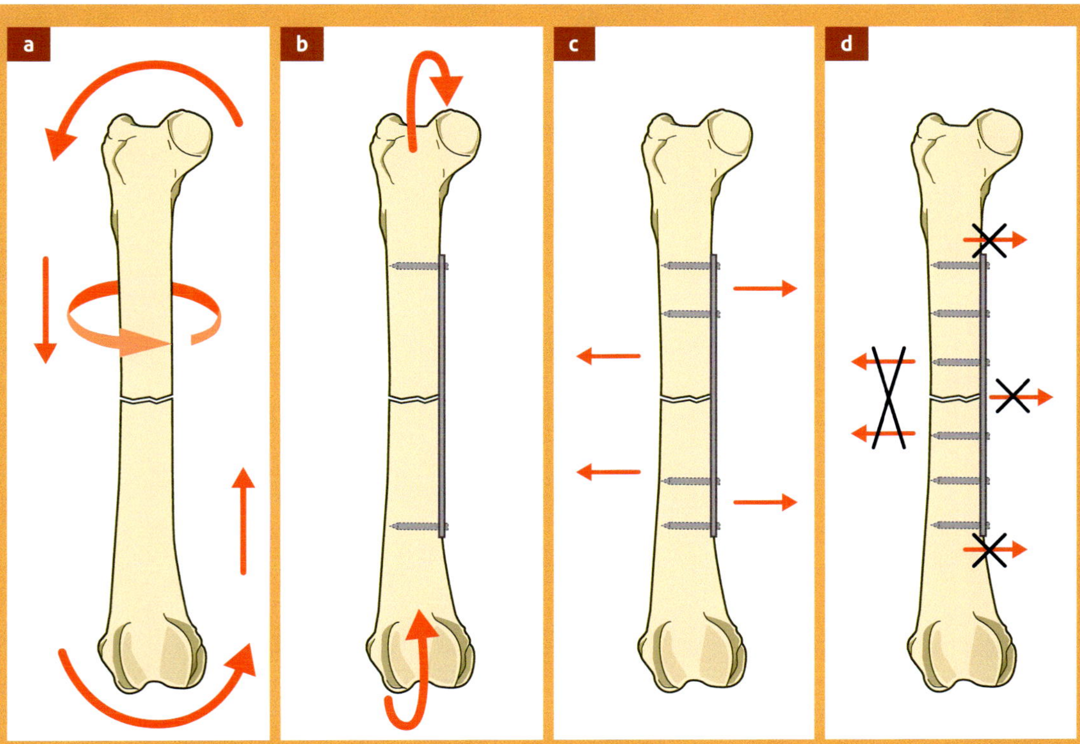

FIGURE 143. Representation of the action exerted by the screws according to the number. Representation of all possible moments of bone fragments (a) effect of the insertion of one screw per fragment (b); of two screws per fragment (c); and of three screws (d). The arrows indicate the possible movements.

highly malleable, a "mould" can be made of the exact shape that the definitive implant will have. Once removed from the bone, they serve as a reference to mould the plate (Fig. 144).

The instruments needed to bend the implants is varied: wrenches, clamps and bending pliers make the adjustment of the plate to the bone possible (Fig. 145). Said adjustment should be achieved by smoothly curving the implant, always avoiding angles in the metal. This is because the sharp points of flexion (the angles), are weak areas given that the metal structure has been damaged. Pliers and clamps partially prevent these issues.

The bending should be done progressively. If not, and if the bending is excessive, the implant would have to be "unbent", which would also damage the metal structure.

In the case of plates made of titanium, more care must be taken to avoid the previously mentioned mistakes as this metal, which is less flexible than steel, suffers more from structural damage. Avoiding the correction of over bending is especially important.

The correction of over bending titanium plates is significantly more critical due to their reduced flexibility.

Once the plate is moulded, it is placed in the desired position to proceed with the fixation using screws.

When using compression plates, the two holes closest to each side of the fracture line are perforated, as previously mentioned, using the eccentric perforation guide, and the rest will be made using the neutral guide. The guide, along with orientating the position of the hole in the correct spot, prevents any damage to the surrounding soft tissues that could occur as a consequence of the rotation of the drill bit (Fig. 146).

The steps to insert the screws are the same as those described in the Screws section (page 71). When perforating with the diameter of the nucleus of the screw at low revolutions, saline solution should be used for cooling to avoid overheating (Fig. 147). If a guide specifically for plates is not used, it must be taken into account that if the perforation is laterally displaced in relation with the hole, when tightening the screw, a partial displacement of the bone will take place in the opposite direction due to contact with the head of the screw against the implant. Likewise, this guide prevents the perforation from being excessively inclined.

For neutralisation or supporting plates, all perforations are made using a neutral guide.

Once the hole is made, the length of the screw is measured using a depth gauge (Fig. 148). Generally, a screw that is one size larger than the measured depth should be

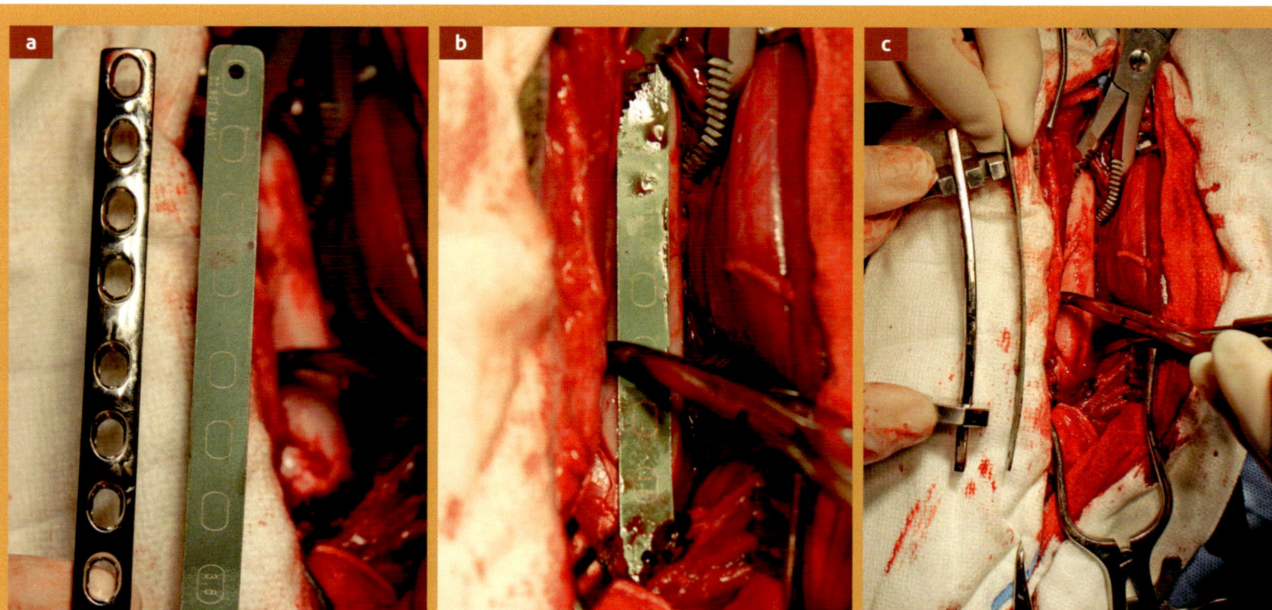

FIGURE 144. Moulding of a plate with the help of an aluminium template. Comparison of both plates (a); moulding of the aluminium plate that is placed in what will be the definitive location of the plate (b); and moulding of the definitive plate using the template (c) as reference.

selected to guarantee perfect anchoring in the cortical surface opposite to the surface where the plate is placed.

Regarding the possibility to carve the threading into the thickness of the cortical bone depends on whether self-tapping screws are used or not. If the threading has to be carved, the thread insert that corresponds with the diameter of the screw should be used.

> *To guarantee perfect anchoring, screws with a length slightly greater than the measurement taken are used.*

A few years ago, the threading of 3.5 screws changed from 1.75 to 1.25 and therefore it is recommended that a thread insert that corresponds with the screw be used.

The thread insert should always be inserted using a guide to protect the soft tissues, as well as to prevent losing the edge of the threading by hitting up against the hole of the plate (Fig. 149). To eliminate the bone "chips" that are produced when carving the threading, three half turns should be made clockwise, and one counter-clockwise, repeating until the threading has been completely carved in both cortical surfaces. Another important detail is to correctly orient the thread insert so that it matches the location of the hole on the second cortical surface. If the diameter of the bone is large, or the cortical bone is thin, it is possible that the when the thread insert is angled, its tip hits up against the endostium and, consequently, it would not be able to continue turning and the threading of the first cortical surface would be lost.

A thread insert is not necessary when using self-tapping screws. In certain bones that have an excessively hard

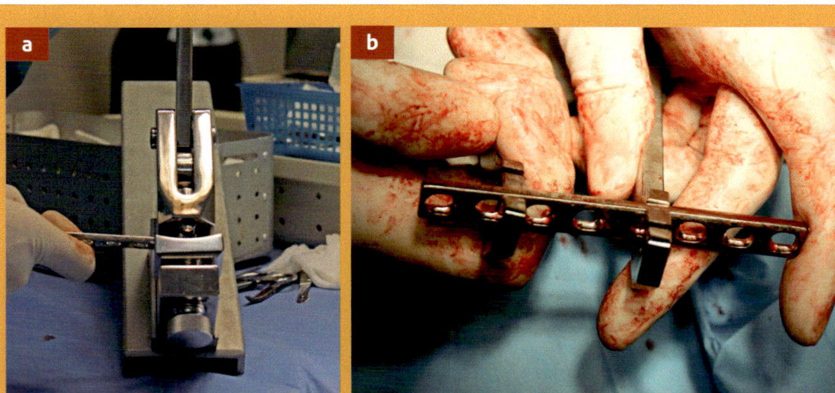

FIGURE 145. The moulding of the plates is done with the help of different instruments such as the clamp (a) or wrench (b), among others.

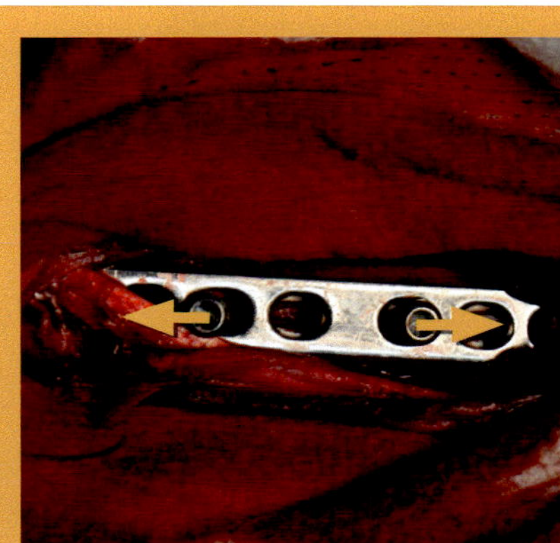

FIGURE 146. Eccentric screws set in place before tightening. Take note of the displacement in the opposite direction from the fracture.

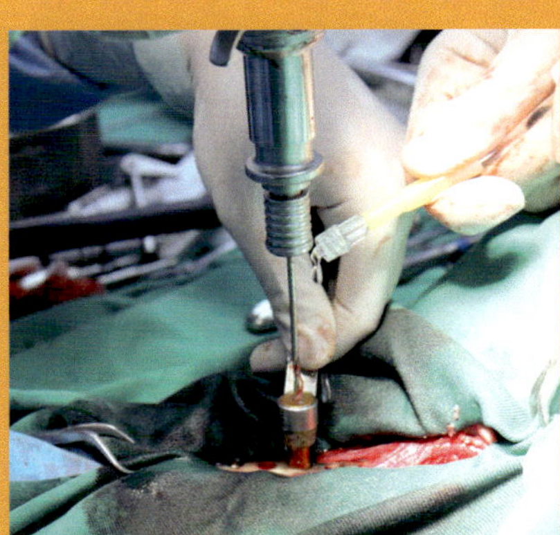

FIGURE 147. Perforation using a guide. Here you can see how the operation is performed with a cooling system, pouring saline solution over the area.

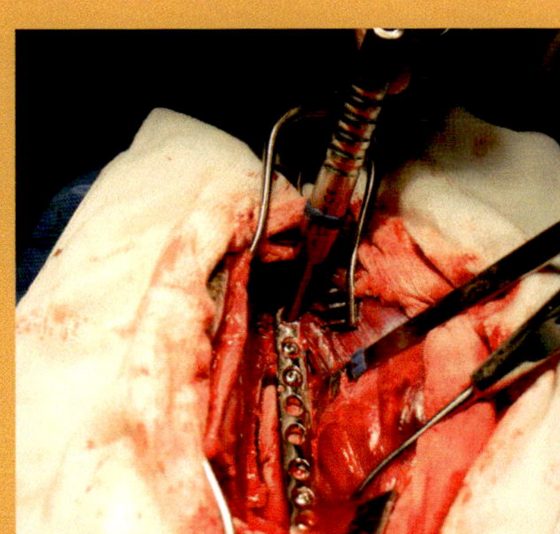

FIGURE 148. Determination of the length needed of a screw using a depth gauge.

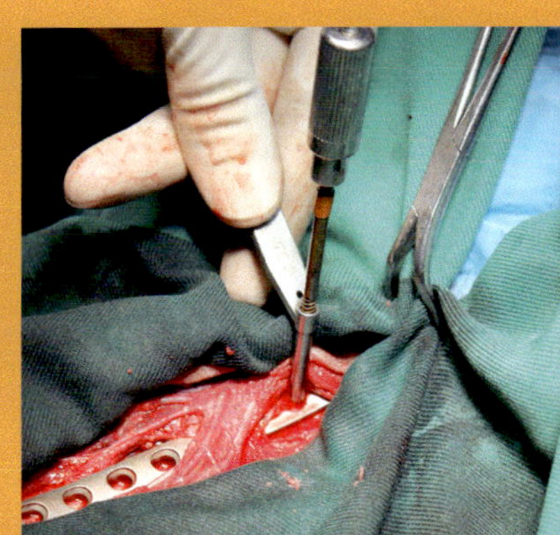

FIGURE 149. Carving threads using a guide.

cortical surface, and in cases in which excessive pressure should not be exerted by the screw, it may be useful to carve one thread first using the thread insert and later use the screw itself to finish the threading.

The order to insert the screws is not important except for with eccentric screws. However, alternating from one primary fragment to another is recommended, assessing the effect that the screws produce on the fracture site as the screws are tightened.

Alternating the insertion of the screws between one bone fragment to the other is recommended so that their effect on the fracture site can be assessed as they are tightened.

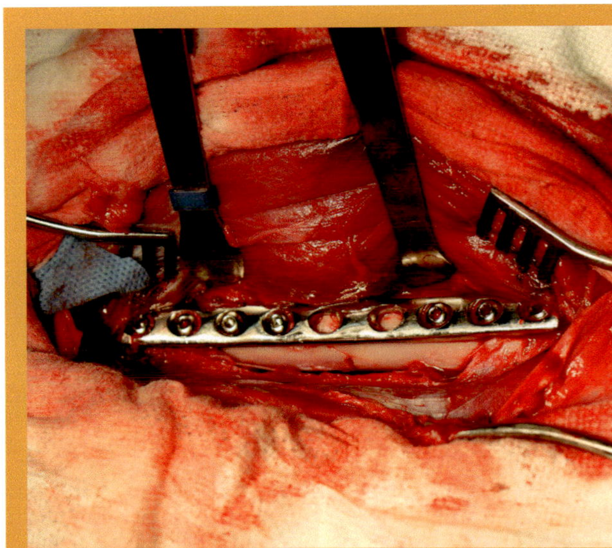

FIGURE 150. Plate stabilised with all of the necessary screws set in place. Note that the two central holes remain free to cruciate the tension in the weak points of the plate (edges near the fracture).

It should be kept in mind that the moment when two screws per fragment have been inserted, the position of the implant cannot be modified. Therefore, before perforating the hole for the second screw of each primary fragment, it must be confirmed that the ends of the plate are over the bone. This is because in the case of long implants, any angle in the area close to the fracture site can cause one of the ends to move off of the bone making it impossible to insert the screws in their corresponding holes.

Once the screws have been inserted, they should be tightened again as each screw inserted moves the plate a little bit closer to the bone and one of the previously inserted screws may have loosened slightly (Fig. 150).

To conclude the surgery, sutures should be used to close the soft tissues, while avoiding direct contact of the plate with the skin to avoid healing problems.

Locking plates

As mentioned at the beginning of this chapter, the plates are fastened to the bone from the pressure exerted by the screws as they are being tightened. This pressure causes a loss of periosteal blood supply, directly underneath the implant, as well as the intraosseous blood supply (derived from the mechanical pressure), which leads to a decrease in the bone's vitality.

When the fracture is stabilised, the implant (especially compression implants) modifies the forces that act on the fracture site, subjecting the bone to a series of artificially created anomalous forces. That is, bone healing is produced under the effect of forces that are not exclusively physiological, and thus the newly formed bone, meant to tolerate physiological forces, is sometimes unprepared to adequately tolerate said artificial forces without the support of the implant. Overtime the bone will readapt its structure until it creates mechanically-adequate tissue.

This phenomena does not occur when the bone heals by means of a conservative treatment or biological osteosynthesis. In these cases, the bone tissue is created under conditions that are considerably natural, so that the bone that forms is prepared to tolerate physiological loads much sooner. This is why, in certain occasions, an external fixator can be removed one month after surgery, while in adult patients, the plate should not be removed until six months have passed since the surgery.

As discussed in the External Fixators section (page 58), the locking plates are most likely the most biological system that exists as they avoid undesirable forces and allow for those of axial compression. However, they have a series of external structures with certain disadvantages, one of them being the distance between the rigid structure and the bone axis (Fig. 151).

As a solution to these issues, locking plates have been developed that combine two concepts: create an external fixator that allows for biological healing that reduces the distance between the rigid system and the bone, and avoids the loss of blood supply both outside and inside of the bone. The result is the creation of a plate that is not fastened to the bone by pressing the implant on the cortical surface but through the locking of the screws against the plate itself (and thus gives it its name). That is, the screws are screwed into the bone and to the plate (Fig. 152).

The locking plates avoid the disadvantages of external fixators and plates as they allow for biological healing with a greater proximity between the bone and the fixator and they do not alter the periosteal or intraosseous blood supply.

Consequently, the result offers various advantages. On the one hand, when introducing the plate under the soft tissues, the rigid system is brought closer to the bone and the structure is thus much more effective (biomechanical aspect); on the other hand, the system allows for certain movements, and as the loads are not entirely neutralised, the formation of significantly more physiological tissue is favoured; and lastly, as the plate does not apply pressure to the cortical surface, the periosteal and intraosseous blood supplies are not affected (Fig. 153), and for this reason, the periostium can develop around the entire bone perimeter, accelerating the healing process.

Different plate designs have been developed over the last few years based on the same principle: the head of the screw is locked into the hole in the implant.

The technique to apply these plates varies slightly depending on the manufacturer, as there are differences in the design of each model. In this section, each one will not be explained, but rather the bases regarding their functioning and the difference between the most-used plates.

In most of the existing systems, the threading is previously carved in the head of the screw as well as in the hole in the implant. The strength of the anchoring between the screw and the plate is slightly greater in this system. However, the surgeon is forced to place the screws in a predetermined position, normally in a 90° angle from the plate, which means that the possibility to place the screws in the position that best suits each situation is restricted.

To overcome this issue, certain manufacturers design their plates so that in one hole, a screw can be inserted on an angle or not. In the case that the surgeon wants to insert on an angle, the screw should not be locked. Other

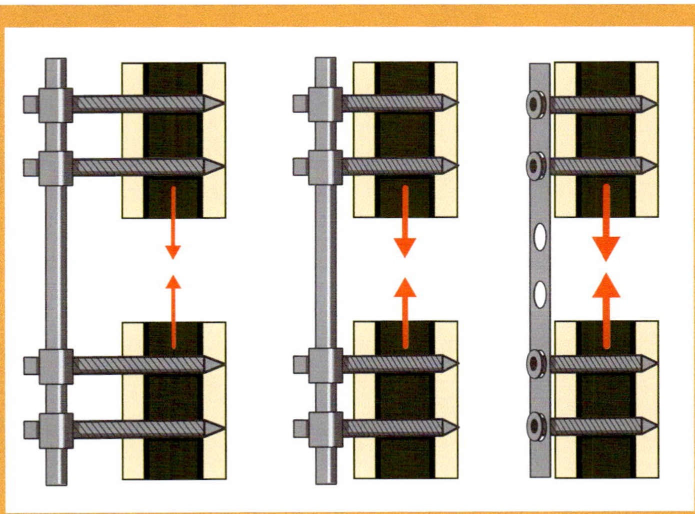

FIGURE 151. The rigidity of the fixator-bone combination depends on the distance between the fixation system and the bone. Said rigidity is proportional to this distance, cubed.

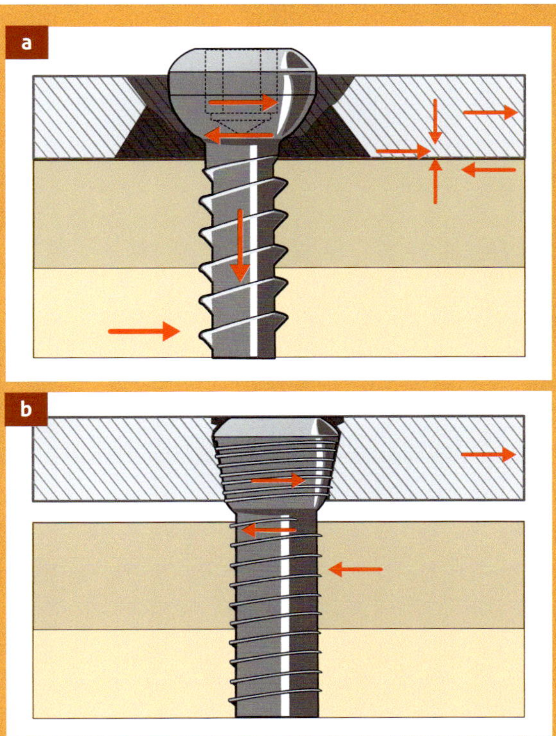

FIGURE 152. Representation of the difference in the fixation with screws from traditional plates (a) and with locking plates (b).

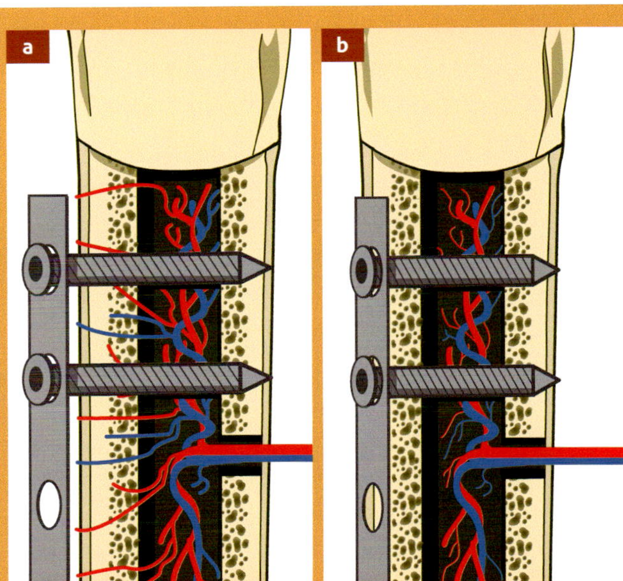

FIGURE 153. Graphic representation of the effect on the periosteal and intraosseous blood supplies of a locking plate, located very close to the bone, without coming into contact with it (a), and a traditional plate that compresses the bone (b).

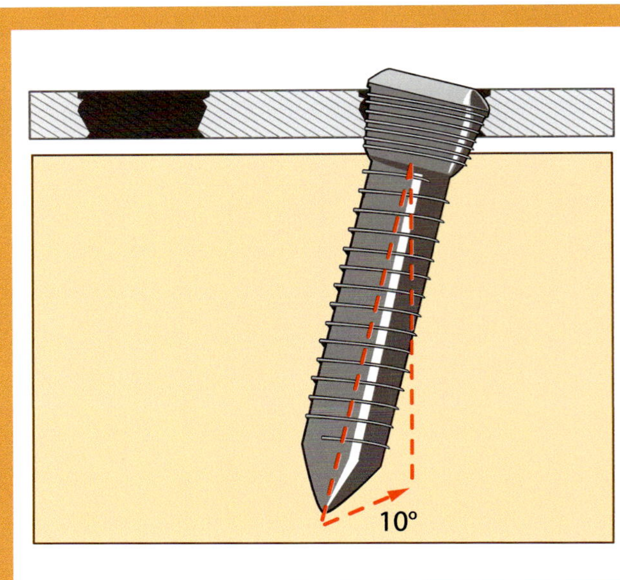

FIGURE 154. Representation of a polyaxial system that shows the angle of the insertion of the screw. Said angle gives the system more purchase.

manufacturers allow for the screw to be inclined 10 %, as the head of the screw itself carves the threading in the thickness of the hole in the plate. These are called polyaxial systems and they allow more freedom in the placement of screws (Fig. 154). The angulation of the screw can be increased, but the strength of its grip is lost progressively in relation to the increase in its inclination.

> *The polyaxial locking plates allow for the inclination of the screw to be oriented to a certain degree because the head of the screw itself carves the threading in the hole in the plate.*

Most locking plates are made of titanium, a metal that along with providing great resistance to infection, it possesses a greater rate of osteointegration. However, if certain norms are not followed, it breaks more frequently than those made of steel as it is less flexible. Regarding the recommendation to leave no holes open, the surgeon must leave at least two to disperse the cycles of flexion. In the particular case that the plate is made of titanium, at least three should be left open (Fig. 155).

Although locking plates can be used perfectly as a rigid osteosynthesis system, when applying screws close to the fracture site, its characteristics adapt better to biological osteosynthesis (Fig. 156). That is, they are implants that are normally fixed to the bone using screws located on its ends for which the problem of the concentration of cycles of flexion is not usually produced.

Another significant difference between traditional plates and these plates are the points where they are fastened. In the first case, the ideal condition for the plate to tolerate the forces that tend to rip them out of the bone is that each bone fragment be anchored in at least five cortical surfaces (see page 91). In the case of locking plates, as the screw is firmly fastened to the implant, it serves the same purpose as the cortical bone and thus, hypothetically, one bicortical screw and one monocortical screw would be enough to achieve the adequate strength.

One monocortical locking screw has the same resistance to being ripped out of the bone as one traditional bicortical screw. The grip strength increases by 30 % when the locking screw is bicortical. This allows for the use of monocortical screws which avert risks in situations in which long screws cannot be applied (Fig. 157).

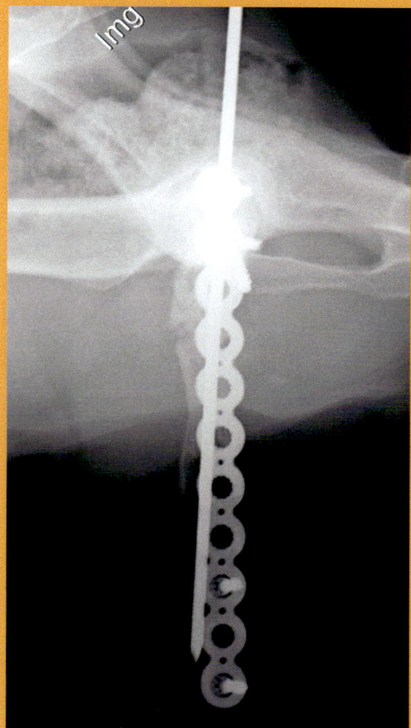

FIGURE 155. X-ray image showing various holes without screws on the fracture site in a titanium plate.

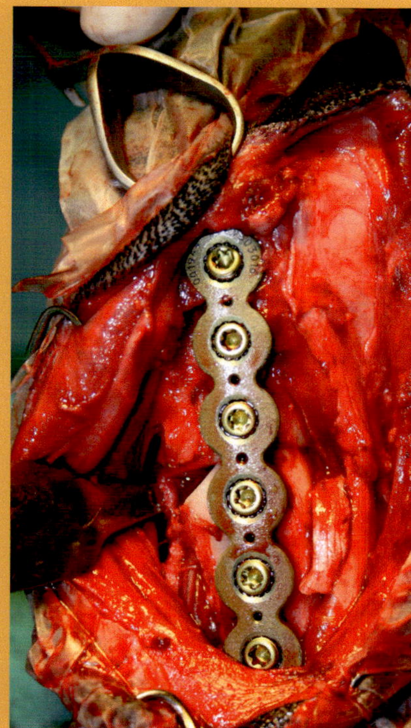

FIGURE 156. Locking plate applied as a compression plate in a corrective osteotomy.

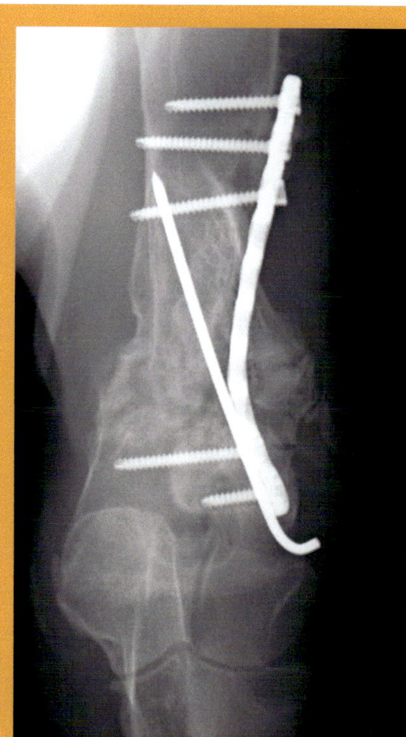

FIGURE 157. X-ray of the distal epiphysis of the humerus showing how the screw is only anchored to one cortical surface (monocortical) to avoid interfering with the anconeus muscle.

The monocortical locking screw exerts greater resistance to being ripped out of the bone than a traditional bicortical screw; its grip strength increases by 30% if the screw if bicortical.

The greatest difference in relation to traditional plates, without a doubt and as previously mentioned, is how they are fastened to the bone. In normal plates, the fastening is produced by the friction between the metal and the bone. This way, when a screw is inserted in a plate, the head eventually comes into contact with the edges of the hole. From that moment on, as the screw is turned, the bone is tractioned until its cortical surface is in intimate contact with the plate. However, in the case of locking plates, when the head of the screw comes into contact with the hole, it screws into the plate and into the bone until the plate itself stops it. The threading of the screw itself serves for locking in certain systems.

The maximum torque of a screw in a traditional plate is given by the resistance of the bone, while for locking plates, the torque is limited by the resistance of the metal itself. It is thus very difficult to strip the threads in a locking plate no matter how weak the bone is. That is, the bone does not move towards the implant with locking plates, rather it stays in the original position as when the screw was locked in the hole of the plate. Consequently, when the first two screws begin to lock the fracture, they must be set in the definitive position.

Another advantage of the locking plates is that their moulding is moved to a second plane and becomes less critical to the success of the intervention, which is contrary to what occurs with traditional plates.

When traditional plates are used, the surgeon will find him/herself with a new limiting aspect, which is the moulding of the plate. When this is not done correctly, it could lead to the intervention failing. With locking plates, however, the moulding becomes a secondary issue (Fig. 158), for which this option is usually chosen. This fact, together with the ideal characteristics demonstrated for biological osteosynthesis, converts locking plates into a suitable alternative to perform MIPO techniques (page 89).

This position of the screws in relation to the implant is easily achieved with the polyaxial systems. For the rest of the systems, this possibility is only feasible if the plate is pre-designed with the holes oriented in a non-perpendicular manner. This way, the screw will be set in an oblique manner, for which along with the strength of the fastening provided by the threading, its position prevents it from loosening (if the anchoring of the screws in the bone is lost, their inclination impedes the plate from separating from the bone). If the screws were arranged in a parallel fashion, the implant could separate from the bone. In traditional plates, this option does not provide many benefits as, given the head is not fastened to the hole, it may oscillate and therefore, separation from the bone is not prevented.

There are implants available designed specifically for certain surgeries in which both the form as well as the inclination of the screws is predetermined. In polyaxial systems, however, the screws can always be introduced on an angle.

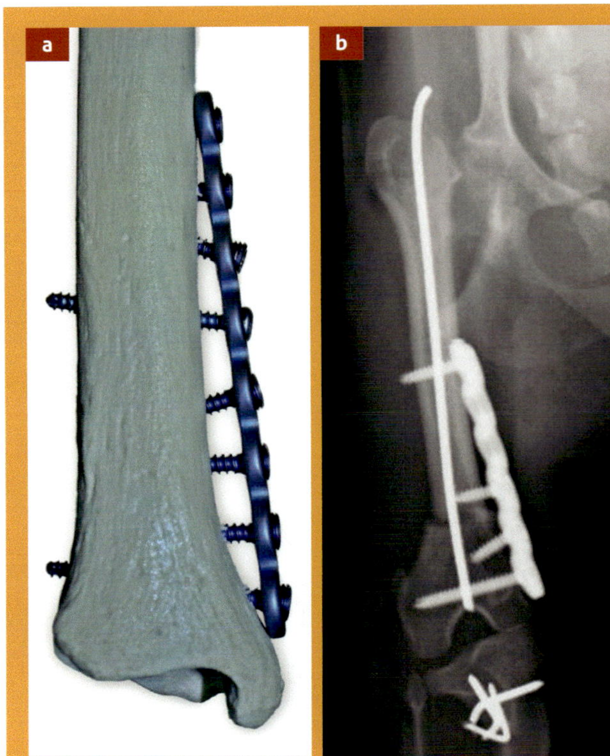

FIGURE 158. Moulding is not a critical issue with locking plates. Recreation of a locking plate where it is clearly visible that it does not adapt to the bone's shape (a). X-ray of a locking plate without moulding in the treatment of a corrective osteotomy of a femur (b).

Complications in the bone healing process

6

The most frequent complications that a clinician will be faced with in bone surgery, as well as their possible treatments, will be discussed in this chapter.

It should be taken into account that the vast majority of complications are a consequence of improper examination of the fracture, poor choice of osteosynthesis systems, or deficient application of said systems. That is, although it is unpleasant to admit, most complications related to osteosynthesis are caused by the surgeon.

The problems that arise in the treatment of fractures are not usually produced as a consequence of a single significant mistake. Generally, the problem arises as a result of a series of small mistakes made throughout the selection process of the osteosynthesis system and its application, as well as during the post-operative period. The sum of all of these small mistakes, together with the lack of collaboration by patients, is what sometimes leads to failed osteosynthesis.

There are various possible complications. However, the primary ones are the following:

- Fracture disease.
- Contracture of the quadriceps femoris muscle.
- Delayed union - non-union.
- Defective consolidation (malunion).
- Osteomyelitis.

FRACTURE DISEASE

Fracture disease is considered as the undesired effects produced on the joints of a limb as a consequence of atrophy of the bone, soft tissues and skin, resulting from prolonged immobilisation of a limb during the treatment of a fracture.

Aetiopathogenesis

These effects are primarily produced by the use of cast type external immobilisations, although they may also result from the application of other osteosynthesis systems.

Nonetheless, there is no single cause that justifies the appearance of this problem, rather it is a consequence of the combination of a series of predisposing factors.

One of the causes that produce bone atrophy, that is, osteoporosis, is the absence or decrease of the forces applied to the bones. These forces are produced by bearing weight on the limb as well as from the effects of muscle contraction (Fig. 1).

Osteoporosis is produced by a modification of the piezoelectric behaviour of the bone. As previously mentioned, the bone areas that no longer bear weight suffer halisteresis with the respective loss of bone mass. A phenomena of bone reabsorption that would act on the entire bone would be produced in some way.

Fortunately, these processes of osteoporosis and muscular atrophy revert as soon as the limb recovers its normal functioning. However, the production of bone tissue in the fracture of a bone with fracture disease is ten times slower than that of a normal bone.

The greatest disadvantage of fracture disease is that it affects joints, where many of the alterations produced are irreversible.

The changes in the joints include contracture, of both the capsule as well as the surrounding tissues, and the proliferation of intra articular connective tissue. On the other hand, prolonged inactivity of a joint leads to a decrease in the supply of nutrients to the cartilage, which eventually causes modifications of the cartilaginous tissue structure itself that can lead to permanent modifications with ankylosis of the joint (Fig. 2).

Joint movement is needed to produce a pumping effect responsible for making the synovial fluid circulate correctly within the joint and providing nutrients to the cartilage.

As deduced from the aforementioned, fracture disease is a consequence of the prolonged immobilisation of a limb. Fortunately, treatment of fractures using external immobilisation methods such as casts is less and less frequent.

Current systems usually allow for the quick recovery of movement of the affected limbs which is the foundation for ideal osteosynthesis. That said, inadequate knowledge of the application of internal fixation methods may also lead to the appearance of fracture disease.

The inadequate application of fixation systems may lead to the appearance of fracture disease.

The most frequent example is the incorrect placement of intramedullary fixation systems that cause pain (Fig. 3). This pain impedes early mobilisation which triggers the previously explained processes.

Other osteosynthesis systems that cause this pathology are external fixators applied as temporary joint stabilisation systems. If a joint is kept immobilised more than three or four weeks, the possibilities that ankylosis, the loss of the physiological range of motion of the joint, is produced are very high. If the immobilisation is made in growing patients, this ankylosis can occur in a short period of time, and may reach a point where it becomes irreversible.

CONTRACTURE OF THE QUADRICEPS MUSCLE

Among the orthopaedic problems that affect soft tissues and lead to functional impediments of the extremities, contracture of the quadriceps muscle should be highlighted. This pathology is one of the surgical complications with the worst prognosis that a surgeon can be faced with. Said pathology basically consists of a loss of the elongating capacity of the quadriceps femoris muscle.

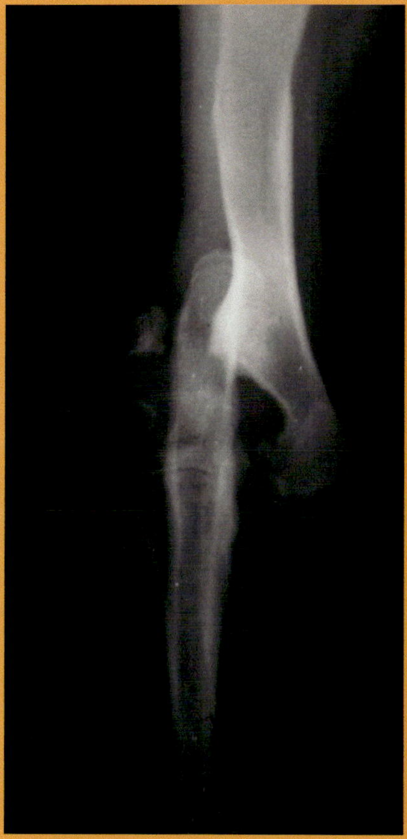

FIGURE 1. Salter IV fracture of the lateral condyle of the humerus, as a consequence of a process of osteoporosis due to lack of use.

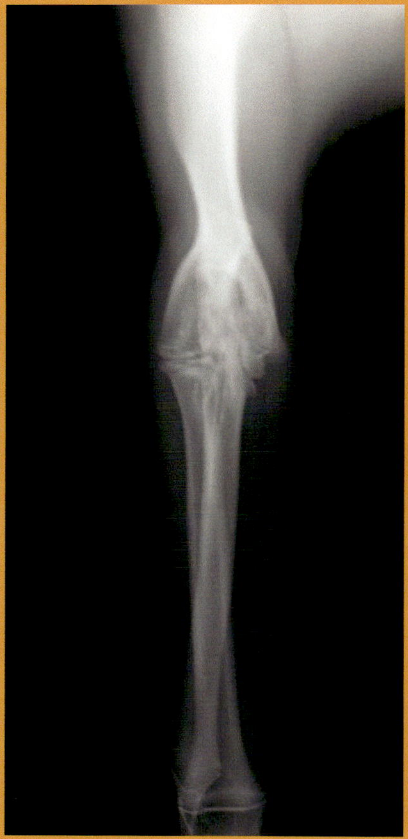

FIGURE 2. Ankylosis of the elbow as a consequence of prolonged fixation in a puppy. Take note of the decrease in the joint space.

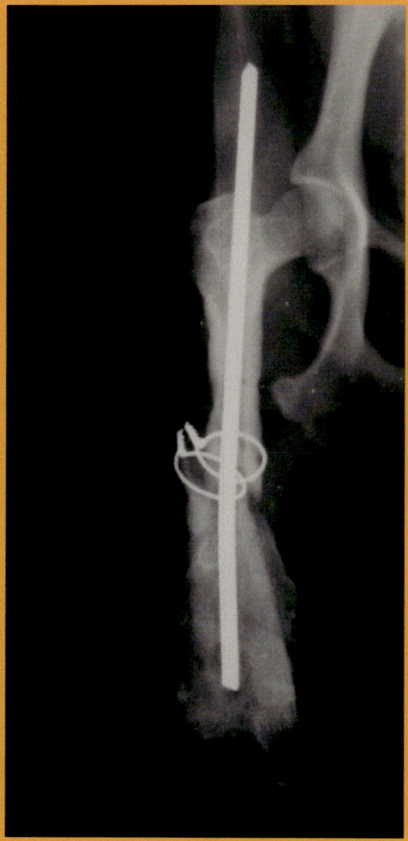

FIGURE 3. Intramedullary pin incorrectly inserted. The pain caused reduces its use and the lack of weight bearing that leads to less bone density.

When a bone fracture takes place, the muscle that surrounds the bone is damaged and, in this case, the anatomical position of the quadriceps femoris muscle is the reason this is the most affected muscle. These lesions at the muscular tissue level produce two effects:

- Substitution of muscle tissue by connective tissue.
- Adherence of the muscle itself to the periostium.

Contracture of the quadriceps femoris muscle has a considerably worse course and consequences when produced in growing animals although it can happen at any age. In these patients, the femur should continue to increase its length along with all of the surrounding tissues.

When the femur is fractured, this muscle (located on the cranial surface of the bone with insertions in the greater trochanter and its tibial crest) suffers modifications in its structure and loses its capacity to grow at the same rate as the femur.

This incapacity of the muscle to continue growing leads to the formation of a fixed tension band at the previously mentioned insertion points leaving the femur without enough space to develop, and the increase in the length of the femur causes a hyperextension of the stifle that becomes more accentuated as the bone grows.

Aetiopathogenesis

The exact cause of this pathology is unknown although there are two theories that attempt to justify its appearance:

- **Compartment syndrome theory**. This occurs when the injury is not accompanied by a tear in the fascia that envelops the quadriceps femoris muscle. The haematoma that forms as a consequence of the lesion of muscle fibres is retained inside of the muscle mass. Given that this tissue has a very limited capacity to regenerate itself, it is substituted by fibrous tissue with a lesser capacity of elongation than the original muscle tissue. Therefore, the previously mentioned band of tension is created.
- **Incorrect handling of soft tissues**. As mentioned above, the periostium in growing animals is a very active tissue. If basic aseptic techniques are not followed, the soft tissues are not handled with care and the periostium is not left intact during the surgical intervention, adhesions between the femur and the muscle in question, primarily the vastus intermedius, may take place. This leads to the incapacity of the quadriceps to make movements of extension.

Clinical process

Clinically, two to three weeks after surgery, and depending on age, the patient presents with a total incapacity to bend the stifle joint, walking with the limb in complete extension and making a movement of abduction with each step (Fig. 4).

Treatment

Logically, the best treatment option is to prevent this problem from appearing. If the fracture site is exposed, a great increase of the volume of the quadriceps can be observed, and if the fascia of said muscle remains intact, an incision can be made to evacuate the haematoma. The transformation of the muscle into connective tissue can thus be partially avoided.

Regarding the handling of soft tissues and the periostium, great care must be taken. This is how the adhesions between the muscle and the bone are kept from becoming extensive enough to cause a contracture of the quadriceps. On the other hand, the early reestablishment of joint movement also prevents the formation of adhesions.

That said, if the pathology already exists, the solution is very difficult. Acting quickly as soon as the first signs of contracture are diagnosed is of utmost importance. This will hopefully reduce the problems that could appear in the stifle joint.

To solve the problem, there are two techniques that we describe briefly as follows:

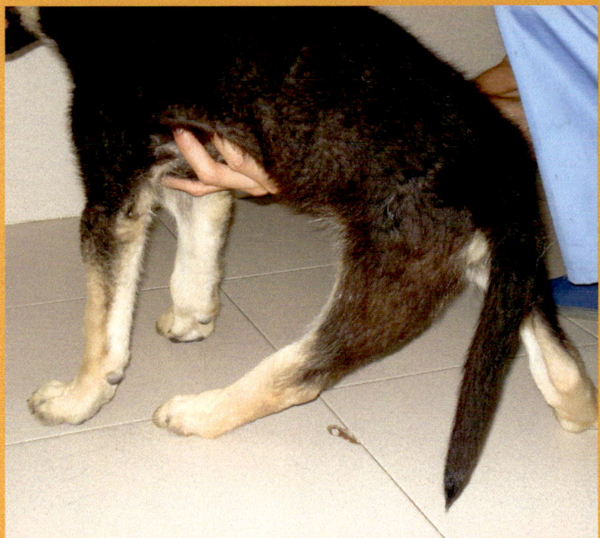

FIGURE 4. Hyperextension of the stifle due to a contracture of the quadriceps femoris muscle.

Elongation of the quadriceps femoris muscle

This technique consists of making a series of cuts, alternating on each side of the muscle to increase its length. The cuts, once the quadriceps femoris muscle has been separated from the bone, should cover approximately one third of the width of the muscle mass.

Separation of adhesions between muscle and bone

This technique consists of completely separating the quadriceps from the adhesions that have formed between the muscle and the femur to allow for the physiological movements of the stifle. First, the four heads of the quadriceps must be located to then detach the muscle mass from the femur. To perform this intervention, a Hohmann elevator, or surgical scissors, are inserted between the muscle and the bone, and moved in a proximal and distal direction from the bone, until completely separating the quadriceps femoris muscle.

Preventing the repeated formation of an adhesion between the muscle and the bone is of great importance in both techniques. One possibility consists of interposing a portion of fascia between the bone and the muscle that serves as a barrier and a surface for the muscle to slide over the bone.

The formation of new adhesions between the muscle and the bone must be avoided.

In some cases, a transarticular external fixator should be used to keep the stifle hyperflexed while allowing for some range of joint movement to avoid the appearance of fracture disease. To do so, a good option is to use elastic structures that force the stifle to remain flexed, allowing for a small degree of extension.

During the postoperative period, the patient should move the stifle joint as soon as possible, not only to avoid adhesions, but also to recover joint mobility. For this reason, the patient should begin to walk again as soon as possible. In this sense, starting physical therapy sessions in which the animal makes passive movements of extension and flexion of the limb is ideal.

On the other hand, it must be taken into account that when a contracture of the quadriceps takes place, the rectus femoris muscle is also affected. When a muscle presents with a contracture, a force is created that displaces the femur in a proximal direction, pushing it against the acetabulum. If this force is produced during the development of the joint, it causes a deformity of the head of the acetabulum that leads to juvenile arthritis and even dislocation of the hip (Fig. 5).

To avoid this problem, a tenotomy of the rectus femoris muscle at the level of its insertion into the ilium should always be performed. In cases of advanced arthritis, the only option is to perform a coxofemoral joint replacement.

In many patients, the degree of arthritis and periarticular fibrosis found in the stifle makes its functional recovery impossible. In these cases, aside from amputation of the limb, there is only one alternative: performing an arthrodesis of this joint (Fig. 6).

DELAYED UNION - NON-UNION

Delayed union

A delayed union is when the time needed for bone healing increases beyond that expected, taking into account the type of fracture, bone and area affected, age of patient and fixation system used (Fig. 7).

The estimated ossification times for bone healing to take place depending on the patient's age and the fixation system used are listed in the Table below:

TABLE 1. Estimated ossification times for bone healing depending on the patient's age and the fixation system used.

Age of patient	Ossification time	
	Extra and intramedullary fixation	Plates
< 3 months	2-3 weeks	4 weeks
3-6 months	3-4 weeks	2-3 months
6-12 months	4-6 weeks	3-4 months
> 1 year	6-8 weeks	5-8 months

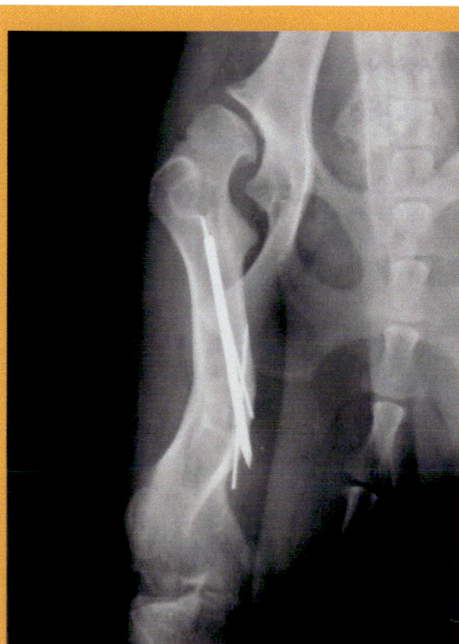

FIGURE 5. Deformation of the coxofemoral joint due to a contracture of the quadriceps femoris muscle.

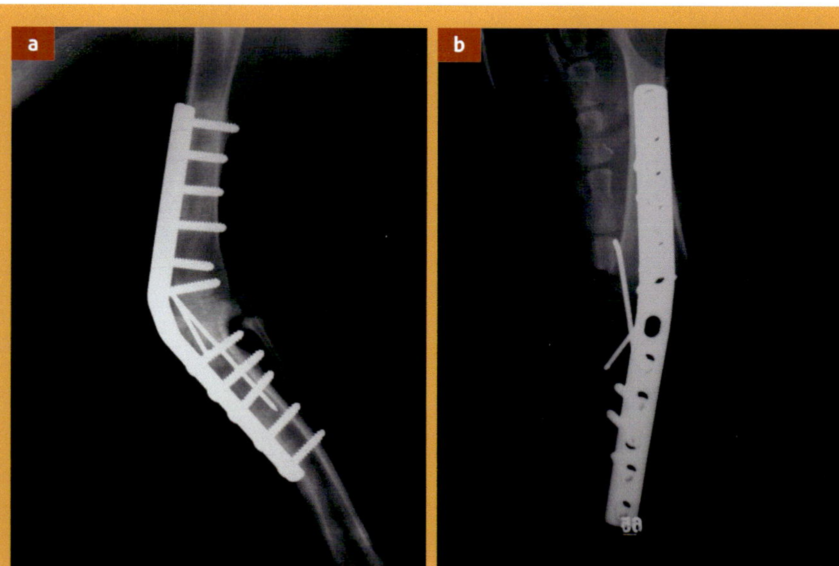

FIGURE 6. Stifle arthrodesis in a patient with advanced arthritis of the joint, secondary to the contracture of the quadriceps femoris muscle.

Non-union

A non-union is when the bone healing processes fail. More specifically, a non-union is considered when none of the bone healing processes have achieved the recovery of the continuity of said tissue (Fig. 8).

Aetiopathogenesis of the delayed union and the non-union

There are many predisposing factors that can lead to a delay or failure in the bone healing process. Traditionally, they are attributed to various causes: inadequate reduction of the fracture, application of an immobilisation system that is not stable enough, decrease in blood supply and infection.

A poor reduction together with the application of rigid osteosynthesis systems usually leads to an inadequate transmission of the weight bearing in the fracture site, needed for healing.

Another possible cause is the interposition of soft tissues in the fracture site, which interferes with the healing processes.

Insufficient immobilisation, as previously mentioned, interferes in the biomechanical processes of ossification. It must be kept in mind that the smaller the separation of the fragments in a fracture line, the greater the damage done by these micro-movements. That is, in cases where ossification by first intention is desired (minimal inter-fragmentary separation), achieving perfect immobilisation is of utmost importance. However, when ossification by second intention is desired, these micro-movements are well-tolerated given that they are the foundation of biological osteosynthesis.

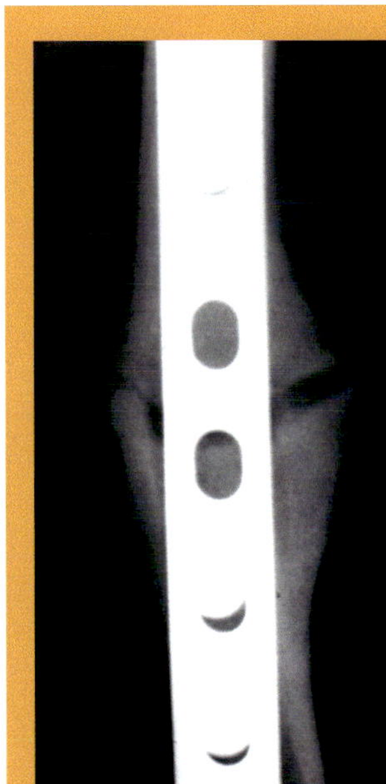

FIGURE 7. Delayed union caused by instability of the implant.

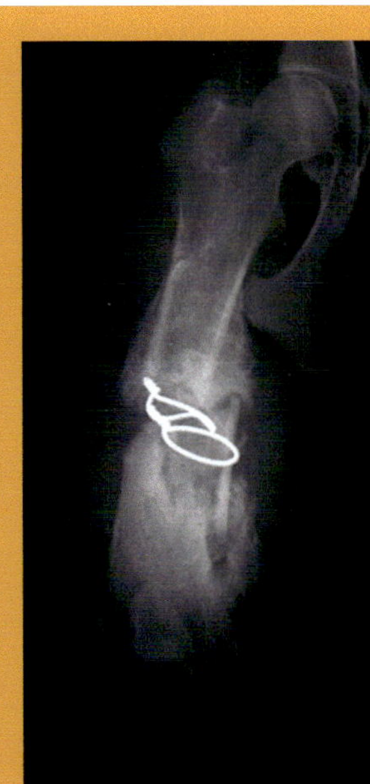

FIGURE 8. Non-union caused by a poor choice of implant.

As mentioned previously several times, preserving the soft tissues around the fracture is fundamental, as well as the adhesions of these tissues to the periosteum in the first phases of bone healing. In areas of large muscle masses, revascularisation is easily compensated. Nonetheless, in areas with little muscle mass, such as the distal third of the radius, the new formation of vessels is slow, increasing the possibilities of a non-union (Fig. 9). Consequently, great care must be taken with the soft tissues when performing surgical interventions, and especially in bony areas with little muscle coverage.

Non-unions are divided into two large groups depending on the blood supply that reaches the fracture edges, that is, of the viability. Therefore, the viable non-unions can be considered as delayed unions, and the non-viable non-unions as the non-unions, strictly speaking (Fig. 10).

In human medicine, the term "non-union" is applied to cases in which more than three months more than the time considered as normal have passed for bone healing.

The difference between a delayed union and a non-union is frequently a mere question of time, given that the non-union always starts as a delayed union. For this reason, being able to anticipate the identification of a case of a delayed union is fundamental to establish adequate treatment to avoid its transformation into a non-union.

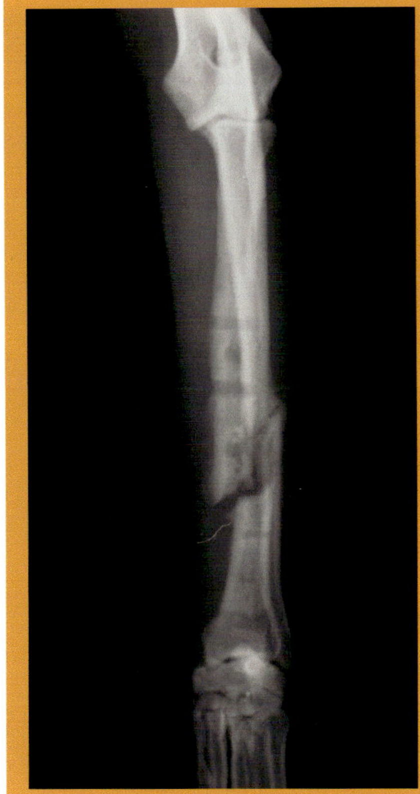

FIGURE 9. Non-union of the distal third of the radius in a transversal fracture insufficiently stabilised using external fixation.

Clinical process

The clinical symptoms of a patient with a delayed union are varied; they may present with anything from no limping whatsoever to the complete lack of use of the limb with the non-union. In the case of a delay in the use of the limb, an X-ray exam should be performed in the first month after the surgical intervention.

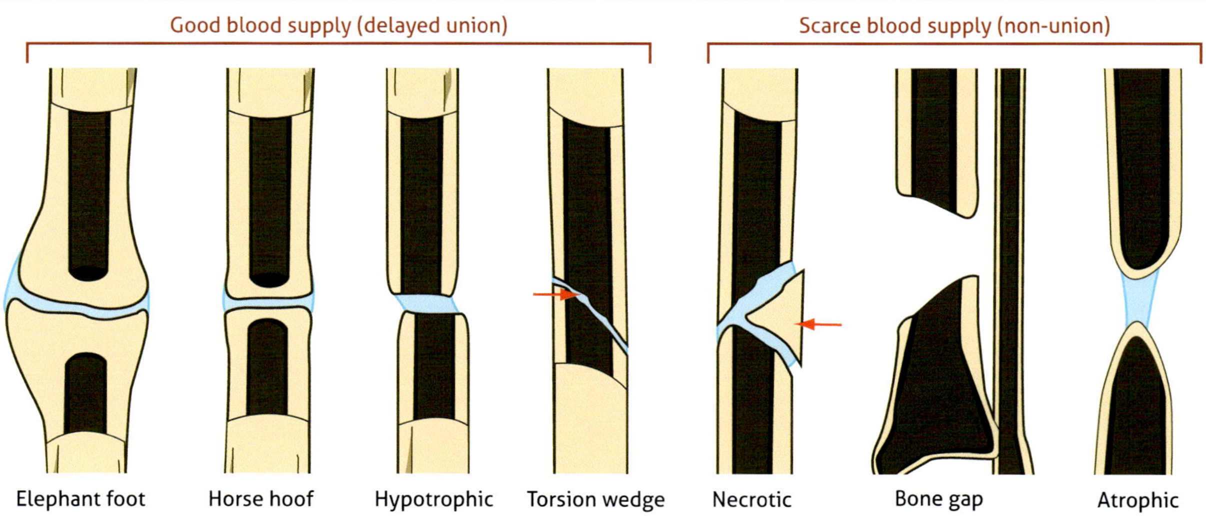

FIGURE 10. Representation of the different delayed unions and non-unions. Weber Pseudoarthrosis Classification.

X-ray signs of a delayed union

In greater or lesser degree, the following is observed:

1. Persistence of the fracture line.
2. Irregular or well-defined fracture edges.
3. Excessive formation of bone callous around the fracture site.
4. Sclerosis of the edges of the fracture line.
5. Obturation of the medullary cavity (non-union).

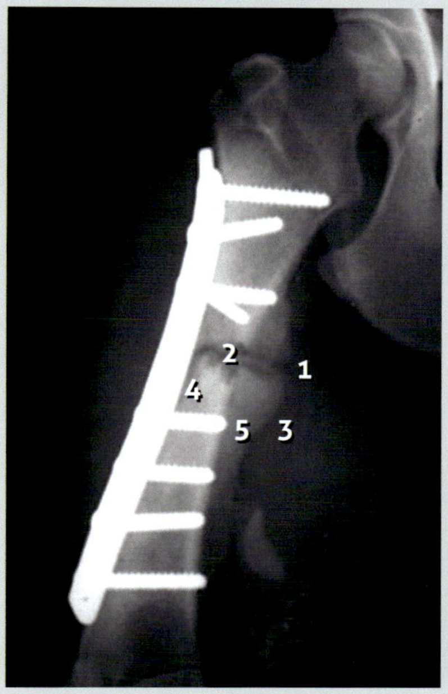

FIGURE 11. Delayed union caused by a lack of weight bearing on the cortical surface opposite the implant.

When a true non-union has occurred, the clinical signs are much clearer (no weight bearing on the affected limb, pain when palpated and even muscular atrophy). In some cases, if the osteosynthesis system does not block visibility, instability can be observed in the fractured area.

The signs are much clearer in X-rays as well. However, the formation of bone callous may vary greatly depending on the type of non-union. Generally, it is not limited to the area of the fracture, but the organism frequently attempts to form a bridge "jumping" above the actual area of the fracture (Fig. 12).

In the last two types of pseudoarthrosis (with bone and atrophic defects), which present the worst prognosis, the formation of bone callous is practically non-existent; as the bone does not heal, the organism reabsorbs it.

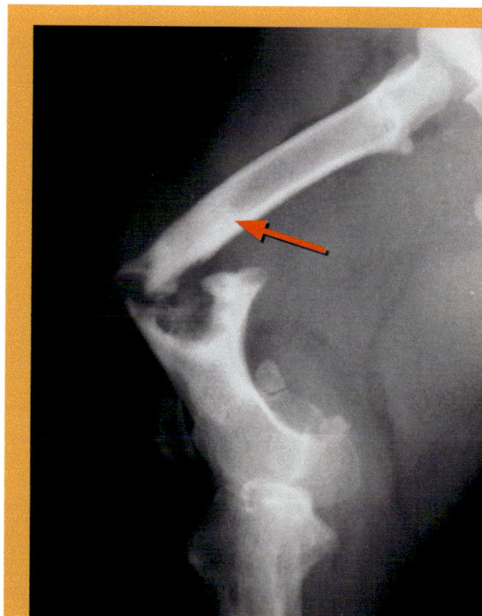

FIGURE 12. Non-union in the femur. Note the obstruction of the medullary cavity (arrow).

Treatment

The best therapy to correct a non-union is to identify the delay in the ossification process as soon as possible and apply the most suitable treatment depending on the type of non-union.

All treatments are based on achieving perfect stability of the fracture site, as well as reactivation of the healing processes. In this sense, neutralising movements of rotation is fundamental as they cause the most damage.

It is important that the limb recovers its functionality as soon as possible for the weight borne by the limb causes micro-compressions at the level of the fracture site that accelerate the bone healing processes. Similarly, the processes of muscular atrophy, adhesions and joint ankylosis will be minimised. This also favours blood circulation which will prevent the appearance of fracture disease.

When a delay in ossification is quickly diagnosed and there is good blood irrigation to the fracture site, various treatments can be implemented, depending on the osteosynthesis system used:

a. If it is foreseen that the osteosynthesis may provide stability for a long period of time (for example, osteosynthesis plates without any loosening of the screws), bone healing can be achieved by simply restricting movements (Fig. 13). Attempts should be made to have the patient use its limb gently to favour healing, but without straining the osteosynthesis system. This is achieved by walking

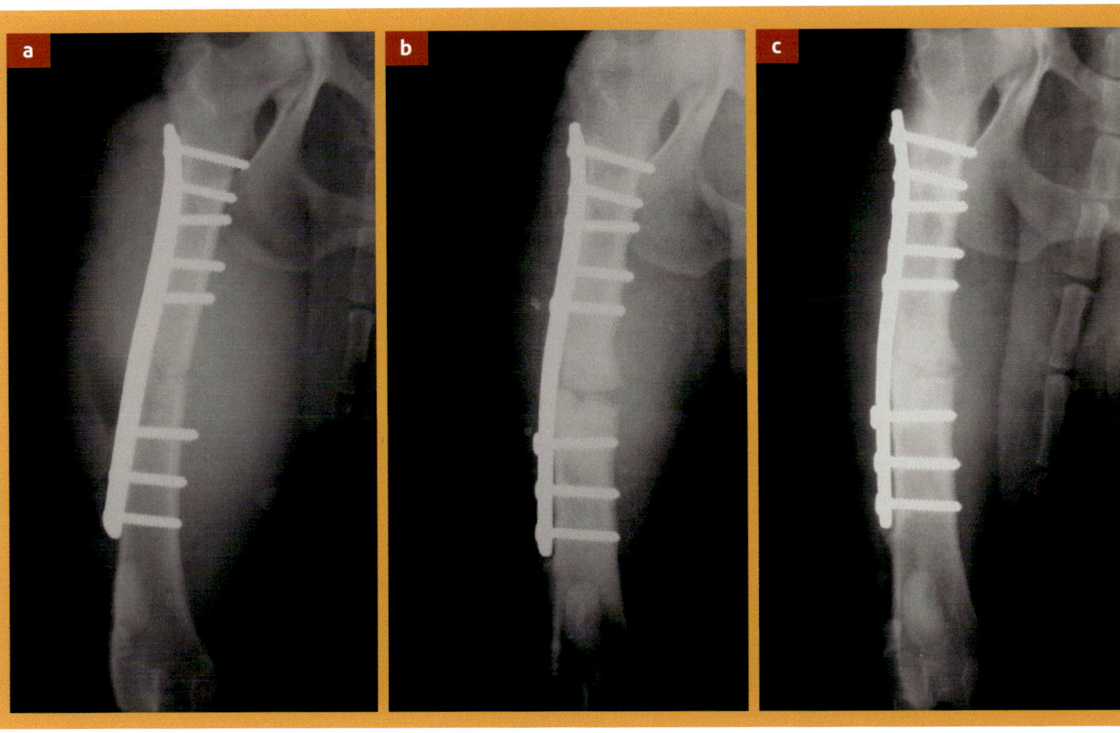

FIGURE 13. Treatment of delayed healing through rest. Postoperative X-ray (a). In the control X-ray one month after surgery, widening of the fracture site can be observed (horse hoof) (b). Nearly complete consolidation after 15 days of rest (c).

the animal on a short leash several time per day for short periods of time.

b. The osteosynthesis system used should be substituted is there are suspicions that it may progressively lose its stability (for example, external fixation without threaded percutaneous pins or intramedullary fixation). In these cases, the ideal treatment consists of the application of an osteosynthesis plate (Fig. 14).

c. Providing greater stability to the fracture site, reinforcing the osteosynthesis system by applying a fixation system that prolongs its "service life". The ideal option if to apply some kind of simple external fixation configuration, or in some cases, a cast-type rigid bandage.

On the contrary, if dealing with a non-union with insufficient blood supply of the fracture site, or complete lack of stability, a new surgical intervention should always be performed to resolve the problem by changing the osteosynthesis system and adapting it to the type of non-union (Fig. 15).

The medullary cavity is usually destroyed by the bone callous itself in all non-unions. Once the old implants have been removed, it is important in these cases to reopen the medullary cavity to allow for new formation of blood vessels. This can be done using a curette, a simple Steinmann pin or a drill bit (Fig. 16). The bone tissue with no blood supply must then be removed from the edges of the fracture using rongeur forceps.

If the surgeon encounters bone sequestrum, all devitalised bone fragments must be eliminated (Fig. 17).

In some cases where a certain amount of time has passed or in young patients, the organism attempts to isolate the bone fragments by forming what is known as an *involucrum* (formation of new bone tissue completely surrounding the fragments for their elimination by osteoclasts, Fig. 18). In these cases, along with removing the fragments, the internal walls must be completely scraped to eliminate the fistula tract. If possible, the walls of the *involucrum* should be left intact as they are made of highly vascularised bone tissue that provides stability to the fracture site.

In all non-unions, except for dystrophic non-unions, there is a varied amount of a lack of bone tissue. In these circumstances, the surgeon has two options: perform a cortico-cancellous bone transplant or shorten the length of the bone with the possibility to lengthen it in the future.

In veterinary medicine, shortening the length of a limb is well compensated through partial hyperextension of the joints of said limb. The capacity to compensate said shortening in the hindlimb is greater than that of the forelimb as the presence of three joints allows for greater modification of the angle

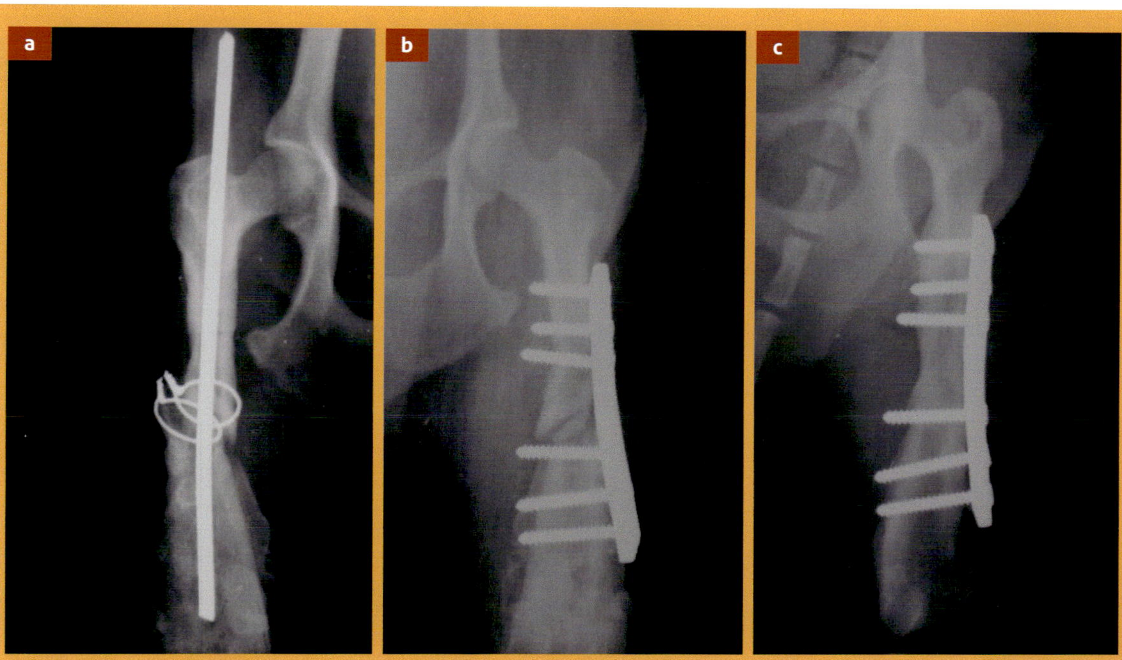

FIGURE 14. Substitution of a defective fixation using an intramedullary pin and cerclage for a plate. Take note of the defective reduction of the fracture (a), resolved with a plate (b) and the progress of the non-union (c).

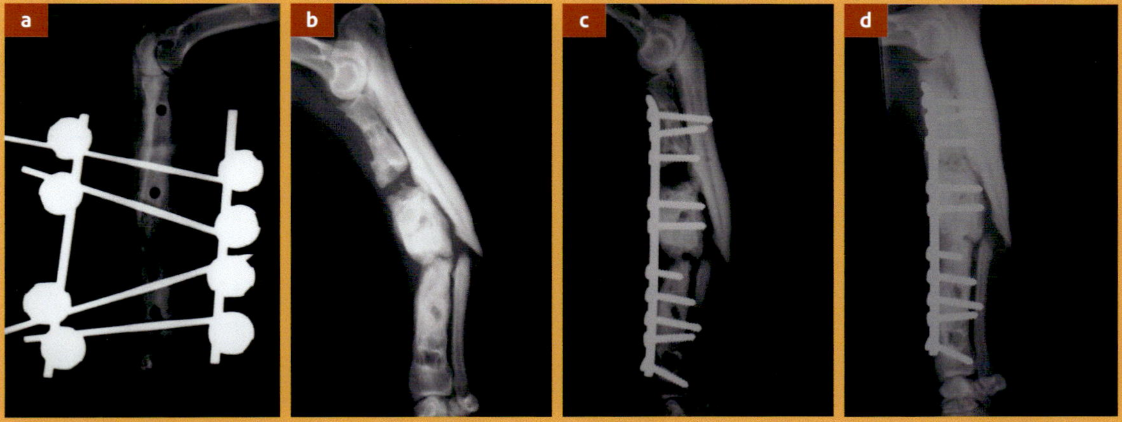

FIGURE 15. Non-union initially treated with an external fixation system (a). After its removal, the non-unions are clearly visible (b). Application of an osteosynthesis plate (c) and progress of the fractures (d).

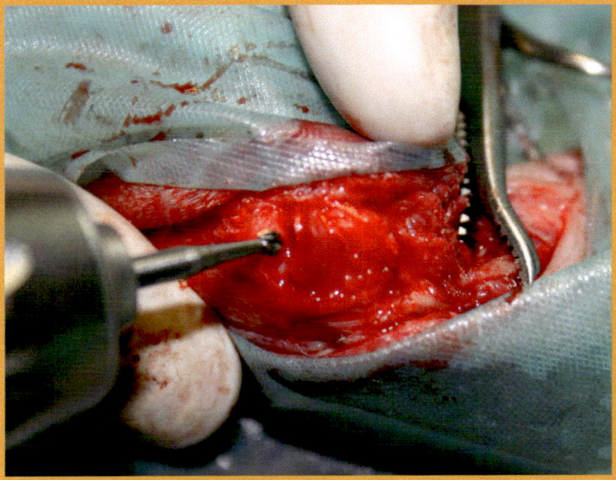

FIGURE 16. Reopening of the medullary cavity with a drill.

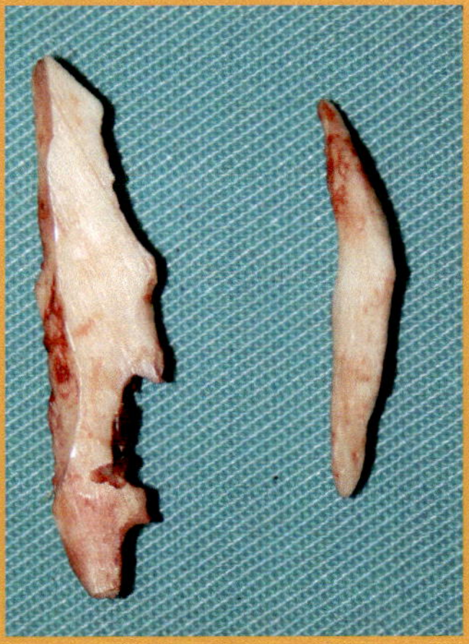

FIGURE 17. Bone sequestrum removed from fracture site.

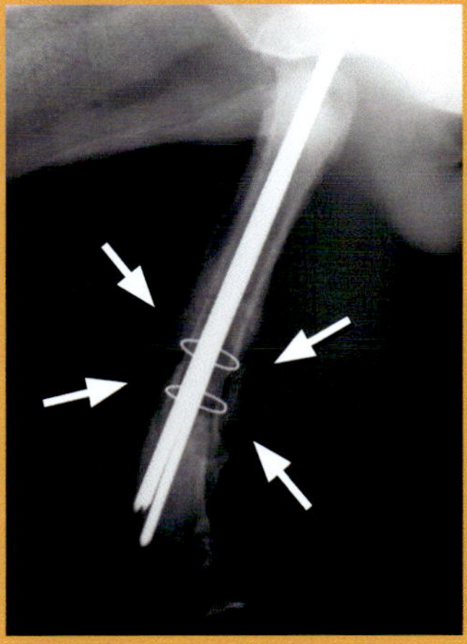

FIGURE 18. Bone sequestrum without periosteal reaction compared with the bone proliferation on the edges of the primary fragments.

of flexion, while the forelimb have only two joints and the carpus cannot be extended any further. In dogs, for example, a shortening of the femur of up to 25 % of its length can be compensated while maintaining good functionality of the limb.

In the treatment of a non-union that presents a loss of bone tissue, a perfect reduction of the fracture edges will most likely be impossible and therefore attempts should be made to achieve the most anatomical alignment of the limb possible. In this regard, it is important to keep in mind that patients compensate from better to worse the following angular defects: cranio-caudal or caudo-cranial angulation, latero-medial or medio-lateral angulation and rotations (internal rotation of the limb is the worst compensated).

> *When cases of a delayed union or non-union or resolved surgically, bone healing must be stimulated.*

In all cases of delayed unions or non-unions that are treated surgically, bone healing must be stimulated. To do so, there are various options to reactivate the bone's osteoblastic function (see Bone Stimulation chapter, page 27).

DEFECTIVE CONSOLIDATION (MALUNION)

Consolidation of a fracture is considered when bone healing processes have been successful without reestablishing the anatomical functionality of the bone. That is, the bone has ossified with some kind of incorrect angle (Fig. 19).

When dealing with a defective consolidation, surgical correction should first be considered. This is only necessary in cases in which the limb presents some kind of dysfunction, that is, when the joints adjacent to the bone are not capable of compensating for the bone angle formed. If there is no dysfunction, the angle can usually be corrected using remodelling processes.

> *Generally, a defective consolidation should only be surgically corrected if it causes a functional alteration of the limb.*

Aetiopathogenesis

The causes of a defective consolidation are always a consequence of an inadequate surgical technique: poor reduction of the fracture, application of an osteosynthesis system that provides little stability, or the premature removal of the osteosynthesis material.

When selecting the most suitable osteosynthesis system, certain details must be taken into account such as the type of bone and fracture, weight and age of the patient, as well as if the animal is very active with little possibilities of complying with adequate rest during the postoperative period.

In the Bone Growth and Healing chapter (page 8) it has been discussed how in the first phases of healing by second intention, the fracture site is replenished with a pseudo-cartilaginous tissue that is capable of tolerating deformations in its structure without this interrupting the healing processes. It is for this reason that in some cases, if the implant fails, or when an osteosynthesis system is removed too soon, the ossification continues without any problems, but the bone, due to the weight it bears, curves (Fig. 20).

It is thus very important to know how to recognize by X-ray what is known as a mature callous, a stage in which the bone no longer deforms itself. By X-ray, it is characterised by a soft and continuous outline in the shape of a spindle with no clear edges of the cortical bone surfaces. A fracture line can be observed, but healing continues with no problems (Fig. 21). However, and when in doubt, it is best to remove the stabilisation system when there is clear evidence that the ossification process has terminated. The need to remove an osteosynthesis system too soon is usually due to the poor choice or application of the system.

Typical examples of errors when selecting the fixation system are intramedullary pins that invade joints or protrude from the skin, external fixators used in older animals, or configurations of the osteosynthesis system that interfere with the patient's gaits.

Treatment

The treatment of a defective consolidation always consists of performing an osteotomy or ostectomy and correcting the existing angle. In certain cases, depending on the severity of the problem, perfect alignment of the longitudinal axis of the bone is not always achieved. However, this is not important as the purpose of the surgery is to achieve functionality of the limb. To do so, once the osteotomy is performed, special attention should be paid to the orientation of the adjacent joints.

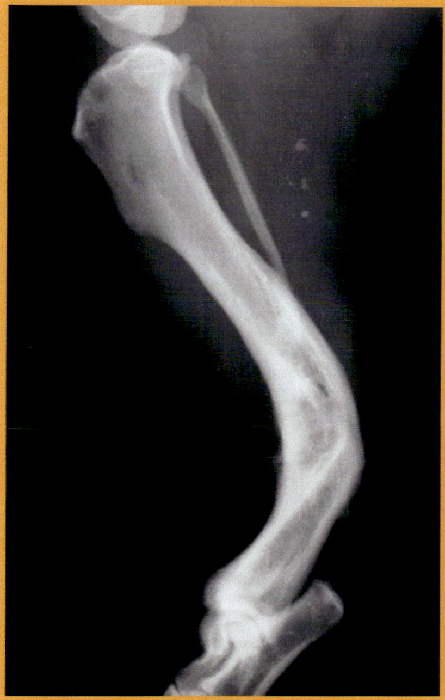

FIGURE 19. X-ray image of a defective consolidation of a tibia. Take note of the abnormal angle of the middle-distal third.

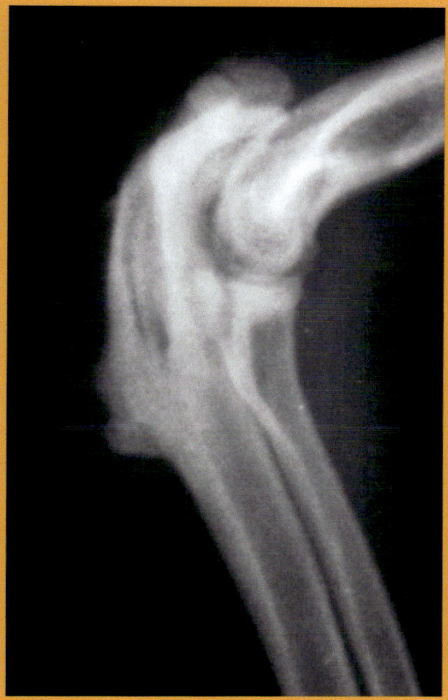

FIGURE 20. Defective consolidation in the ulna of a cat caused by the premature removal of implants.

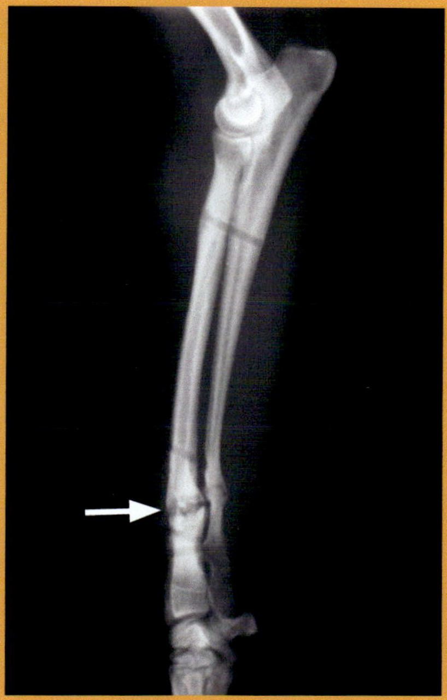

FIGURE 21. X-ray image of a mature callous; although the fracture line is visible, the outline of the cortical surface is lighter (arrow).

Before performing the intervention, this should be planned for. In many cases, it may be necessary to correct not only the lateral or medial angles, but also the rotational angles (Fig. 22).

Planning surgery should ideally include a CT scan of the bone. The three-dimensional reconstruction enables the measurements of the angles that need to be corrected (Fig. 23). If this test cannot be performed, an in-depth X-ray study should be carried out. The line of the osteotomy or the wedged bone fragment to be eliminated to correct the angle can be traced over the X-ray (Fig. 24). The slice should always be made in the area of the bone where the angulation is greatest in order to respect the axial axis of the bone as much as possible (Fig. 25).

The intervention should be performed using the measurements taken over the X-ray as a reference. To reduce the fracture to a correct position, the surgeon palpates the bone protrusions, which serve as a guide, orientating the joints in what he/she considers to be the most adequate position. Once this is done, movements of flexion and extension of the extremity should be made along with a comparison with the other limb to ensure that they follow the same direction. The reduction of a fracture is frequently incorrect, however, the surgeon must focus on the functional aspect of the limb (Fig. 26).

Stabilisation is implemented using the osteosynthesis system that the surgeon deems suitable. The best system for this type of interventions is the use of osteosynthesis plates, or, if the error is greatly complicated, to perform postoperative corrections.

When the bones affected are the radius or the tibia, one solution is stabilisation by means of external fixation which allows for small corrections of the erroneous orientations that are detected through control X-rays taken after surgery.

Among the external fixations, one system that allows for various options are the Ilizarov-type circular fixator (Fig. 27). The advantage of this system resides in the possibility to correct angular (Fig. 28) or even rotational deviations (Fig. 29).

Healing problems should never be stabilised by means of intramedullary fixation.

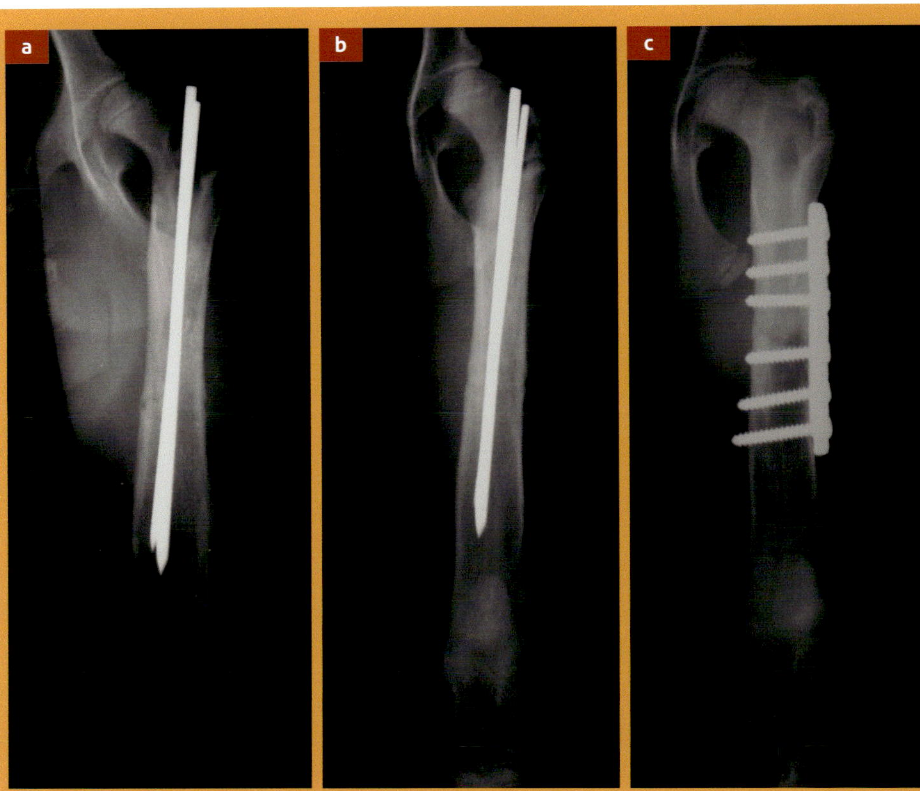

FIGURE 22. Defective rotational consolidation in a femur. Compare the orientation of the head of the femur and the position of the patella (a and b) with the postoperative X-ray (c).

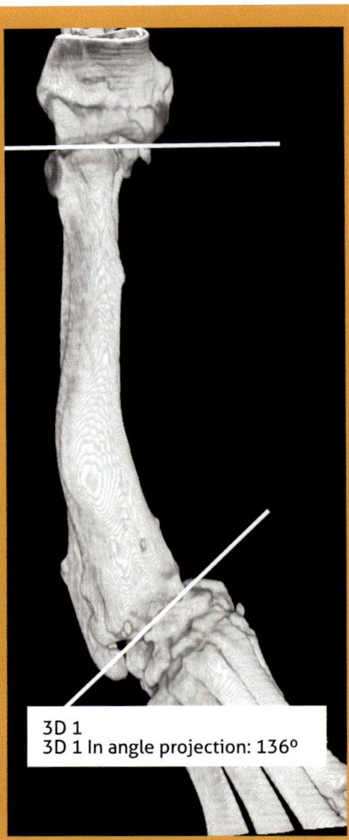

FIGURE 23. Measurement of the angles over a reconstruction using a CT scan.

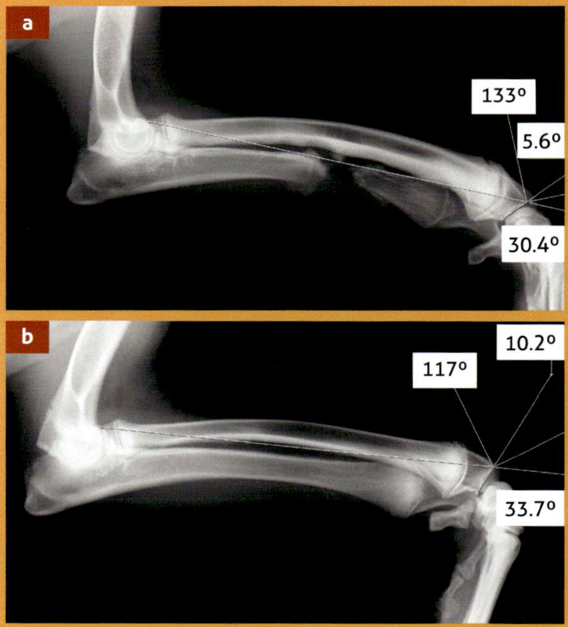

FIGURE 24. Measurement of the angles using an X-ray (a) and comparison with the X-ray of the healthy limb (b).

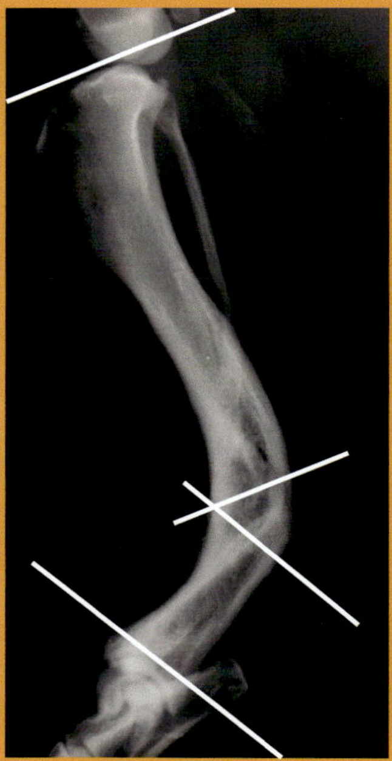

FIGURE 25. Tracing of the ostectomy located in the area of maximum curvature (ideal).

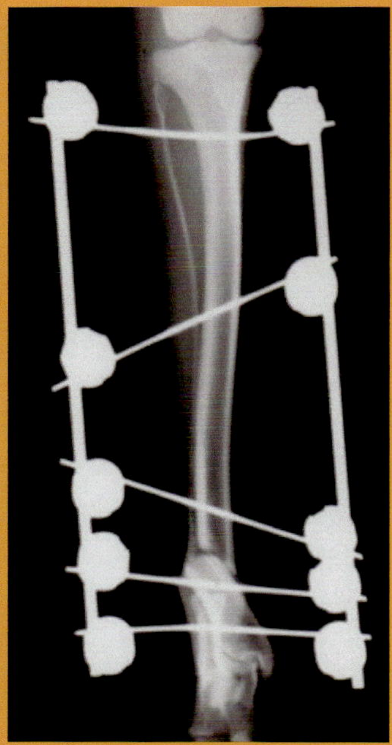

FIGURE 26. X-ray that shows the result of an ostectomy for correction of the tibia. Joint alignment is correct even if the reduction of the fracture site is not.

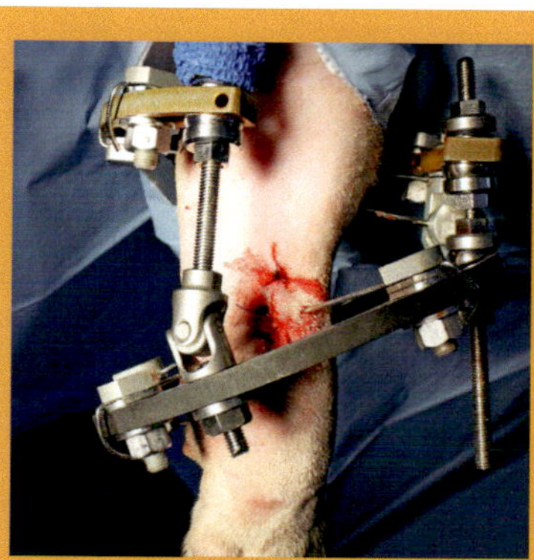

FIGURE 27. Ilizarov-type external fixator to perform an angular correction. Results of the intervention, after placing the fixator in its position.

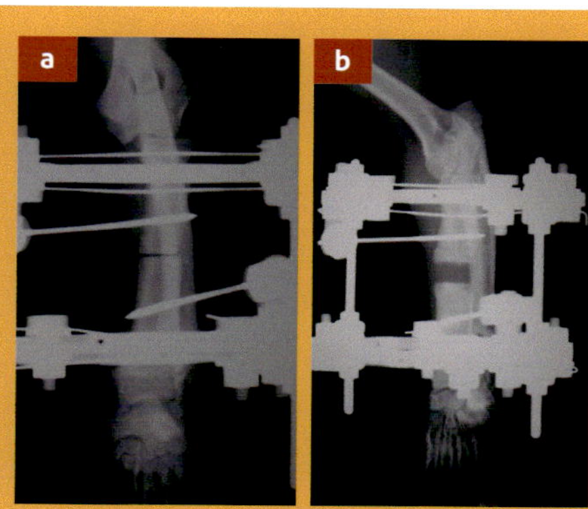

FIGURE 28. Longitudinal elongation using an Ilizarov-type external fixation system.

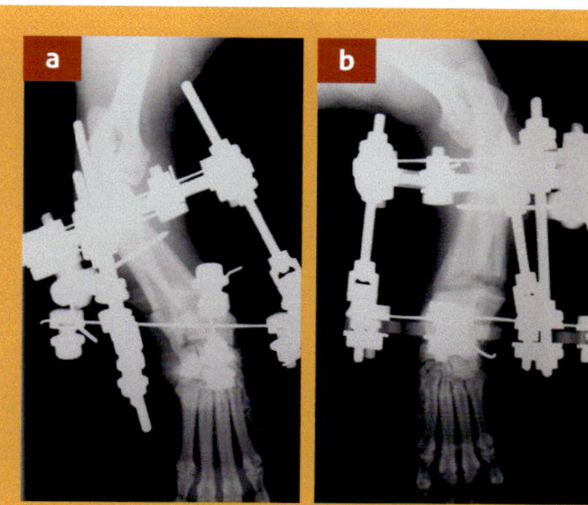

FIGURE 29. Angular correction using an Ilizarov-type external fixation system.

OSTEOMYELITIS

Osteomyelitis is defined as the infection of all elements of a bone, medullary cavity, cortical surface and periostium.

Aetiopathogenesis

The most frequent cause of osteomyelitis is contamination by bacteria, although it can also be caused by fungus. Approximately between 50 and 75 % of the cases of osteomyelitis are caused by *Staphylococcus* spp. Other micro-organisms that frequently cause these infections are: *E. coli*, *Proteus* spp. and *Pseudomonas* spp. The possible implication of anaerobic or facultative anaerobic organisms should be kept in mind such as *Bacteroides* spp. and *Peptostreptococcus* spp.

The existence of anaerobic organisms should be suspected and specific cultures taken for the following circumstances:

- Bad odour.
- Chronic osteomyelitis.
- Osteomyelitis from a dog bite.
- Osteomyelitis after an open fracture.
- Observation after a Gram stain of bacteria with varied morphology.
- Absence of growth in aerobic mediums after having identified bacteria by staining.

The contamination of the fracture may take place during the surgical act, when it is exposed to the exterior (open fractures) or through haematogenous dissemination. Unfortunately, the most frequent cause of osteomyelitis is iatrogenic, that is, from surgery. The predisposing factors of contamination of a bone during surgery are described below:

- **Poor aseptic conditions**. A lack of aseptic conditions is likely the most frequent cause leading to surgical complications leading to osteomyelitis. The presence of some bacteria in the surgical field will obviously not cause an infection alone. For this reason, a series of basic aseptic norms should be followed to decrease the bacterial load that is spread to the surgical field. On the other hand, to avoid the bacteria that reach the bone during the intervention from colonising the tissue, correct antibiotic coverage should be administered prior to surgery.

Antibiotics should be administered before surgery so that the blood contains an adequate concentration at the fracture site during the intervention.

- **Excessive surgery duration**. The intervention time is also an important factor; the more time that the surgical field is exposed to the exterior, the greater the bacterial load. If a surgery takes longer than one and half hours, the intravenous administration of a new dose of antibiotics may be advisable.
- **Inadequate haemostasis**. The existence of a good microbiological culture around the bone favours the proliferation of bacteria. It is thus of utmost importance that correct haemostasis is followed during surgery to impede the formation of haematoma. When soft tissues are sutured,

attempts should be made to avoid leaving dead spaces as these can fill with blood and exudate. In those cases in which there is a great laceration of the soft tissues, it may be helpful to apply a suction drainage that should be removed 24 hours after surgery.

- **Aseptic techniques**. In bone surgery, aseptic techniques must be strictly followed given that the blood supply of bone tissue is very precarious (reduced supply of organic defences) and the velocity of healing is very slow. These two particularities imply a much lower capacity to fight infection than that of the soft tissues (in the chapter on Bone Growth and Healing it was already mentioned how the vascularisation of a fracture depends on soft tissues during the first moments). For this reason, keeping said tissues as intact as possible is fundamental as it is during the first moments of healing when the organism has to fight against bacteria.
- **Weakness of patient**.
- **Incorporation of foreign materials**. In bone surgery, a series of foreign materials are introduced into the organism in most surgical interventions that will complicate the organism's fight against infection. This is especially the case with plates that may decrease the bone's peripheral blood supply by up to 25 % as they are inserted between the soft tissues and the periostium.

  On the other hand, certain bacteria are capable of attaching themselves to the implant and even creating a layer of protection around themselves called a glycocalyx that impedes the action of the macrophages, lymphocytes and neutrophils making it difficult for the antibacterial substances to penetrate.

  To avoid interrupting the correct vascularisation of the cortical bone surface and avoid sub-clinical infections, low-contact plates have been developed. These implants rest only on certain spots of the cortical bone surface, like the pillars of a bridge, thus leaving a space between the plate and the bone, allowing for proper vascularisation.

  Another type of plates that preserve the vascularisation under the implant are the locking plates (see page 94).

For all of the previously mentioned reasons, it is easy to see how osteomyelitis is hard to treat in many cases.

> ***The best treatment against bone infection is prevention.***

Diagnosis

A series of details that help to identify osteomyelitis via X-rays are listed below.

Areas of lysis associated with processes of periostitis can be observed on the cortical bone surface. That is, the characteristic signs of osteomyelitis are the appearance of processes of reabsorption in the affected area associated with other processes of bone formation (Fig. 30).

However, it must be taken into account that these X-ray signs are also characteristic of other noninfectious processes, for example, situations of instability or incipient bone tumours. Therefore, the diagnosis of osteomyelitis should be made taking into account the clinical signs along with those found in the X-rays.

A difference between instability and osteomyelitis resides in that the areas of bone reabsorption in cases of instability are usually more defined, primarily located around the implant and the fracture lines (Fig. 31). That said, in cases of infection, these radiolucent areas are distributed irregularly along the bone and the signs of sclerosis are less manifested.

Another typical sign of osteomyelitis, especially in its chronic form, is the formation of what are known as *involucrum* (page 106). In X-rays, a bone fragment with a greater bone density than that of the surrounding bone is observed with no signs of periosteal reaction (Fig. 32), because ultimately it is dead avascular bone tissue.

Classification of osteomyelitis

There are two forms of osteomyelitis: acute and chronic.

Acute osteomyelitis

The symptoms appear soon after the surgical intervention. The patient presents with acute inflammation of the area operated on, with limping, pain, accumulation of liquid and increased temperature. Frequently, it is difficult to differentiate this from a deep infection of the incision. To determine the presence of bacteria and make a diagnosis, a culture of the liquid accumulated should be taken. In an X-ray study, a periosteal reaction can sometimes be observed, depending on the time passed since the process began.

Treatment depends on the severity of the process, ranging from simple administration of antibiotics, cleaning the fracture site and drainage, to having to replace the osteosynthesis material.

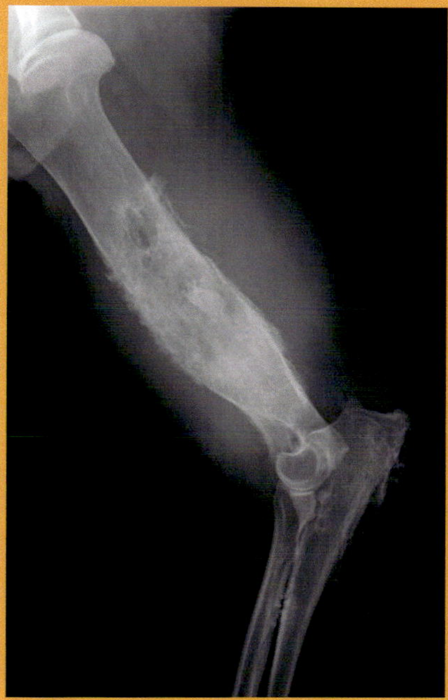

FIGURE 30. X-ray image of the humerus showing the osteomyelitis.

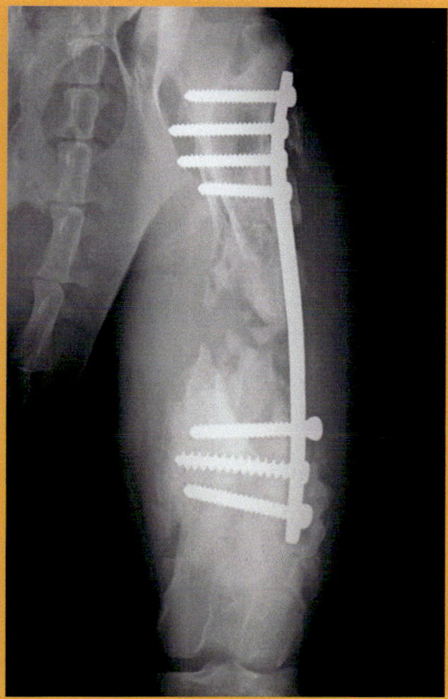

FIGURE 31. Area of reabsorption derived from a situation of instability.

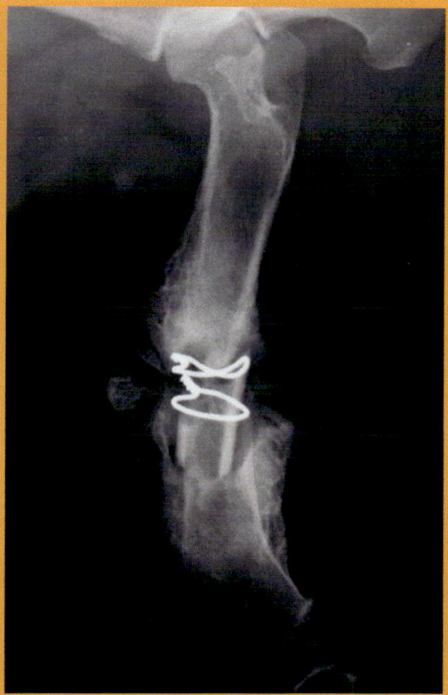

FIGURE 32. Bone sequestrum that is being surrounded by bone tissue (involucrum).

Basically, it consists of eliminating the liquid retained and administering long-term antibiotic treatment. In most cases, if proper treatment is started quickly, the infection can be controlled. If there is not an excessive accumulation of liquid, it can be evacuated by aspiration with a syringe. If the patient's condition does not improve, a suction drainage will have to be inserted by accessing the fracture site.

Throughout the entire treatment period, the patient must be kept on antibiotics that will be established depending on the results of the antibiogram (for aerobic and anaerobic organisms). The sample for the culture must be taken from the fracture site. If there are fistulae, the liquid extracted is not adequate, as it is always contaminated by saprophytic bacteria from the skin. Until the results are obtained from the antibiogram, antibiotics effective against streptococcus and staphylococcus such as cephalosporins, clindamycin or a combination of amoxicillin and clavulanic acid should be administered.

Chronic osteomyelitis

Chronic osteomyelitis is usually due to inadequate treatment of the acute form. The patient presents with a limp that may be slight to completely avoiding bearing weight on the affected limb. There is usually muscular atrophy, as well as fistulae with purulent discharge (Fig. 33). A definitive diagnosis is made by X-ray where an increase in the periosteal reaction is observed that in very chronic cases acquires a characteristic appearance known as a "moiré" pattern.

Treatment must always be surgical in these patients. To clean the fracture site, strict aseptic techniques must be followed before debriding, eliminating any dead tissue along with any unnecessary external material without causing excessive damage to the soft tissues. The surgical field must be washed continuously during the entire process, using an isotonic saline solution. It must be taken into account that the volume of liquid used is more important than the type of solution used as the treatment is primarily based on the mechanical flushing action and dilution of the contaminated fluids. Some kind of antibiotic can also be added, but the amount should never exceed the amount that would be used intravenously. This is especially important in the case of using aminoglycosides, due to their cytotoxic potential.

Once cleaned, the stability of the fracture site should be assessed. If mobility is detected, and depending on its degree, another type of supplemental stabilisation can be used, for example, external fixators, or, if deemed necessary, the entire fixation system can be changed. Weakening of the anchor points of the osteosynthesis system frequently takes place due to the infection. For this reason, any fixation system that is not firmly attached should be removed (Fig. 34).

Likewise, all of the devitalised bone tissues, both bone sequestrum and devascularised edges of the fragments, should be eliminated. A transplant of cancellous bone can be performed which, on one hand, induces the formation of new bone, producing immobility of the fracture site faster, and on the other, favours early revascularisation of the fracture site, allowing for the organism's immune system to act more efficiently, and achieve a greater concentration of the antibiotics administered intravenously.

In the case of an active infection, the best bone stimulator is an autologous transplant of cancellous bone.

Perfect stability should have been achieved during the intervention, of both the components of the fixation system as well as that of all the bone fragments. The absence of movement is vital to cure the infectious process.

In the case of injuries with a high degree of contamination or if there is too much tension to suture, it is preferable that the incision be left open even if the implant and bone are left exposed. In these cases, the area should be covered with a moist bandage which should be changed once or twice every 24 hours. When the incision presents good granulation tissue, ideal for closure by second intention without contamination, performing some kind of skin flap may be considered.

Given that one of the primary causes of osteomyelitis is open fractures, a series of recommendations and care techniques to avoid them are described below.

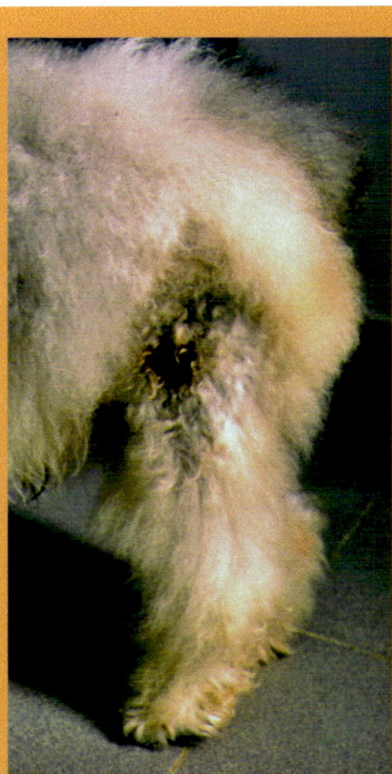

FIGURE 33. Fistula in the femoral region of a dog with chronic osteomyelitis.

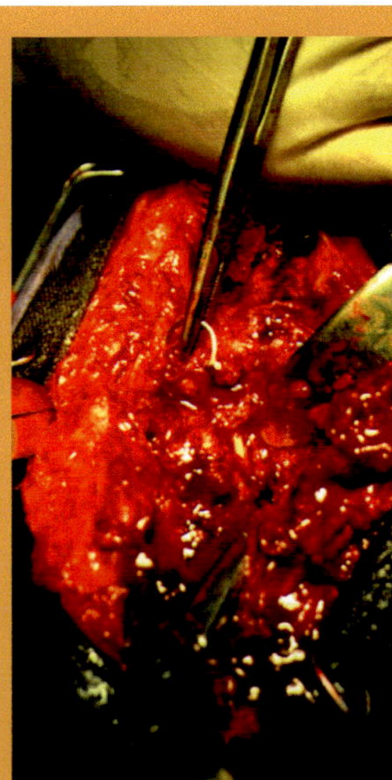

FIGURE 34. Removal of a cerclage wire from an infection site.

Treatment of the open fractures

As previously mentioned, achieving proper stability of the fracture site is primordial; otherwise, mobility together with an external supply of bacteria could cause osteomyelitis.

Treatment of open fractures depends on two factors: the grade of the open fracture and the time passed since the fracture occurred.

Grade I and certain grade II open fractures can be treated like a closed fracture. This is possible as long as more than six or eight hours have not passed since the fracture occurred. This period is called the "golden period", when bacterial colonisation has not yet taken place.

Aseptic preparation of the surgical field

The purpose of the initial treatment of open fractures is to avoid the prognosis from worsening. Therefore, when the animal arrives to the clinic, the clinician should proceed as follows: first, the injury should be carefully covered with sterile bandages and attempts should be made to temporarily stabilise the limb to avoid greater damage to the soft tissues as well as pain.

If the vital signs of the patient allow for it, the animal should be sedated or anaesthetised to be able to perform a more in-depth study of the injury as well as an X-ray study.

The limb should be prepared for the surgical intervention following strict aseptic techniques. First of all, the injury is debrided. In this step, all remnants of necrotic tissues, both soft as well as bone splinters that appear to be devascularised, should be removed. The entire process is performed while flushing with isotonic solution. As previously mentioned, the mechanical flushing action and dilution of the bacteria is essential. Once the fracture site is free of necrotic tissues, it is then stabilised.

To implement proper antibiotic treatment, as well as to prevent bone infection, the clinician should take a bacterial culture from the fracture site. Ideally, two samples should be taken, one before cleaning the fracture area, and one afterwards. Of the two samples, the second is usually more representative.

Foundation for correct stabilisation

The stability of the fracture site is the foundation to achieve fast ossification as well as to avoid greater damage to the soft tissues. It must be kept in mind that the fixation system to be used must allow for the care of the soft tissues in certain cases. The systems that are normally used are plates and external fixators.

The advantage of the plates is that they provide perfect stabilisation of the limb, and consequently, the animal can use it sooner. This way, the oedema is reduced and, thus, the proliferation of bacteria. However, the direct contact with the bone decreases the vascularisation of the fracture site with its respective alteration in the organic defences of this area.

In the case of infected fractures, the possibility of applying implants made of titanium should be assessed as certain experimental studies have shown that the bacterial load needed for a process of osteomyelitis to take place in fractures treated with implants of this material must be considerably greater than if they are made of surgical steel.

External fixators, on the contrary, do not interfere at all in the fracture site by holding the bone by its ends. They also allow for easy handling of the soft tissues (Fig. 35). Given that its application is fast, it is the ideal system in cases in which the patient is very weak.

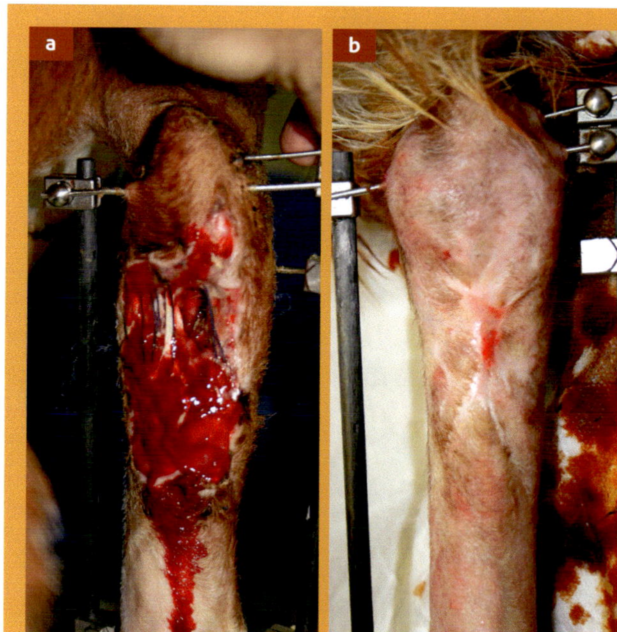

FIGURE 35. Open fracture site stabilised by external fixation (a). Progress of the previous case after seven weeks (b).

No other osteosynthesis systems should be used in open fractures. Intramedullary pins do not provide good stability and they favour the propagation of infection through the medullary cavity. Fixation using plaster is not adequate as the stability achieved is not optimal. Also, it has to be changed with relative frequency which implies a greater risk of infection, as well as the need to anaesthetise the animal several times.

Prevention of osteomyelitis

To avoid infection in the treatment of open fractures, the following measures should be applied:

Grade I and II fractures

- If less than eight hours have passed: treatment same as that for a closed fracture.
- Stabilisation with plates.
- If more than eight hours have passed: treat as a grade III open fracture.

Grade III fractures

- Stabilisation with plates. Perfect stabilisation must be achieved of all implants used to stabilise the fracture.
- Stabilisation through external fixation, if absolute immobilisation is not achieved with plates. If necessary, a second stabilisation system with a plate can be added as long as the risk of infection has disappeared.

Prolonged antibiotic treatment for at least four weeks should be administered in all cases.

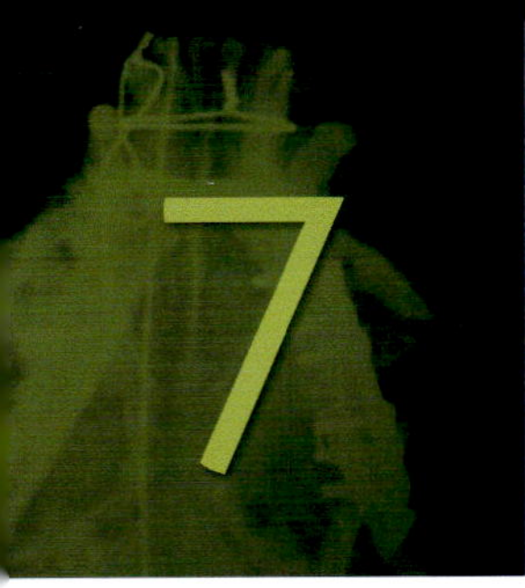

7 Head fractures

Fractures that affect the heads of pets are not excessively frequent. They can be divided into two large groups: those that affect the cranium, strictly speaking, and those that affect the jaw. The second type are more common.

CRANIAL FRACTURES

Cranial fractures are very rare in our patients and, similar to human medicine, when they occur, the consequences are usually fatal (Fig. 1).

If the patient survives, the general condition of the patient should first be stabilised to evaluate the possible damage at a central level. It is essential to attempt to decrease the intracranial pressure and control any haemorrhaging that could affect the brain mass. Fractures that affect the cranium are not usually surgical emergencies and thus, their treatment can be postponed until the patient is in suitable condition. Most of these fractures can be treated conservatively as the cranium is primarily formed by flat bones and the fragments are rarely subjected to loads or forces.

Flat bones present the advantage that they have a high healing capacity. This characteristic, together with the absence of forces that would cause displacement of fragments, are why surgery is only necessary if the fragments affect the brain mass or if haematomas must be eliminated.

To determine the exact scope of the lesion, a computerised tomography (CT) study is the best option. The information provided through said test not only analyses the real scope of the lesion, but also allows for the correct planning of surgical alternatives (Fig. 2).

In certain cases, fractures of the frontal bone need to be stabilised for two reasons: the first, because the communication between the nasal cavity and the sinuses allows for the passage of air during respiration which causes displacement of the fragments, impeding the fracture from healing; and second, because the air could pass through to the subcutaneous tissue, causing it to separate from the bone and form subcutaneous emphysema that at times cannot be resolved with conservative treatment.

Regarding the stabilisation systems used for fractures, it should be highlighted that the cortical bone of the frontal

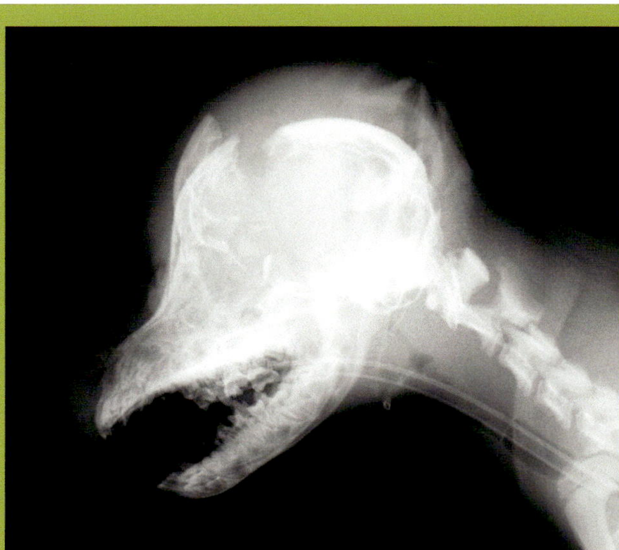

FIGURE 1. Avulsion of frontal bone from an animal bite.

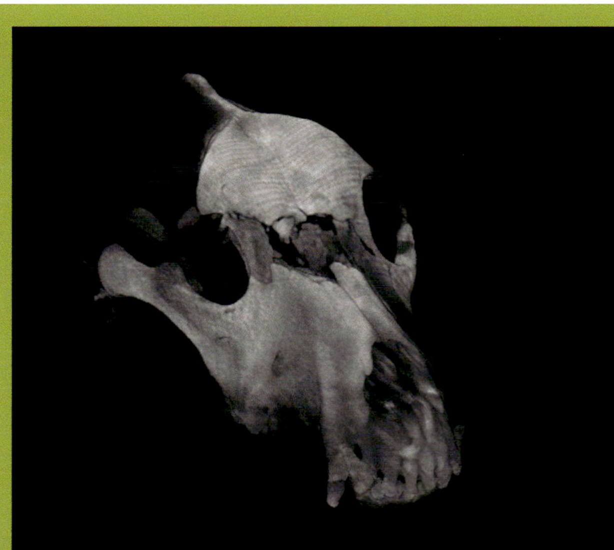

FIGURE 2. Cranial fracture from being run-over by a vehicle Three-dimensional reconstruction using CT.

and nasal bones is very thin and thus treatments using traditional implants do not always achieve adequate stability. For this reason, special implants that consist of very thin sheets of perforated metal can be used on the entire surface which can be easily moulded as needed (Fig. 3). As the forces that need to be neutralised are of little intensity, these implants provide sufficient resistance. On the other hand, as the screws can be placed anywhere, the larger fragments can be stabilised regardless of their distribution.

Once the fracture is reduced, the metal sheet is cut into the needed size and shape (the fragment must be big enough to cover all of the healthy edges of the bone, Fig. 4). Next, the fragments are fixed in their position using screws and, finally, the implant is anchored to the edges of the fracture (Fig. 5).

These implants are manufactured in titanium which favours their osseointegration, facilitating the intramembranous ossification inherent to flat bones (Fig. 6).

FRACTURES OF THE ZYGOMATIC ARCH

Among cranial fractures, the most frequent is probably those affecting the zygomatic arch (Fig. 7). Almost always, conservative treatment can be implemented for this type of fracture, however, surgical treatment is recommended if the eyeball is affected. Also, given that this arch gives the shape and expressiveness to the cranium, surgical treatment is often implemented for aesthetic reasons.

If the eyeball is affected, surgical treatment is recommended for fractures of the zygomatic arch.

The X-ray diagnosis is simple by means of an X-ray of the dorsoventral view of the head.

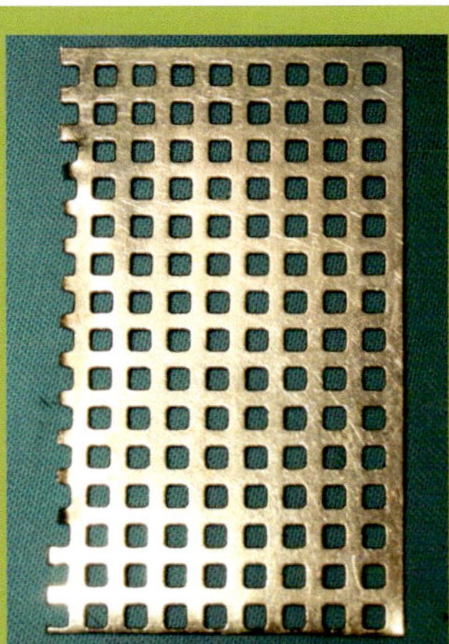

FIGURE 3. Cuttable plate.

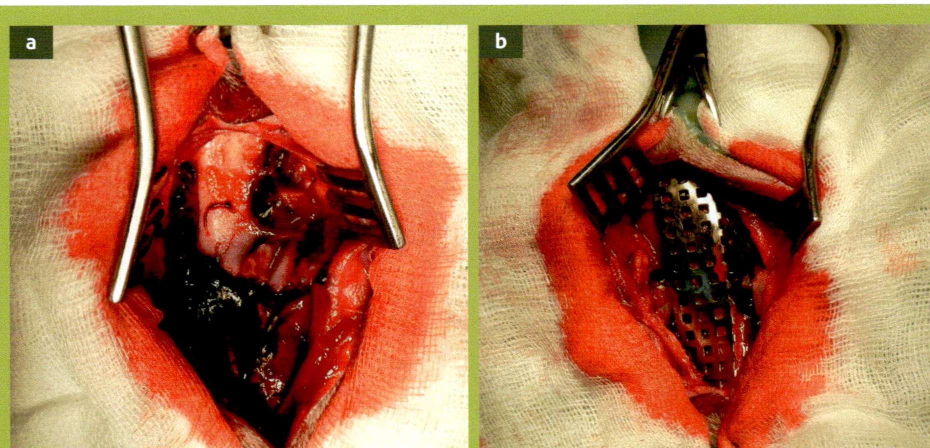

FIGURE 4. Cranial fracture. The loose fragments (a) and the osteosynthesis plate that has been moulded and placed (b) are visible.

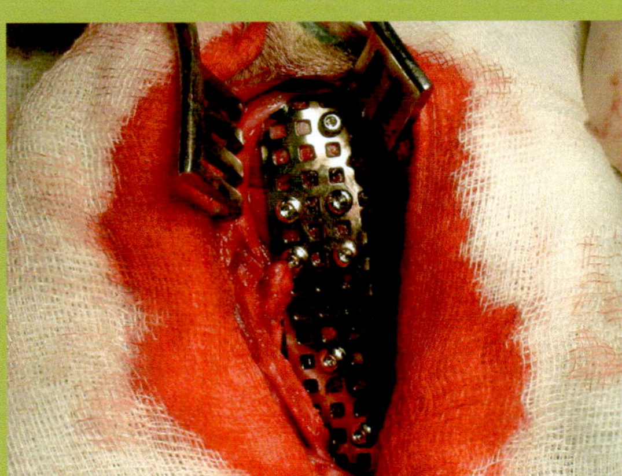

FIGURE 5. Anterior fracture, with the screws placed lifting the fragments.

FIGURE 6. Three-dimensional reconstruction using CT. Note the osteosynthesis plate 2 years after surgery.

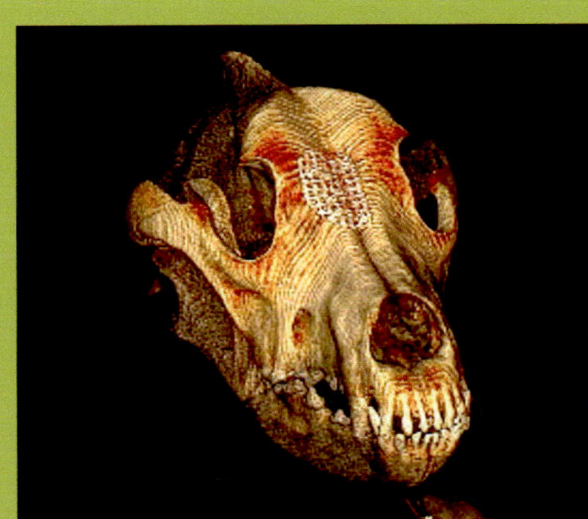

Similarly, surgical treatment presents no complications and the prognosis is excellent. Once the approach is performed and the fracture is reduced, stabilisation is simple by applying an osteosynthesis plate (Fig. 8).

FRACTURES OF THE JAW

Without doubt, these are the most frequent within the group of fractures that affect the head.

The X-ray diagnosis of jaw fractures can be complicated due to the overlapping of bone structures (similar to cranial fractures). X-rays must be made of specific positions of the head. The oblique view is one of the most useful, keeping the mouth open and inserting a separator between the two canine teeth, that ideally is radiolucent; this prevents the overlapping of the jaw branches that is observed in the lateral view (Fig. 9).

In highly rostral fractures, occlusal X-rays are also recommended. A corner of the chassis should be inserted into the mouth, so that when taking the X-ray, the mandibular bone does not overlap the maxillary bone. The disadvantage of this technique is that due to the thickness of the chassis, it cannot be inserted as much as needed (Fig. 10). Only the most rostral portion can be assessed if special odontological films are used which are prepared in envelopes that act as a chassis. In other cases, without doubt, a CT scan is the test that provides the most information.

Regarding the application of one osteosynthesis system or another, almost all can be used as long as they comply with two fundamental premises: achieving correct occlusion of the dental pieces (Fig. 11) and not damaging the tooth roots.

In the case of simple fractures of only one branch, when reducing the fracture lines, it is easy to align the dental pieces. However, when dealing with multiple fractures, as

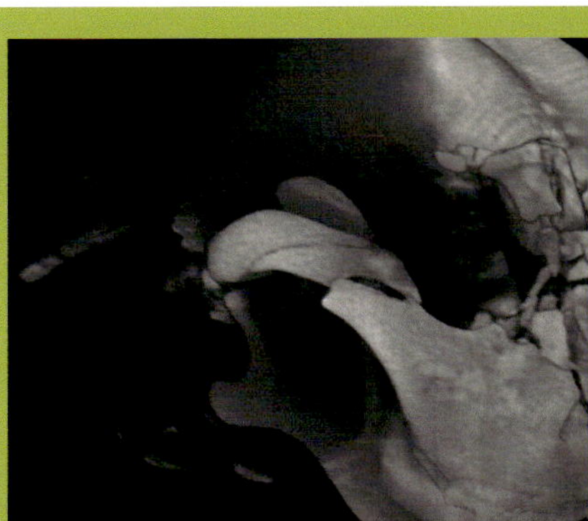

FIGURE 7. Three-dimensional reconstruction using CT that shows a fracture of the zygomatic arch.

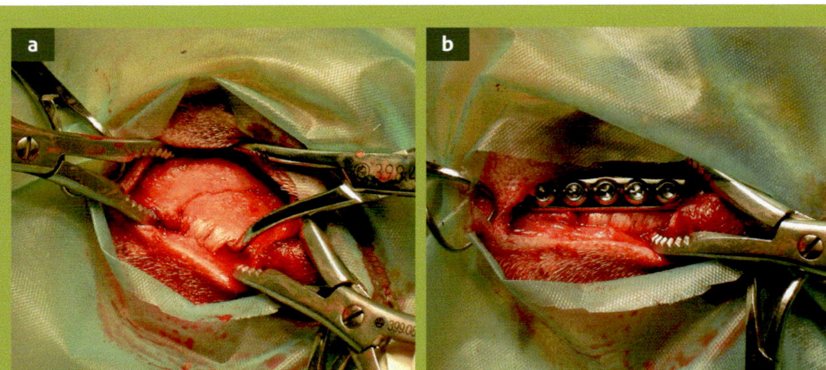

FIGURE 8. Stabilisation of a fracture of the zygomatic arch. Reduction of the fracture (a) and placement of the osteosynthesis plate (b).

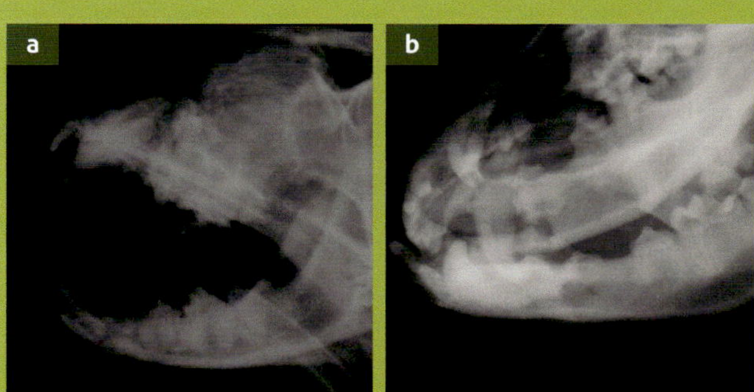

FIGURE 9. X-ray of a jaw fracture. Note how in the latero-lateral view (a) the branches of the mandible overlap making it hard to see the fracture. In the oblique view, the cortical bone of both branches is visible (b).

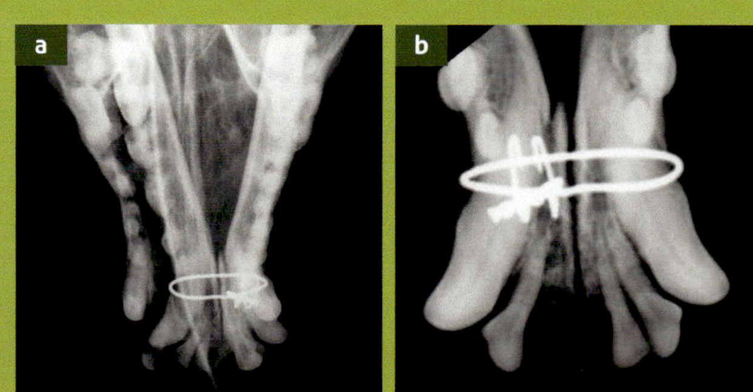

FIGURE 10. Comparison between a standard X-ray (a) and an occlusal X-ray after the intervention (b). Note how the visibility of the structures is better in the occlusal X-ray.

reduction is more difficult, any rotation of a fragment may make it impossible for the patient to close its mouth correctly; consequently, chewing becomes difficult and the purpose of the surgery will have failed.

The respiratory tract must be kept permeable during surgical interventions through the use of tracheal tubes. Complete occlusion will thus be impossible and the success of the intervention cannot be evaluated until it is finished. If the surgeon is not sure of being able to correctly reduce the fracture, it is preferable that the patient is intubated using a pharyngostoma. This way, the mouth can be closed completely and the occlusion can be evaluated with greater precision.

To perform the pharyngostomy, once the patient is anaesthetised, an incision is made in a spot identified by inserting a finger under the tongue of the patient to locate the point where the soft tissues are thinner. The incision is made to the oral cavity where the end of the tracheal tube will stick out to be connected with the anaesthetic circuit (Fig. 12). Once the intervention is done, the tube can be removed and only the skin needs to be sutured.

In some cases where the stability of the osteosynthesis systems is not ideal, it may be helpful to feed the patient through a feeding tube for a few days; in this case, the incision of the pharyngostoma can be used to insert the gastric feeding tube (Fig. 13).

In the case of simple fractures, a correct reduction of the fracture guarantees perfect occlusion without having to perform a pharyngostomy.

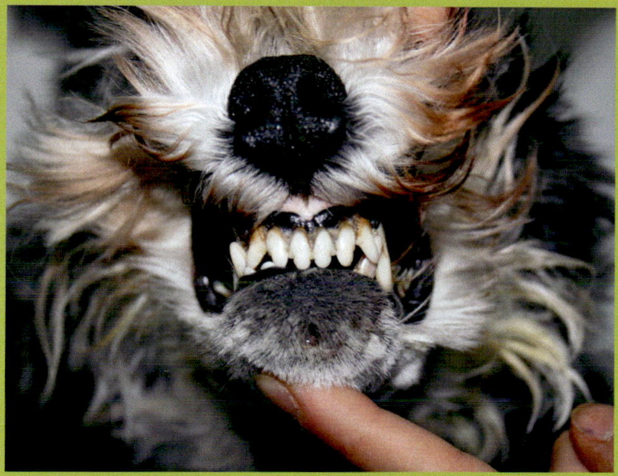

FIGURE 11. Note a slight lateralisation of the jaw with adequate occlusion after removal of the osteosynthesis material in a jaw fracture.

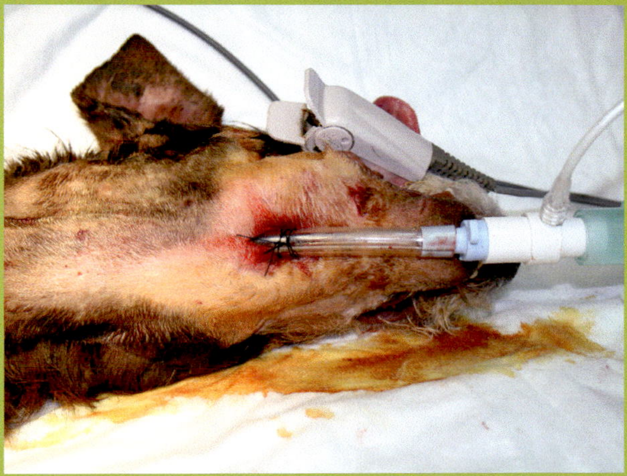

FIGURE 12. Tracheal tube introduced through a pharyngostoma.

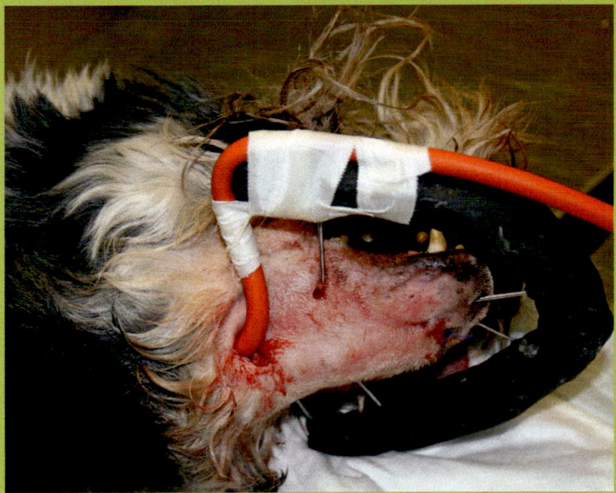

FIGURE 13. Feeding tube introduced through a pharyngostoma.

The most used fixation systems for these kinds of fractures are described below.

External fixation

This is most likely the most used osteosynthesis system for jaw fractures thanks to its versatility and easy application. However, it does present disadvantages: it can be cumbersome and in some cases it requires extensive cleaning.

The simplest surgical technique basically consists of applying at least two pins with a threaded tip in each fragment. Care should be taken not to damage the tooth roots. They are much harder than those of the bone and thus it should be easy to notice when the pin does not enter easily. At that moment, the direction of insertion should be altered. The pins should be inserted in such a way that the parts that stand out are on one single plane. Substituting a connective rod with methyl methacrylate may be useful in fractures of this bone as the pins are inserted without prior reduction of the fracture and are thus not aligned in one single plane, which makes their stabilisation using clamps and connecting rods difficult (Fig. 14). Methyl methacrylate can be adapted to the projection of each pin.

Acrylic cements (page 69) can be injected through a tube (Fig. 15) or the pins can be bent and it can be applied like modelling clay.

Once the percutaneous pins are inserted, a simple system that guarantees correct occlusion is to close the patient's mouth completely and keep the pieces fitting together when the cement is applied, allowing it to dry in this position (Fig. 16).

Cerclages

A cerclage wire can be of great use in the treatment of jaw fractures, used alone or with other systems.

This system basically consists of introducing a surgical wire between the dental pieces and stabilising the fracture through them. Although it is somewhat unstable, it presents the advantage that as it is fixated to the dental pieces, it is located on the tension-bearing face of the mandibular and maxillary bones. When the patient bites down, the load is reoriented towards the opposite cortical surface of the dental pieces.

The fastening of the wire depends on its location: the area of the incisors, or of the molars and premolars. The best option is to introduce the cerclage between the roots to obtain better fixation. Logically, in the case of the incisors, this is not possible, and the wire will have to pass between them and in front of the canine teeth (Fig. 17). Everything depends on the location of the fracture. The surgeon must create a kind of net that stabilises the movement of the fragments, especially when biting down or chewing (Fig. 18).

First of all, to introduce the wire between the roots, a perforation is made with a fine drill bit or with a Kirschner pin in the appropriate point (Fig. 19) that is determined by X-ray. Later, the wire is introduced and the same is done in a piece on the other side of the fracture line. Finally, with the fracture reduced, the wire is tightened taking care to not tighten it too much (Fig. 20), as excessive tension would cause the fracture line to separate in the bone area.

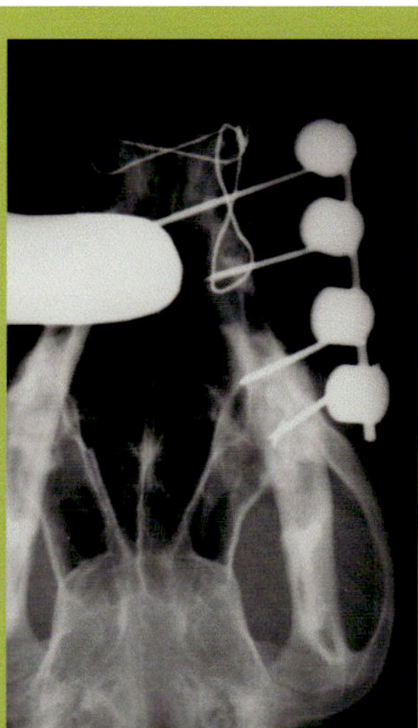

FIGURE 14. External partial fixation system associated with cerclages. The percutaneous pins should be placed on one single plane to be able to stabilise them using clamps and connecting rods.

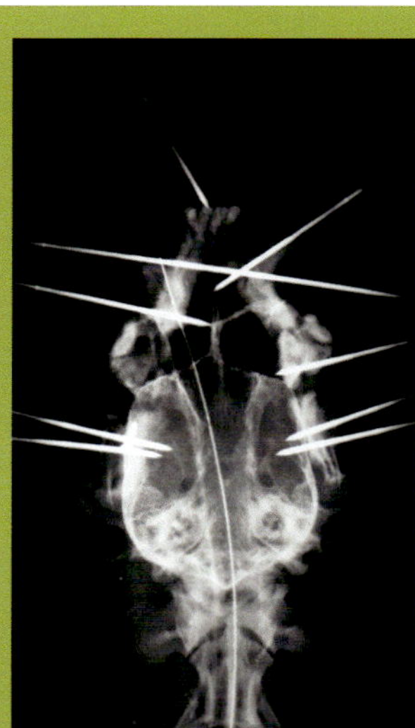

FIGURE 15. X-ray of a fracture of both mandibular branches, stabilised using an external fixator with methyl methacrylate injected through a tube. This system allows for the use of a combination of percutaneous pins with different diameters.

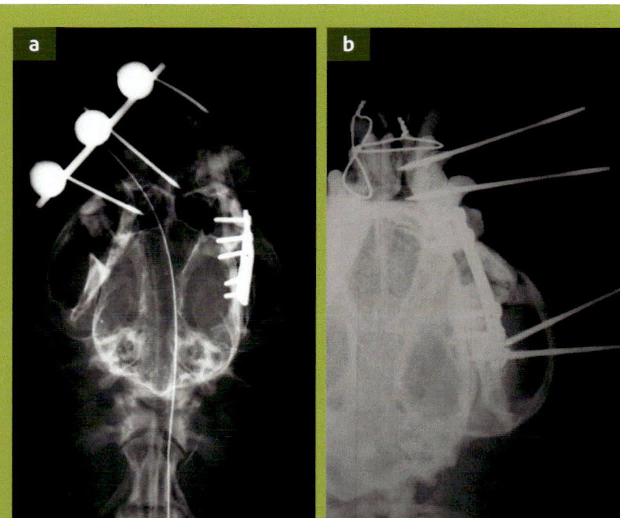

FIGURE 16. Combination of osteosynthesis using a plate reinforced with partial external fixation by means of clamps and a connecting rod (a) and with acrylic cement (b).

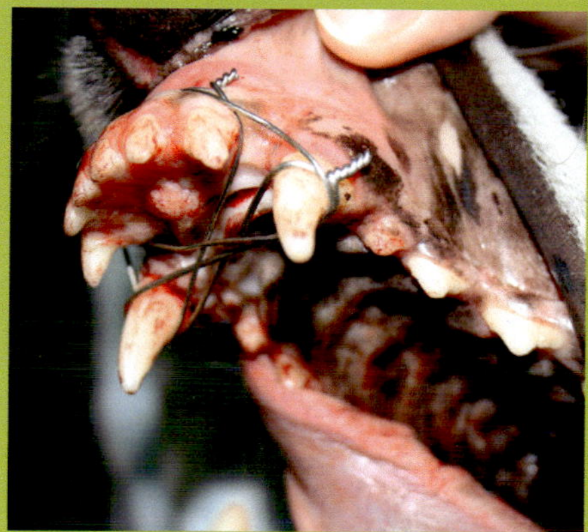

FIGURE 17. Fracture in which the incisors have been torn out. The cerclage cannot be passed between the dental roots.

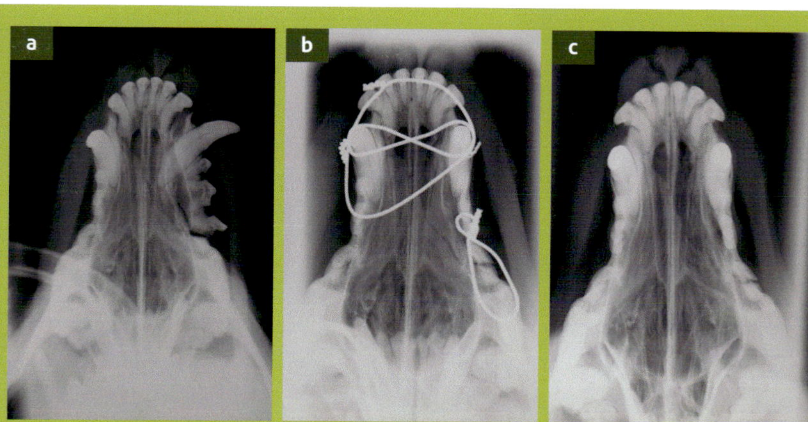

FIGURE 18. Avulsion of a maxillary fragment that has been treated with cerclages, of which some could be anchored between the roots. Sequence of X-rays in which the fracture (a), its stabilisation with cerclage wires (b) and the final result (c) can be observed.

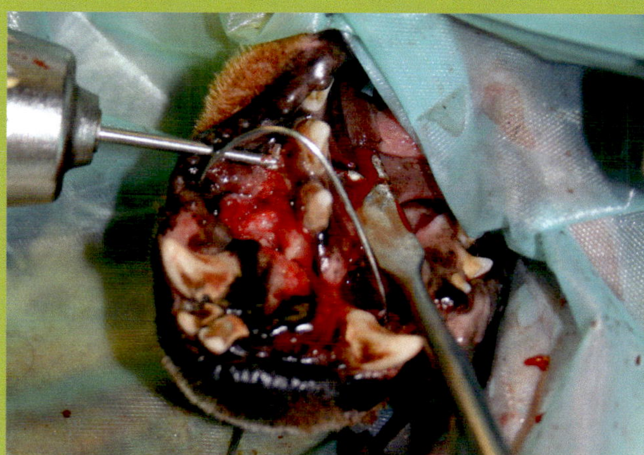

FIGURE 19. Perforation of a hole in each branch of the jaw with a drill bit or a Kirschner pin. The holes are located between the dental roots.

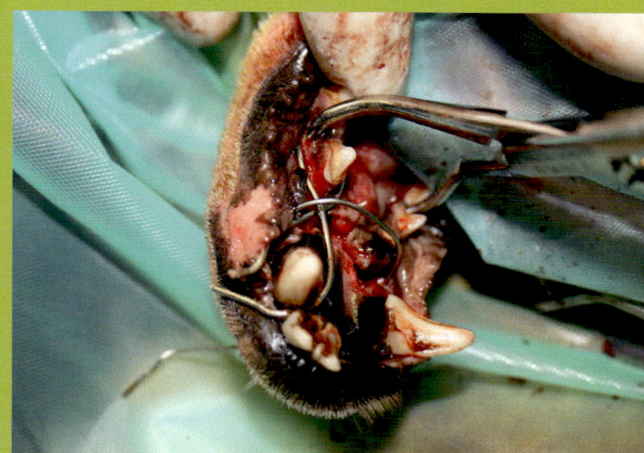

FIGURE 20. The fracture has been reduced and a cerclage has been placed that is shown without tightening.

Fracture of the mandibular symphysis

Fractures of the mandibular symphysis are peculiar as they are not technically fractures, but treated as such. This "fracture" is typical in cats when they jump from great heights. The diagnosis is simple as is treatment, which consists of placing a cerclage around the most rostral area of the mandibular branches, immediately behind the canine teeth.

Once the patient is anaesthetised, all of the remnants of soft tissues are removed from the edges of the symphysis, using a periosteotome to scrape them away (Fig. 21). Next, the fracture is reduced and stabilised using twin point reduction forceps. Special precaution should be taken to place the points in the lower part of the branch as if they were applied close to the canines or, if tightened too much, they would pull the tips of the canines too close together due to their anatomical position (slightly divergent from each other). By closing the patient's mouth, it should be confirmed that they are in the correct position, otherwise they would come in contact with the palate and impede chewing.

When the fracture has been correctly reduced, an incision is made in the chin and two pins (calibre 18 G) are introduced through said incision, sliding along the external cortical surface of both branches until exiting into the oral cavity (Fig. 22). These pins serve as guides for the wire. Each end of the wire is inserted by the tip of each one of the pins and pulled out through the incision in the chin. To remove the pins, they can be pulled out (Fig. 23). The last step is to tighten the cerclage enough to impede movements of the fracture site without pulling the tips of the canine teeth together (Fig. 24). The knot of the wire is adapted to the jaw and the skin is sutured (Fig. 25).

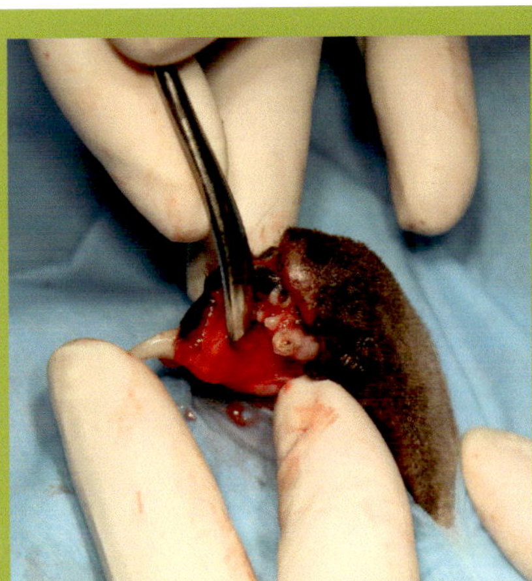

FIGURE 21. Scraping of the mandibular symphysis to remove remnants of soft tissues.

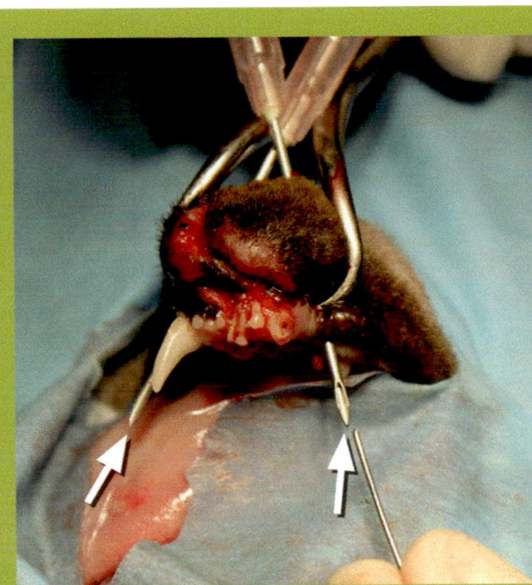

FIGURE 22. Insertion of two pins that serve as guides to introduce the cerclage.

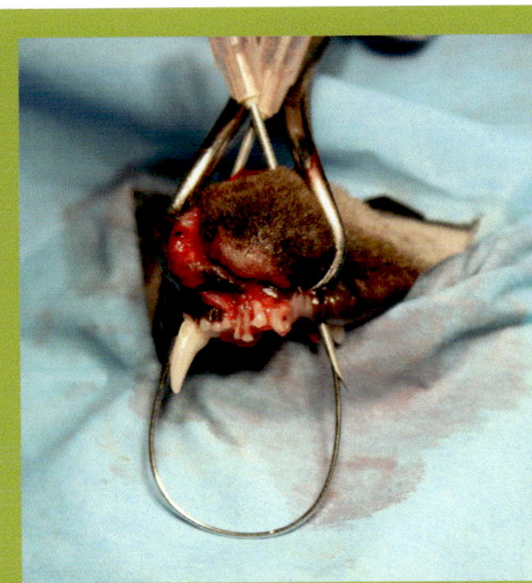

FIGURE 23. Introduction of the cerclage through the holes. Once the wire has been inserted and pulled out through the incision in the chin, pins are removed using traction.

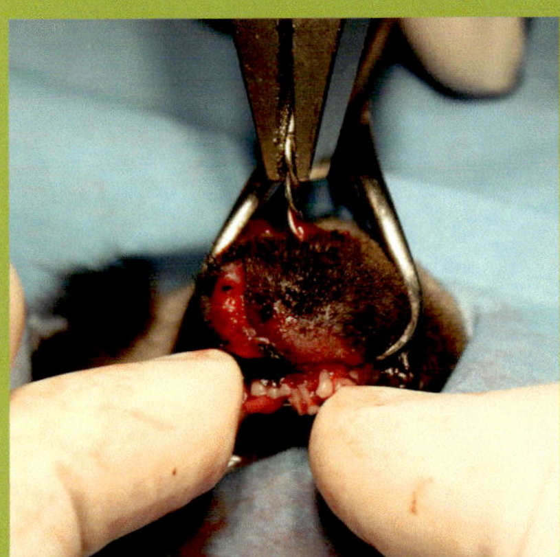

FIGURE 24. Tightening of cerclage.

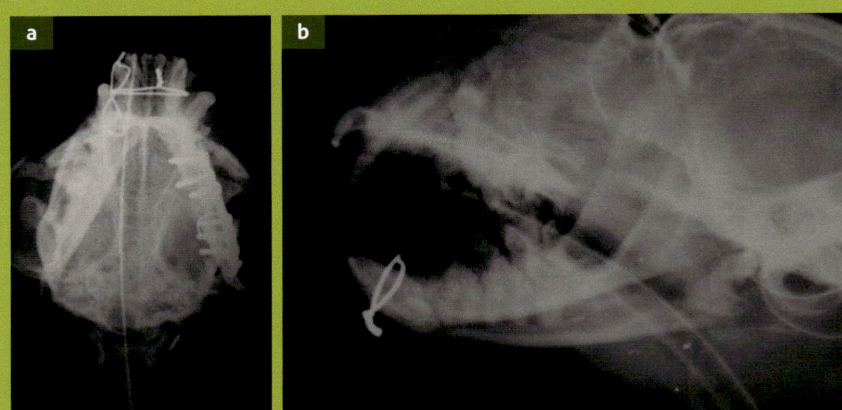

FIGURE 25. Postoperative X-rays showing the placement of the cerclage. Dorsoventral (a) and latero-lateral view (b).

This cerclage is removed after at least one month as passed since the surgery to avoid the accumulation of food on the lingual side of the teeth.

Plates

Osteosynthesis plates are also a suitable system to treat jaw fractures.

The foundation for their use is the same as that for fractures of other bones although there are certain differences that must be kept in mind. First, the plate is located on an angle regarding the direction of the forces that the jaw is subjected to when chewing (forces of pressure when contact is made with the maxillary bone). Therefore, said forces work to separate the fragments from where the dental pieces are located. This allows for the use of plates smaller than those that would hypothetically correspond with the bone's size (Fig. 26).

Due to the fact that the structure is formed by two branches, the lateral displacement forces are scarce, especially when the fractures affect only one branch. This great stability against the lateral displacements favours, if necessary, the correct fixation using only two screws in each primary fragment.

> *Although the effectiveness of the implant would be greater if it were placed close to the dental pieces, this is not feasible due to the fact that the possibility of damaging the root is greater closer to the gums.*

Treatment with plates consists of first reducing the fracture and then applying the plate that is considered most suitable depending on the type of fracture. In the case of fractures that affect the vertical branch, special implants can be used that adapt to the thinness of the cortical bone and the lack of space (Fig. 27). To place the plates, two approaches can be used: making an incision in the skin, just above the edge of the mandibular branch (Fig. 28), or separating and lifting the gums from the jaw (Fig. 29).

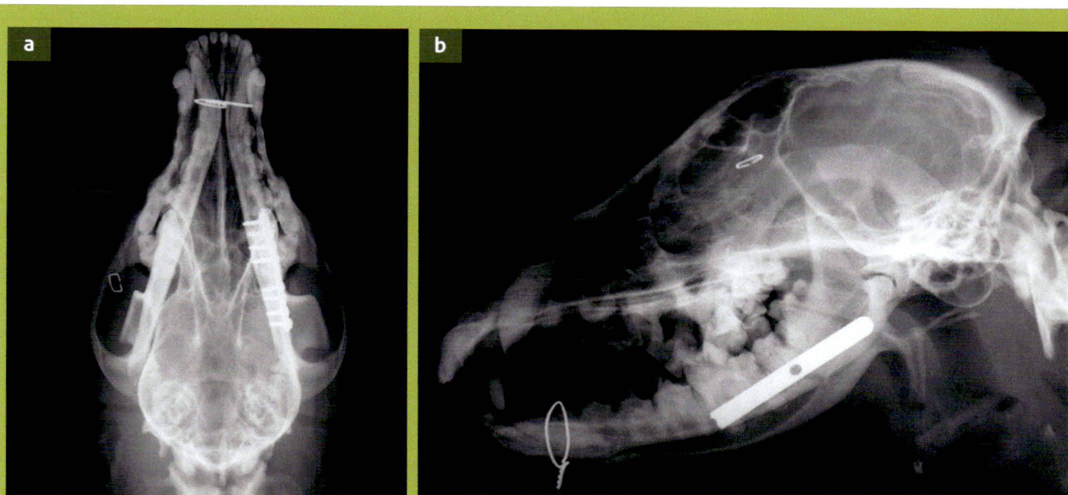

FIGURE 26. Fracture of a mandibular branch stabilised using a plate. Dorsoventral (a) and latero-lateral view (b).

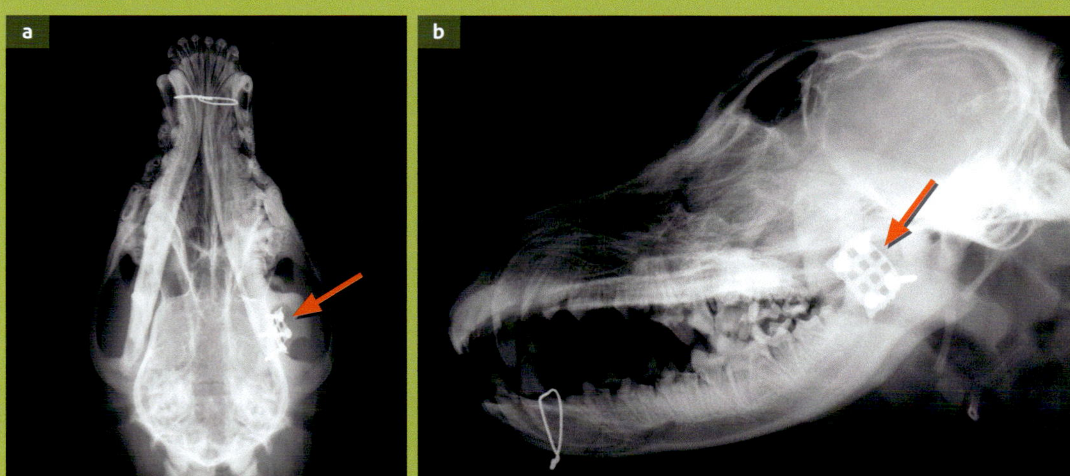

FIGURE 27. Fracture of the vertical mandibular branch treated with a fragment of cuttable plate (arrows). Dorsoventral (a) and latero-lateral view (b).

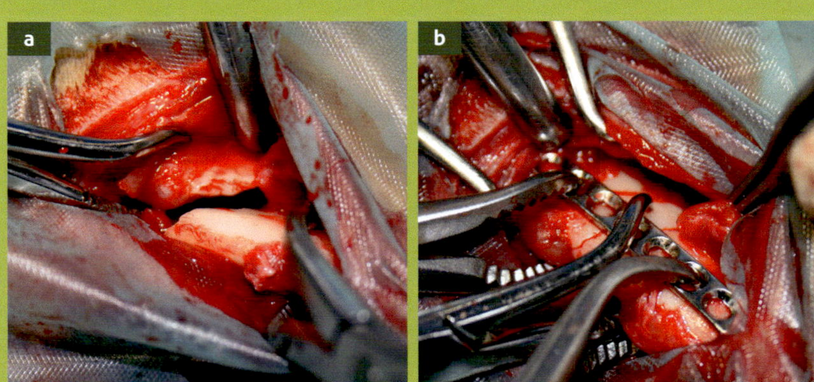

FIGURE 28. Treatment of a jaw fracture with a plate. Treatment approach of the jaw through the skin (a) and reduction of the fracture before inserting the screws (b).

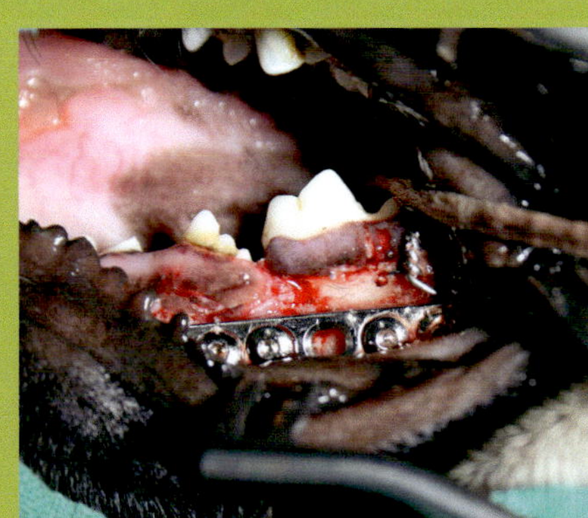

FIGURE 29. Approach used to treat fracture through the gums and stabilisation by means of a plate.

8 Forelimb fractures

SCAPULAR FRACTURES

Scapular fractures are infrequent in pets. This is due to the anatomical conformation and the type of strain that this body part receives. On one hand, as the scapula is not rigidly attached to the thorax, it can float and absorb any impact received, and on the other, it is completely surrounded by a fair amount of muscle mass (supra- and infraspinatus on each side of the scapular spine, and subscapularis and serratus on its medial surface). Said musculature limits the movements of fragments (in the case of fractures) and provides significant vascular support. This, together with its large amount of the spongy tissue, inherent to flat bones, allows for the scapula to have a great healing capacity. In patients with scapular fractures, a thorough general examination must be performed (more thorough than normal) as its anatomical location cushions any blows or trauma, meaning that it must receive a relatively intense impact to fracture. Concomitant wound injuries are frequent, as well as possible rib fractures. An in-depth examination of the peripheral nervous system should also be performed due to the proximity with the brachial plexus which is frequently injured.

Scapular fractures can affect the body, spine, neck and glenoid cavity. Patients with scapular fractures present with a limp that may be from slight to very obvious. In the cases of fractures of the body of the scapula, and especially when the fracture is longitudinal, the limp may be less pronounced as little displacement of the fragments takes place when the extremity is used (this is why these fractures usually respond well to conservative treatment). Fractures that affect the glenoid cavity and the neck, however, are manifested with a pronounced limp due to the great displacement and pain produced by bearing weight on the wounded extremity.

Scapular fractures are diagnosed by means of a two-projection radiography examination. Often, the lateral view does not provide enough information given that there is an overlapping of radio-opaque structures that may mask the lesion (Fig. 2). Therefore, if the fracture is distal, performing a medio-lateral oblique view, is recommended (Fig. 3). The caudo-cranial view is performed under anaesthesia, placing the patient in a supine position and tractioning the affected limb towards the head (this way, the bone does not overlap other structures, Fig. 4). However, this view does not provide enough information regarding the lesions that may have been produced in the body. Performing a computerised tomography (CT) could therefore be a good option.

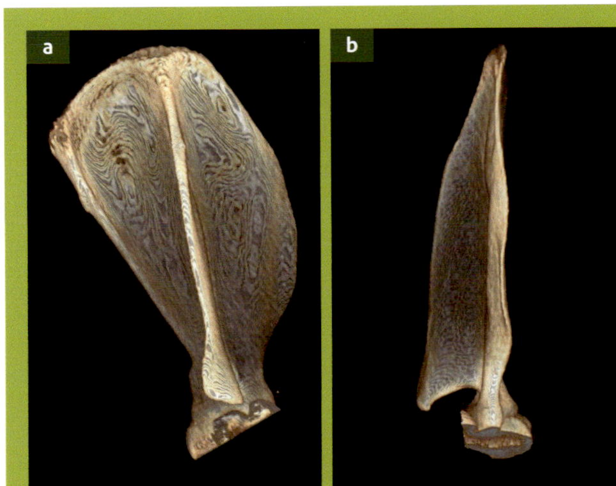

FIGURE 1. Three dimensional reconstruction of the scapula using CT.

Treatment of the most frequent fractures

Treatment of scapular fractures varies significantly depending on where they are located as well as the age of the patient. Usually, plates, pins and cerclages are used.

Body and spine fractures

Fractures of the body of the scapula can be treated with surgery or conservative treatment. Logically, the decision between the two depends on the surgeons criteria, however, the following factors should be taken into account:

The approach is simple as the surgeon only has to press on both sides of the spine and remove the insertion of the cervical portion of the trapezius muscle and the insertion of the infraspinatus muscle, to later separate the supra- and infraspinatus muscles to reach nearly the entire blade (Fig. 5).

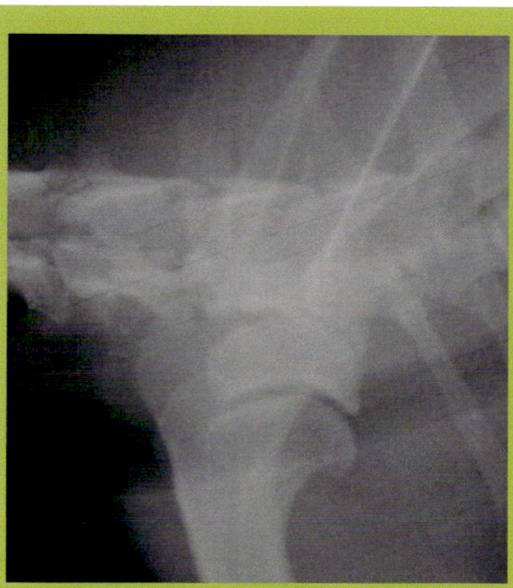

FIGURE 2. Latero-lateral X-ray with scapula fracture (difficult to visualise).

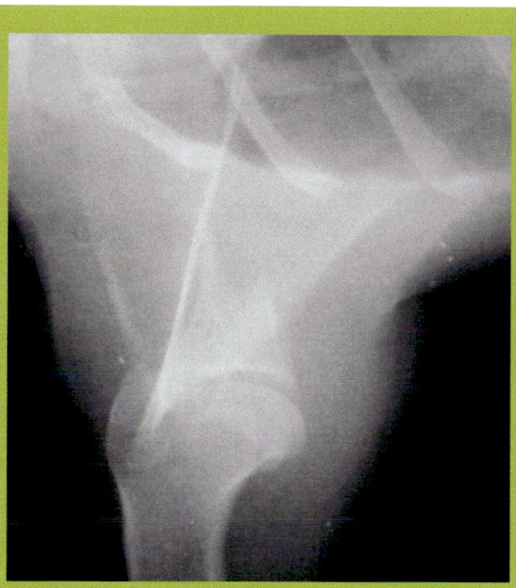

FIGURE 3. Medio-lateral oblique X-ray of the previous case.

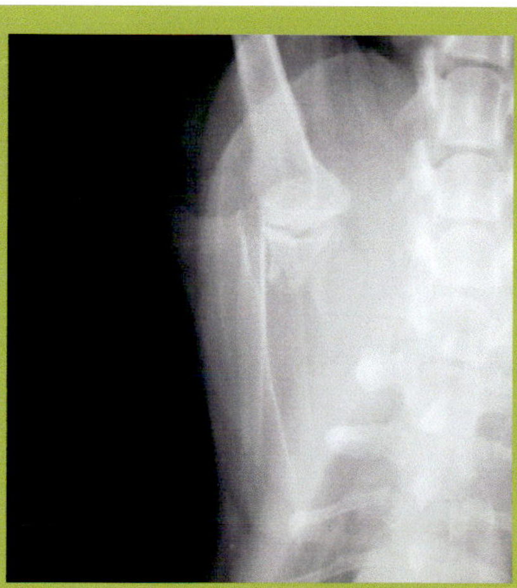

FIGURE 4. Caudo-cranial X-ray fracture of the neck of the scapula.

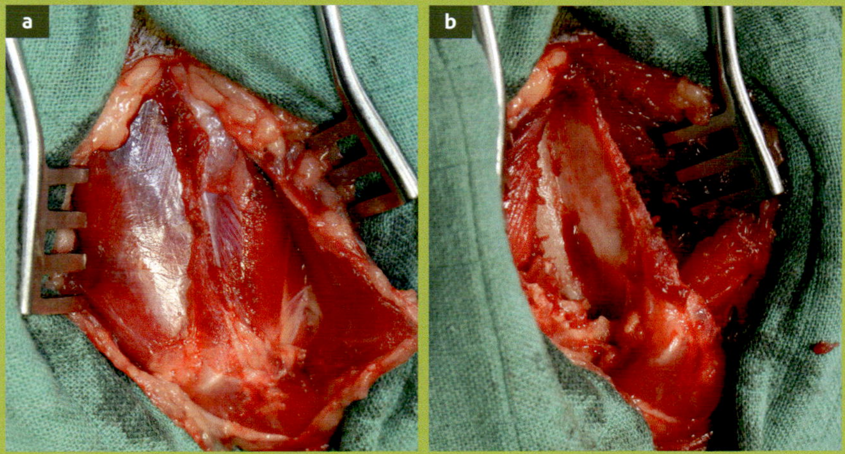

FIGURE 5. Scapular spine approach. Apply pressure on both sides of the spine (a) and separate the supra- and infraspinatus muscles (b).

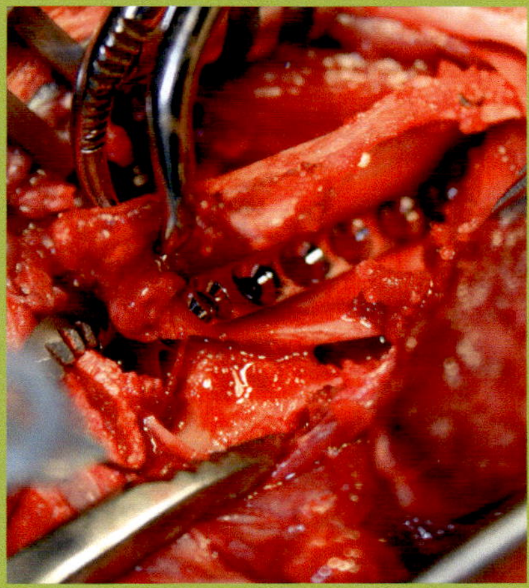

FIGURE 6. The plate is placed in the transition area between the body and the spin, to point the screws towards the origin of the spine.

The most important factor when selecting treatment is probably the direction of the fracture. As previously mentioned, when dealing with longitudinal fractures, the displacement of fragments when bearing weight on the limb, is much less than that of transversal fractures.

Another problem associated with fractures of the body of the scapula is its reduced thickness as well as its small amount of compact bone. Screws easily loosen due to these characteristics. The best way to achieve optimal screw fastening is to place the plate in the transition area between the body and the spine, with the screws in an oblique position. A triangle of thicker bone is created in this area where the anchors are more resistant (Fig. 6).

In certain cases, the fractures that affect the bone lamina can be stabilised using wires. The system consists of passing the wire through a perforation made on each side of the fracture line, that acts as a suture point. This way, the fragments will not be separated while the alignment is maintained thanks to the muscles. This system should primarily be used for longitudinal fractures or partial detachments of the spine.

Regarding transversal fractures, these should be treated using plate osteosynthesis (Fig. 7). If this is not done, it is likely that the extremity will recover its function with time, however, the deformity of the scapula is frequently visible, especially in patients with short hair.

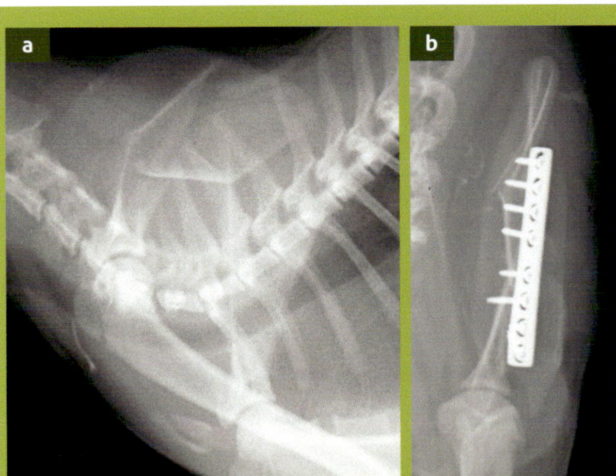

FIGURE 7. Transversal fracture with folding (a). X-ray of the treated fracture using a plate anchored to the base of the spine (b).

Neck fractures

Neck fractures are the most frequent, taking into account that this bone is rarely injured. The signs and symptoms are obvious given that a complete weight-bearing disability is produced as this area is responsible for transferring the weight supported by the humerus towards the body of the animal.

A diagnosis is easily made through a radiology examination, and it is primarily visible in the caudo-cranial view.

Treatment must be surgical in all cases as this is a weight-bearing transition area. Generally, stabilisation is based on the application of plates as the principal problem is the short length of the distal fragment. The use of T or L plates is frequent in this type of fracture to allow for the placement of the greatest number of screws possible, in a distal position from the fracture.

The approach is the same as that previously described, however, to access the area of the fracture, part of the acromion of the deltoid muscle must be lifted. To do so, an osteotomy of the acromion must be performed which will enable the lifting of the muscle by displacing the bone portion where it inserts. To guide the osteotome, it may be useful to place a curved haemostat clamp underneath the deltoid muscle (Fig. 8). Next, the suprascapular nerve is located, which is found above the neck, to avoid damaging it while manipulating the fragments, and lastly, the fracture is reduced.

In certain complicated cases, or when the fracture is located in the caudal portion of the glenoid cavity, it may be necessary to perform a tenotomy of the infraspinatus muscle, and even the teres minor muscle, to increase the space for manipulation (Fig. 9).

Once the fracture has been reduced, it is then stabilised using osteosynthetic plates that can be attached to the spine of the scapula. In order to increase stability, two plates can be used, one placed on each side of the spine, so that the distal fragment can be set in place with a greater number of screws (Fig. 10). Frequently, and with this same objective, L-shaped plates can be used, placing the short end towards the spine (Figs. 11 and 12).

The plates used do not need to be excessively thick as the forces that they are meant to neutralise act mostly in the direction of the wide plane of the plate.

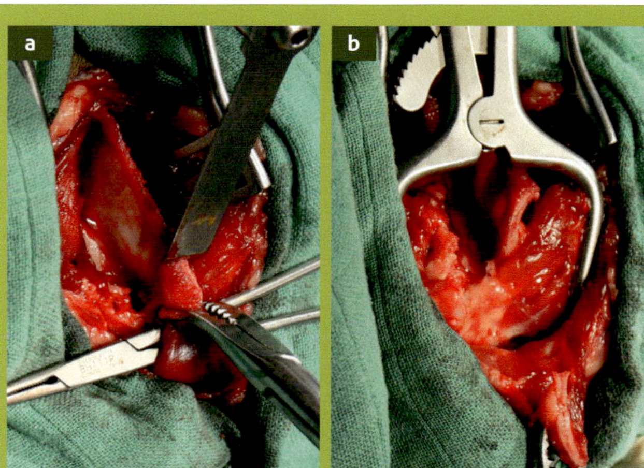

FIGURE 8. Osteotomy of the acromion. A clamp is placed under the deltoid muscle to guide the osteotome (a). Performing the osteotomy (b).

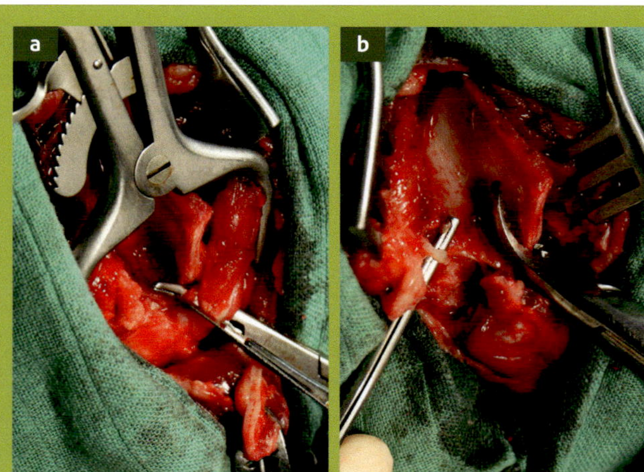

FIGURE 9. Tenotomy of the infraspinatus muscle (a). Detailed view of the suprascapular nerve (b).

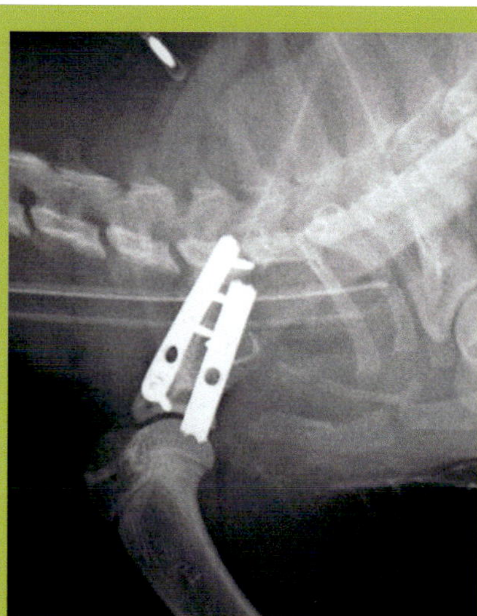

FIGURE 10. Straight plates on both sides of the spin in a neck fracture.

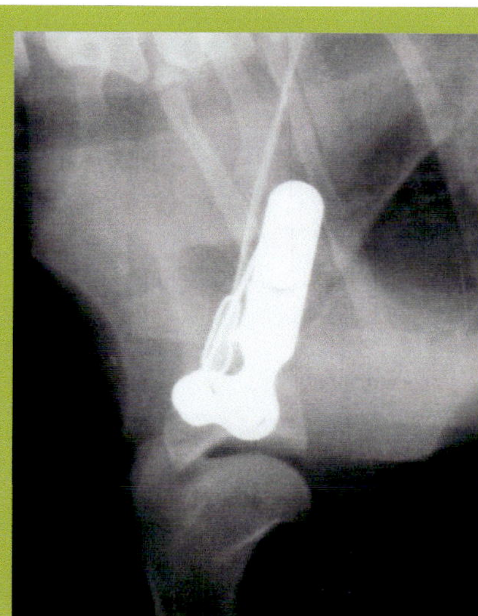

FIGURE 11. L plate in a caudal direction from the spine.

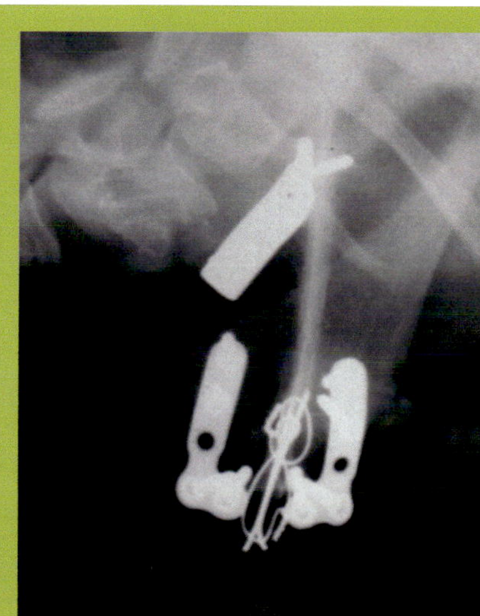

FIGURE 12. L plates on both sides of the spine.

Care should be taken regarding the direction of the screws of the distal fragment as the screw can be erroneously introduced into the joint due to the fact that the glenoid cavity is dome-shaped.

Once the surgery is completed, the osteotomy of the acromion is stabilised. Pins should be inserted with tension bands as this fragment will suffer traction forces. Due to the shape of the acromion and the thinness of the crest, it may be helpful to initially introduce the pins in a retrograde manner, to confirm whether they have been inserted into the proximal fragment or not. Lastly, after the fracture has been reduced, a proximal perforation is made to the incision and the wire is set in place that will act as a tension band (Fig. 13).

Fractures of the glenoid cavity

Fortunately, these fractures are not frequent due to the fact that in cases of trauma, the blows are concentrated in the neck portion. Treatment is based on the principles of joint fractures: emergency surgery, proper reduction and becoming active as soon as possible after surgery.

The approach is similar to that used with fractures of the neck and is normally associated with a tenotomy of the infraspinatus and teres minor muscles to facilitate access to the caudal area of the cavity.

Once the fracture is reduced, and if the size of the fragments allows for it, it should be stabilised, if possible, using compression screws. In other cases, when the fragments are

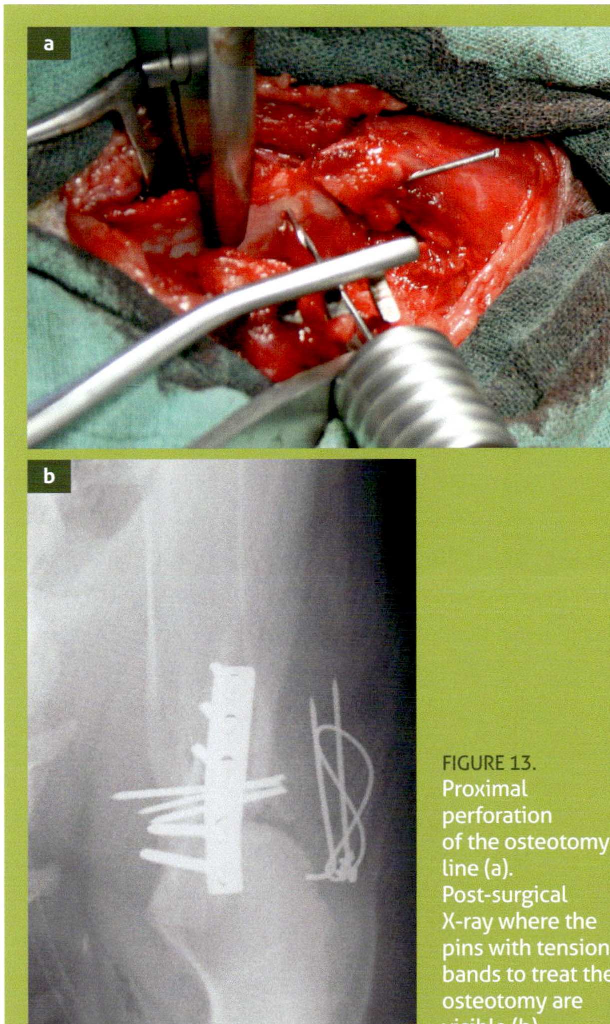

FIGURE 13. Proximal perforation of the osteotomy line (a). Post-surgical X-ray where the pins with tension bands to treat the osteotomy are visible (b).

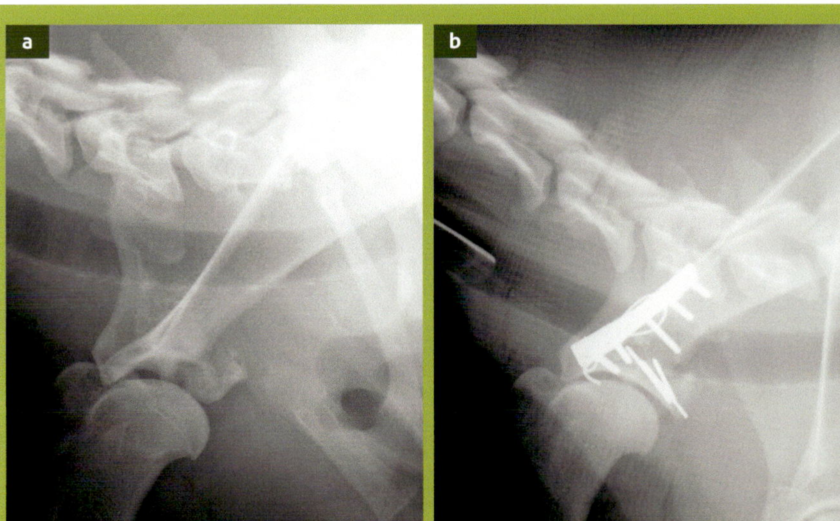

FIGURE 14. Fracture of the neck and glenoid cavity (a). X-ray in which the treatment applied is visible (plates and pins) (b).

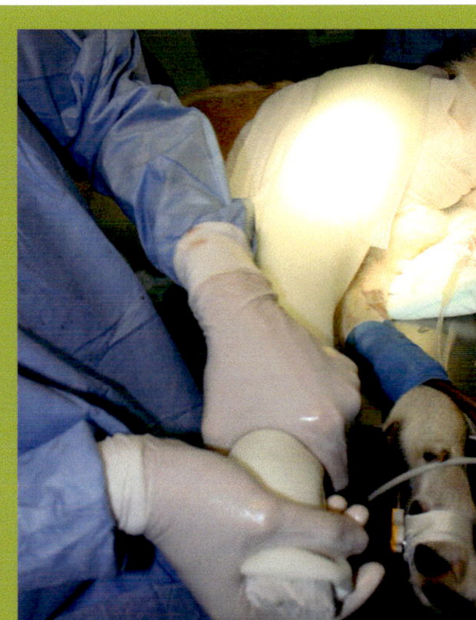

FIGURE 15. Spica cast made with fibreglass.

too small, they must be stabilised using Kirschner pins as there is no other option (Fig. 14).

In most fractures that affect the articular surface, temporary stabilisation of the shoulder may be helpful, especially if the osteosynthesis system used is flimsy. The best option is to apply a Spica cast, made with fibreglass, in a functional position for a few weeks (Fig. 15). Although it is not usually necessary, in some cases of unstable fractures that affect other areas of the scapula, this same system of immobilisation may be needed.

Fractures of the supraglenoid tubercle

The supraglenoid tubercle is the insertion point of the tendon of the biceps muscle. It must be highlighted that there is an independent ossification nucleus in this bone portion during the first months of the patient's life, and thus in young patients the growth line should not be confused with a fracture (Fig. 16). When in doubt, a radiological examination can be performed of the contralateral extremity to confirm the pathological character of the finding.

Although infrequent, this tubercle can be fractured from avulsion. The animal's limp may be slight depending on the course of the process (acute or progressive). On the contrary, as an ossification nucleus, the supraglenoid tubercle has its own growth line that may suffer a progressive detachment that is manifested as a slight limp.

Treatment consists of stabilisation of the fragment using a tension band pin system or a compression screw, given that this type of fracture suffers traction by the biceps tendon.

In older lesions, where the fracture is not likely to heal well, or when surgery has not been successful, the fragment can be removed and a biceps tenodesis can be performed. Similar to that which occurs in cases of chronic lesions of the shoulder extensor muscles, another possibility is to remove the bone fragment and attach the tendon to the capsular portion of the intertubercular groove (Fig. 17).

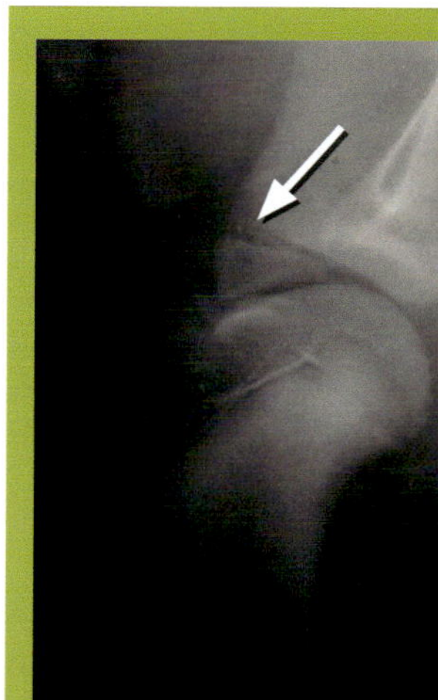

FIGURE 16. Growth plate in the supraglenoid tubercle of a puppy (arrow).

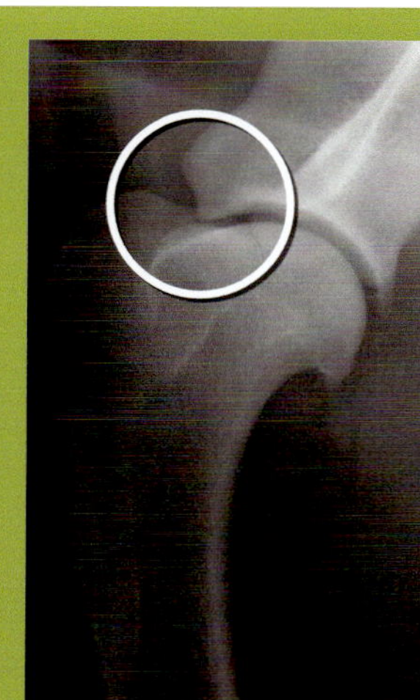

FIGURE 17. Progress of an extraction of the supraglenoid tubercle two years after surgery. Slight osteoarthritis is observed.

FRACTURES OF THE HUMERUS

Of the long bones in the extremities of our patients, the humerus suffers fewer fractures. Statistically, most fractures that affect the humerus are located in the middle and distal thirds. In practice, the most frequent fracture observed is that of the condyle lateral to the distal epiphysis, followed by oblique fractures of the middle-distal third.

Before delving into the study of the surgical techniques that can be applied in fractures of the humerus, certain characteristics of said bone must be understood.

First, the humerus is slightly curved in an "S" shape. This anatomical peculiarity implies a variation regarding the location of the tension-bearing surface that is proximally found located in a cranio-lateral direction, while its distal portion is in a caudo-medial position (Fig. 18). As previously mentioned, the tension-bearing surface is that which bears the partial forces of distraction in the most superficial part of the compact bone when the bone is subjected to forces of longitudinal pressure, that is, when the limb bears weight.

Another characteristic of this bone is the presence of a narrowing of the medullary cavity located between the medial and distal thirds. This narrowing causes the medullary cavity to present an uneven width throughout its length (Fig. 19).

Thirdly, the location of the brachial plexus, which courses through the medial surface of the humerus, forces the clinician to assess its integrity in animals that present with fractures of this bone.

A patient afflicted with a humerus fracture normally presents the limb resting on the dorsal portion of the toes with the shoulder slouching. Frequently, this posture is similar to that found in patients afflicted with paralysis of the radial nerve. Therefore, before proceeding with the stabilisation of the fracture, the integrity of said plexus must be confirmed.

The posture adopted by an animal with a fracture of the humerus is similar to that found in cases of paralysis of the radial nerve, which therefore requires assessment of the integrity of the brachial plexus.

When a surgeon is faced with a fractured long bone, it is nearly impossible to correctly assess reflexes, but not the deep sensitivity. For this reason, before considering any surgical intervention, it is recommended that the last phalanges of the II and IV toes of the extremity be pinched to assess the integrity of the radial, ulnar and median nerves. When performing this examination, precaution should be taken to avoid moving the extremity so that the animal's response will not be from the pain caused in the area around the fracture.

When dealing with a patient with a humeral fracture, a complete assessment of the thorax must be performed to discard the existence of a haemopneumothorax as the humerus is in close contact with the chest cavity.

Stabilisation techniques

The humerus can be stabilised by most of the osteosynthesis techniques currently available on the market: plates, intramedullary fixation and external fixation. External immobilisation using casts or bandages is not usually indicated, however, it will be discussed in the following pages.

External immobilisation

To achieve correct stability of a bone applying a bandage, both joints (proximal and distal) in relation with this bone must be correctly immobilised.

In the specific case of the humerus, achieving proper immobilisation of the glenohumerus joint is impossible due to anatomical reasons. In the hypothetical case that movements of this joint could be avoided, a correct immobilisation of the bone would never be achieved. This is due to the fact that the proximal portion is surrounded by a very strong muscle mass. This musculature acts as if it were made of bandage padding, where it would be impossible to impede the micro-movements of the fracture site, regardless of how well both joints are immobilised.

When external immobilisation is required to add additional support to a minimal osteosynthesis system, a Spica cast can be applied (Fig. 20) that immobilises the limb from the scapula to the toes.

Intramedullary pinning

Although this osteosynthesis system is not the most ideal for the treatment of humerus fractures, there are certain fractures that can be resolved using intramedullary pins.

This osteosynthesis system, with the exception of interlocking pins, is not effective in correctly stabilising the rotation movements of the fracture site. Similarly, it also does not impede collapse, movements of distraction, and compression of the fractured area. Consequently, the only fractures that can be effectively treated with this osteosynthesis system

Special characteristics of the humerus that explain the greater frequency of fractures in its middle-distal third

The tension-bearing surface is found in a cranio-lateral position. In its proximal portion and moving down towards the distal epiphysis, the tension-bearing surface is found towards the caudal area, in a caudo-medial position in its most distal portion (Fig. 18).

The medullary cavity does not present a constant width. It narrows between the middle and distal thirds (Fig. 19).

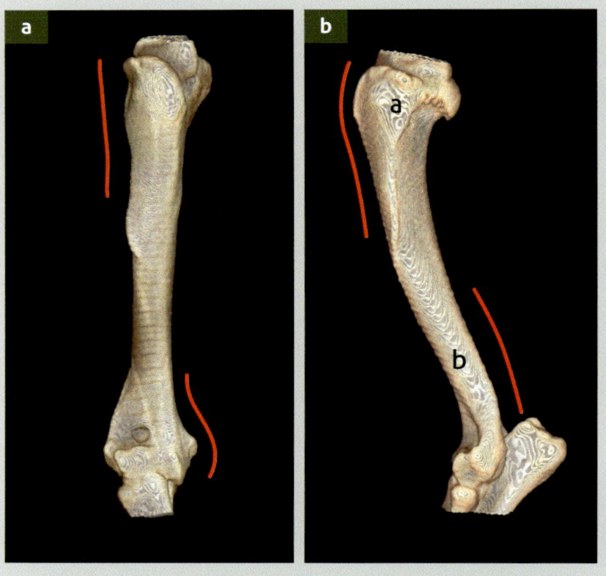

FIGURE 18. Representation of the course of the weight-bearing surface.

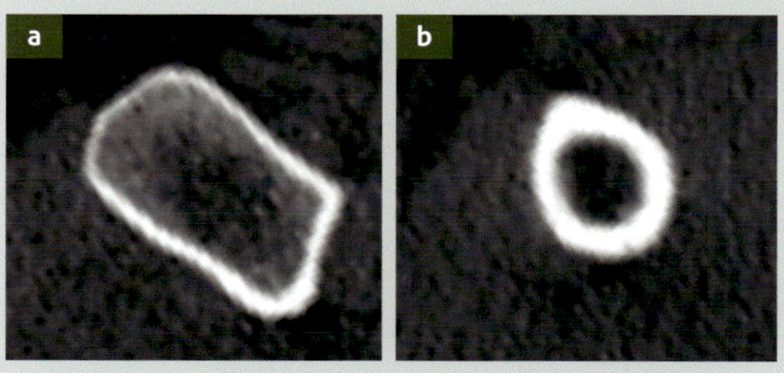

FIGURE 19. CT scan where the narrowing of the medullary cavity can be observed in the areas indicated in Fig. 18. Proximal (a) and distal (b) portions.

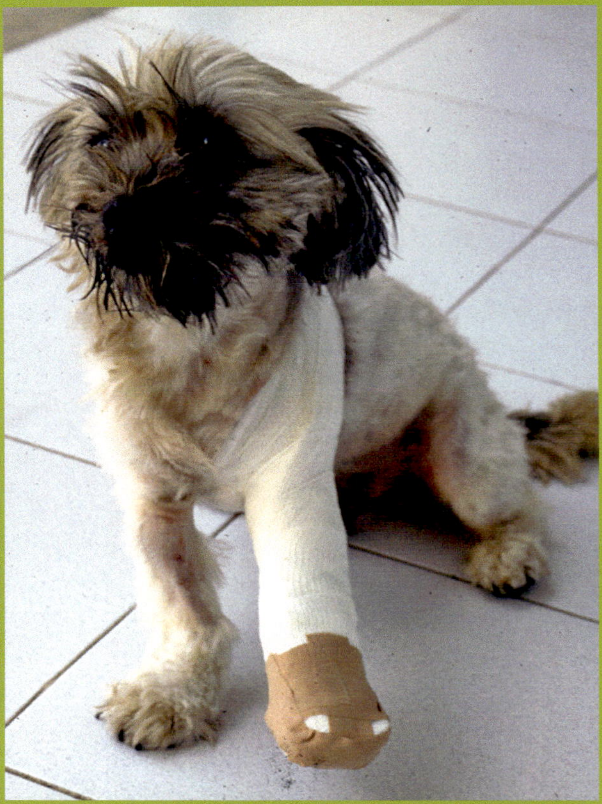

FIGURE 20. Spica cast used to stabilise a humerus fracture.

The intramedullary pinning is not the best option for humerus fractures, except in young patients in which the lack of stability is compensated with the speed of bone healing.

are simple fractures that do not tend to rotate, that is, longitudinal oblique fractures, in which cerclages should be added to provide a certain amount of stability. This type of fracture is infrequent in the humerus.

Another disadvantage is that the immobilisation achieved is not complete. In the particular case of the humerus, due to the narrowing of the medullary cavity, pins with large diameters cannot be introduced. This added difficulty causes the intramedullary pinning in the humerus to be even less stable.

For these reasons, pins should only be used in young patients in which the lack of stability is compensated by faster bone healing mechanisms.

In the humerus, this implant should be anchored proximally on the lateral part of its greater tubercle and distally in the medial epicondyle. The pins should be inserted in a normograde manner, that is, from the greater tubercle to the site of the fracture. This way, the pin will be better anchored to the proximal part of the bone. If this was done in a retrograde manner, firmness would be lost in the fixation of the pin with the proximal epiphysis due to having to move the pin in a proximal direction and later towards the site of the fracture. In order to avoid any movements of rotation, the best option is the insertion of at least two smaller pins instead of one, or, to temporarily associate one with a single plane unilateral fixation system (type I).

The ideal humerus fracture for treatment with intramedullary pinning is a longitudinal oblique or spiral fracture of the distal third of a patient that is still growing.

The ideal fracture for treatment with this osteosynthesis system in the humerus is a longitudinal oblique or spiral fracture of the distal third in a patient that is still growing. This type of fracture is quite frequent in young patients (Fig. 21). In these cases, the association of one or various cerclages to the intramedullary fixation system will help to avoid movements of rotation. Similarly, interfragmentary compression that is achieved using cerclages, will impede micro-movements, and thus provide good stability.

In some patients, the introduction of an intramedullary pin may help to reduce the fracture, especially regarding the alignment and length of the bone. Later, the clinician will only have to orient the rotation of the fragments and apply the osteosynthesis system selected. The high stability of this osteosynthesis system against movements of flexion can be helpful when associated with the use of osteosynthesis plates with monocortical screws, or in the first phases of biological plate systems (Fig. 22).

External fixation

External fixation of the humerus, due to anatomical reasons, is limited to the application of single-plane, unilateral fixation systems with one or two connecting rods. In some cases of comminuted non-reducible fractures, the use of a tie-in type external fixation system or hybrid configurations of said system may be necessary.

This configuration basically consists of fusing the connecting rod of one unilateral external fixator with an intramedullary pin (Fig. 23). This way, the weakness of the pins is avoided and a much more stable structure is created.

One way to achieve faster healing of the fracture site is to place an intramedullary pin in a normograde manner in a closed fracture. This avoids any significant affectation of the vascularisation.

External fixation is frequently associated with other osteosynthesis systems to achieve greater stability.

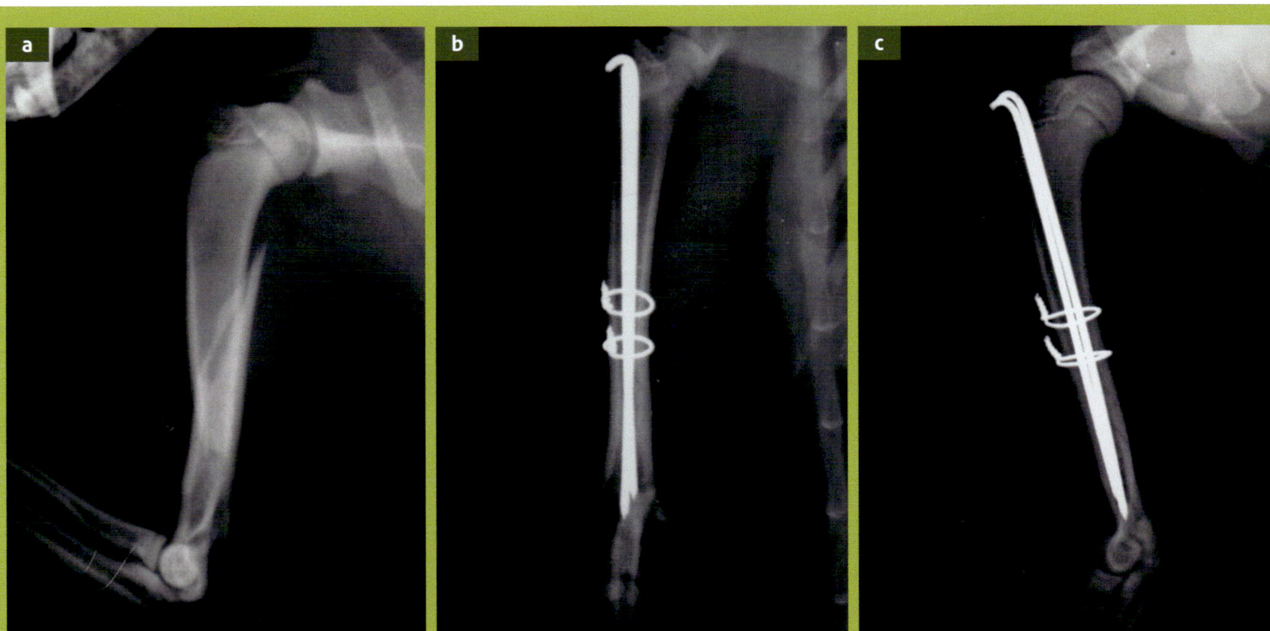

FIGURE 21. Long oblique fracture (a) that has been resolved by placing two intramedullary pins and cerclages that prevent movements of rotation (b and c). The implant does not interfere with the joint area and should not invade the intercondylar space.

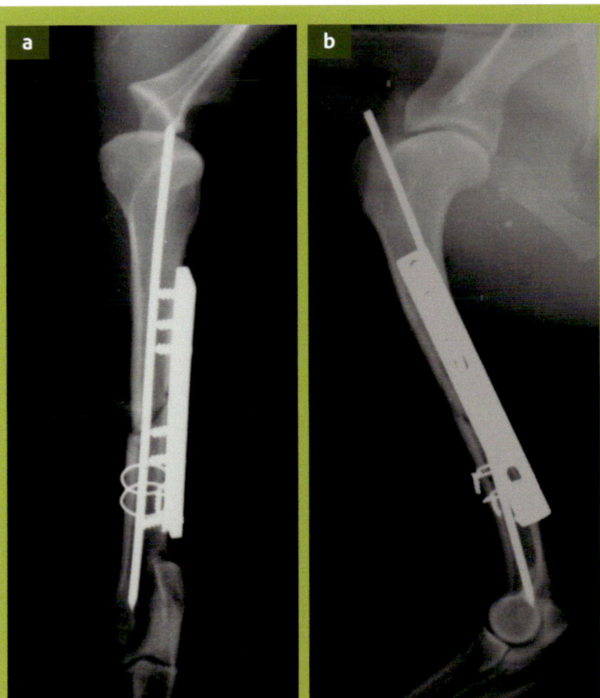

FIGURE 22. Intermedullary pin associated with a plate with monocortical screws to resolve a fracture of the medio-distal diaphysis. Caudo-cranial view (a) and latero-lateral view (b).

In these cases, external fixation is primarily achieved opposing the movements of rotation as well as the approximation of the primary fragments. For these reasons, it becomes an ideal complement to the intramedullary pins and the minimal osteosynthesis systems of the proximal and distal third of the humerus (Fig. 24).

External fixation systems are a great complement to intramedullary pins as they impede any movements of rotation and approximation of the fragments (collapse of the fracture site).

The localisation of the insertion points of the percutaneous pins, located in the ends of the bones, is very simple. The most proximal pin is inserted into the greater tubercle of the humerus, which can easily be palpated. The most distal percutaneous pin is inserted in a slightly cranio-distal position from the most prominent part of the lateral epicondyle of the humerus, facing the medial

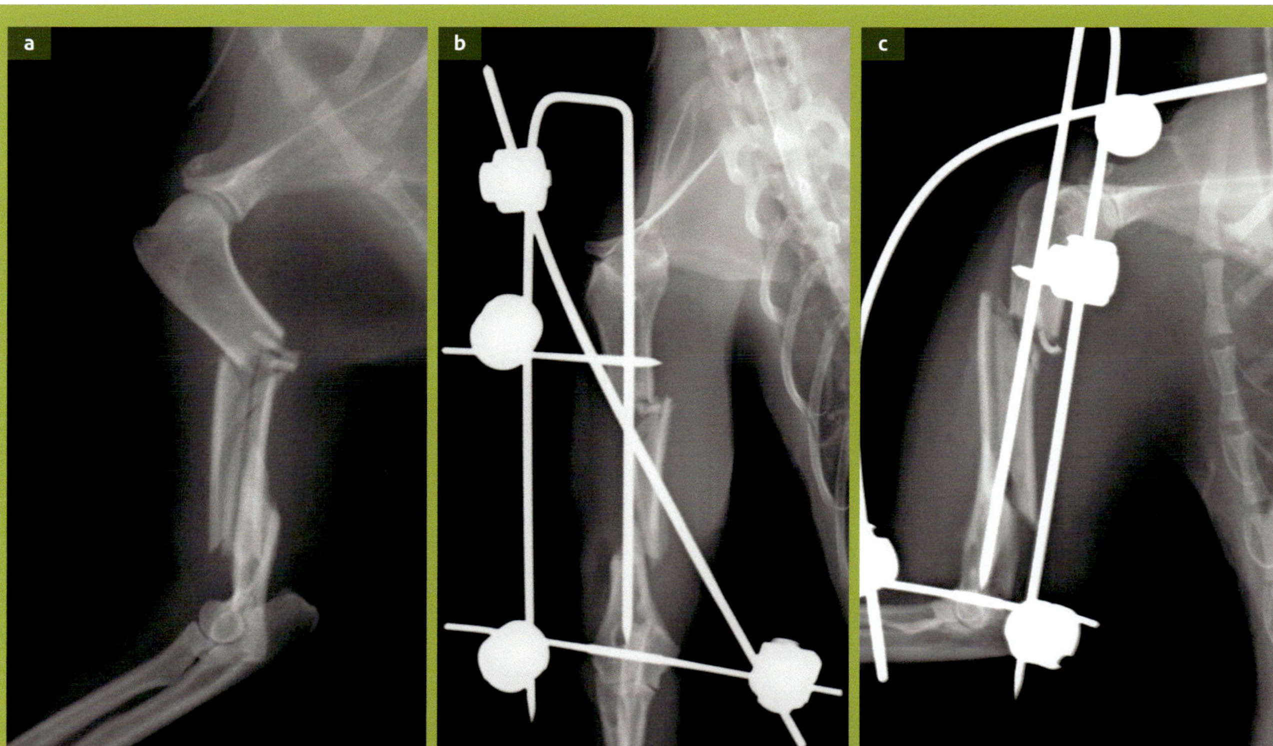

FIGURE 23. Multiple fracture of humerus (a), resolved using a tie-in fixation system; cranio-caudal views with the limb flexed (b) and extended (c).

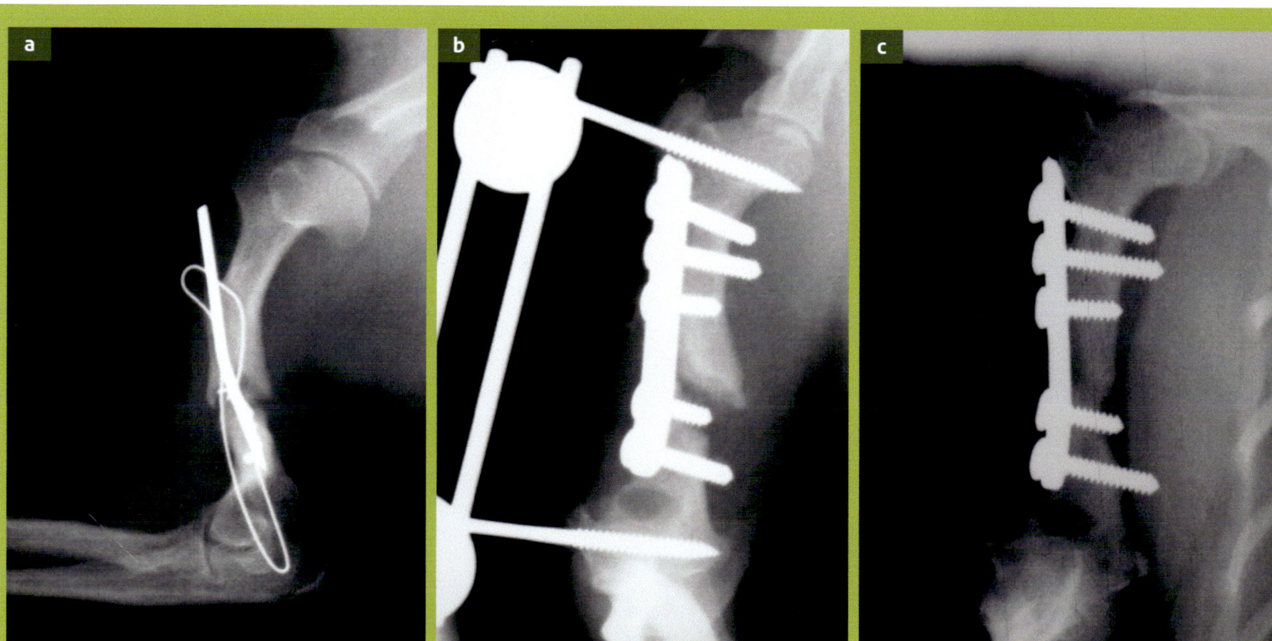

FIGURE 24. X-ray that shows a case of non-union due to the poor use of osteosynthesis systems (a). The fracture is treated with a supporting plate without enough space to insert the screws in the distal fragment, associated with a partial fixation system with a double connecting rod (b). X-ray showing the progress of the fracture once the partial fixation system was removed (c).

epicondyle. This way, there is no risk of introducing it into the joint cavity.

The application of the percutaneous pins of an external fixation system in the humerus at the proximal and distal level presents no complications.

If external fixation configurations that are more complex than a unilateral 1/1 system are needed, certain precaution must be taken when inserting the pins in the middle and distal third to avoid harming the radial nerve (although this happens infrequently).

The application of external skeletal fixation in the humerus as a single osteosynthesis system must be limited to fractures from firearms, open fractures or those in which one of the principal fragments is of a size that impedes the use of plates.

Osteosynthesis plates

Osteosynthesis plates are, without doubt, the best fixation system to treat fractures of the humerus. All fractures, except those that are located on the proximal or distal ends, where there is not enough space to place a sufficient amount of screws, can be treated using osteosynthesis plates as a single system.

Osteosynthesis plates, as much as possible, should be applied on the tension-bearing surface of the bone due to the greater resistance of the metal against the forces of traction.

As previously mentioned, the tension-bearing surface in the humerus depends on the location. For this reason, and in general, the fractures that affect the proximal third must be stabilised by applying an osteosynthesis plate on its craniolateral portion (Fig. 25).

In fractures of the proximal extreme, a plate can be situated in a cranial direction just above the deltoid crest. However, in those located in a more distal area, and due to said location, inserting more than two screws above the distal portion of the previously identified crest is impossible. The plate should thus be placed laterally given that other positions would make it harder to mould the plate.

The humerus, due to the variation of the tension-bearing surfaces, the area where the osteosynthesis plates will be placed varies depending on the location of the fracture.

The plate placement area depends on various factors for fractures that affect the middle third, the first being the extension of the fracture. In transversal and short oblique fractures, a plate can be applied both on the medial and

Applications of the external fixation of the humerus

- Fractures from firearms.
- Open fractures.
- Fractures with one of the primary fragments presenting dimensions that impede the correct anchoring of the plates.

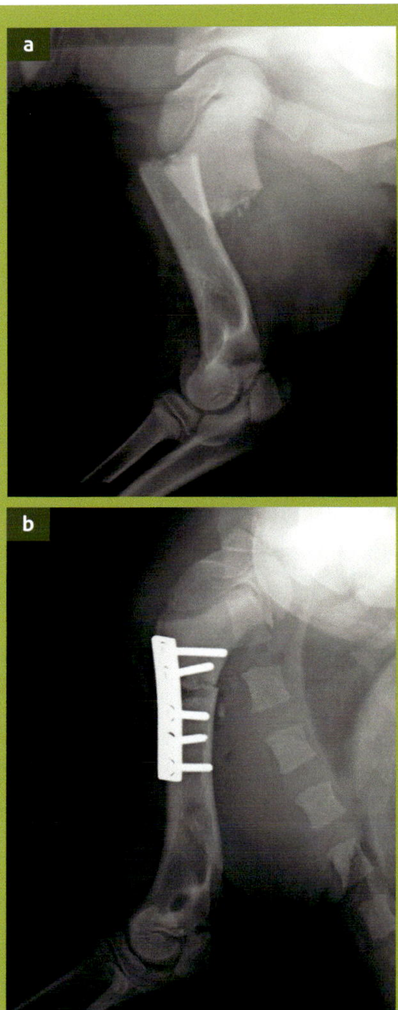

FIGURE 25. Fracture of the proximal third of the humerus (a) stabilised using an osteosynthesis plate in a cranial position (b).

lateral surfaces of the humerus. However, in long oblique, spiral or comminuted fractures, where longer plates are needed for stabilisation of the fracture, the plates must be anchored more distally, and it is recommended in these cases that they be placed on the medial surface of the humerus. Another important aspect to take into account is the breed of the patient; access to the most proximal part of the humerus through the medial surface is very limited in some breeds due to its anatomical position with the thorax, while access is very easy in others. The implant can be placed on the lateral surface of the bone in all breeds; however, as the plate rests on the lateral epicondyle, moulding the plate is much more complicated (Fig. 26).

In fractures located on the distal third, the best area is always the medial portion as the anchor in the medial supracondylar branch is much more effective due to the greater thickness of the compact bone. On the other hand, moulding the plate for its placement in this area is much easier than on the other side (Fig. 27).

In fractures on the distal extreme, as it will be necessary to place screws in the most distal portion of the bone, special attention must be paid to avoid placing any screws in the intercondylar fossa. If this happened, the patient would lose its capacity to fully extend its elbow, resulting in ankylosis of said joint. The following options exist to avoid this problem: only cover the medial supracondylar branch, orient the screw in a sharp cranial direction or towards the lateral epicondyle (Fig. 28).

Surgical approach

There are various surgical approaches to apply different fixation systems to humerus fractures, especially regarding the use of plates. Consequently, the approach should depend on the area where the fracture is located.

If intramedullary pins are used as the osteosynthesis system, or when an open external fixation system is used, the access route is lateral (Fig. 29). This approach is much easier, and it allows for access to nearly the entire length of the bone. Laterally, it should be noted that the radial nerve is a structure that must be avoided. It is easily identified as it is attached to the caudal portion of the brachial muscle. This access route, as previously mentioned, is also an ideal choice when stabilizing fractures that affect the proximal and middle third with plates.

For fractures of the distal third or the middle third, the ideal approach for the placement of plates is medial (Fig. 30). It is significantly more complex, due to the existence of the brachial plexus and the median and ulnar nerves. Both nerves separate at the beginning of the distal third and are accompanied by an important vascular bundle. Sometimes, due to the swollen aspect of all tissues surrounding the fracture site, it may be difficult to locate this neurovascular bundle. To

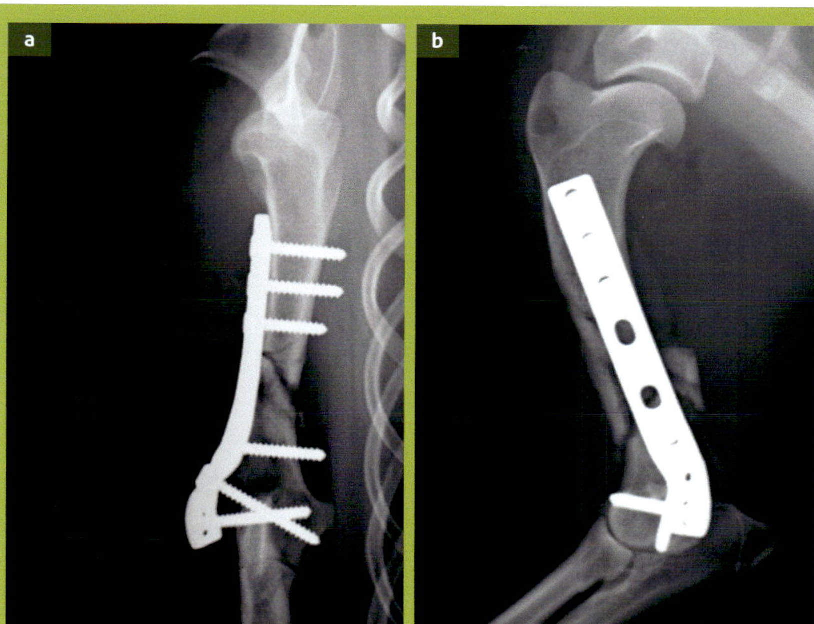

FIGURE 26. Comminuted fracture located in the middle third of the humerus (a) after a few weeks of progress. It is stabilised using a plate placed on its lateral surface (b).

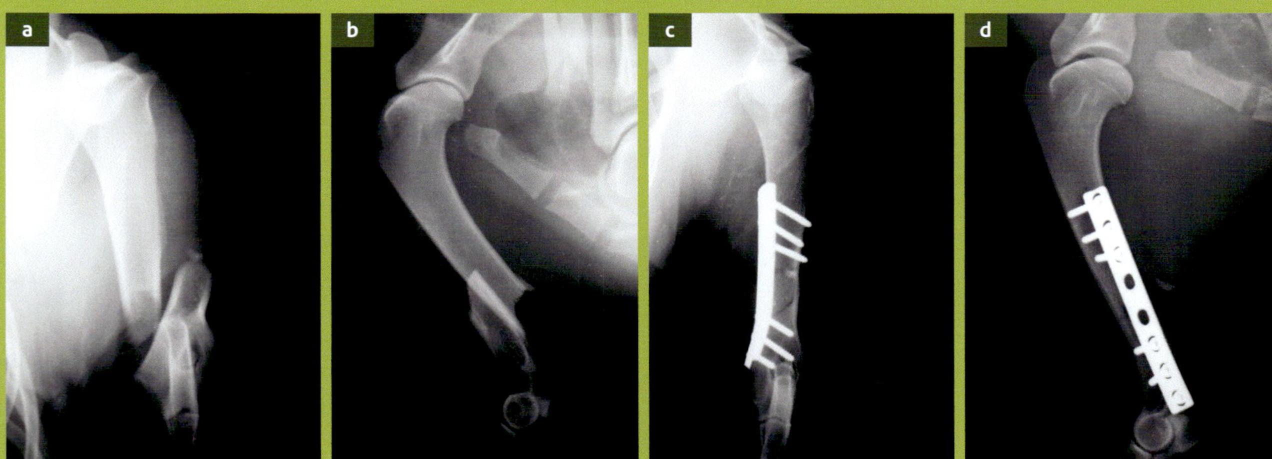

FIGURE 27. Distal short oblique fracture of the humerus (a and b), resolved by placing a plate on its medial surface (c and d).

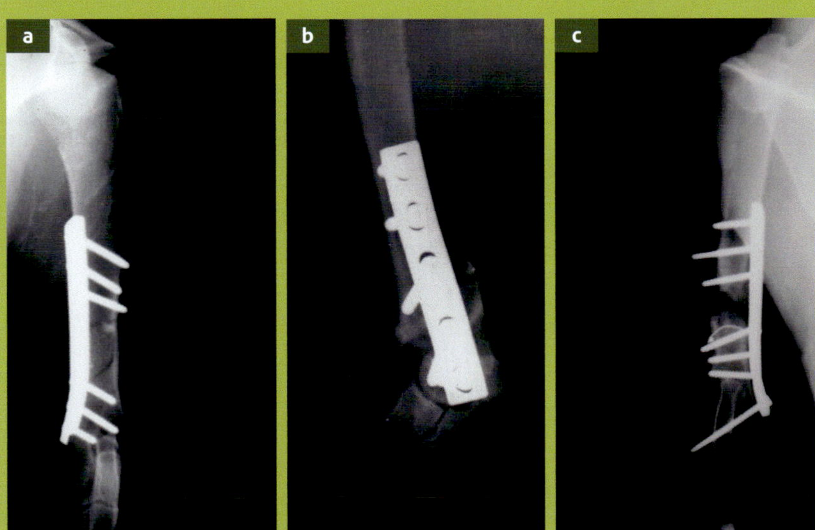

FIGURE 28. Different orientations of the distal screws to avoid the intercondylar fossa and, consequently, a future ankylosis of the joint in different fractures located in the distal portion of the humerus. Spiral fracture, the most distal screw is only anchored to the supracondylar branch (a). Pseudoarthrosis of more than one year of progress in the distal extreme; the distal screws are oriented towards the epicondyle where they cross (b). Pseudoarthrosis, in which the last screw is oriented towards the lateral epicondyle (c).

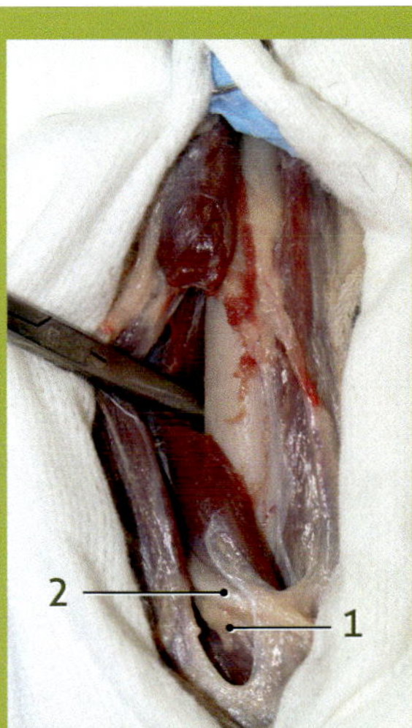

FIGURE 29. Lateral approach of the middle third of the humerus.
1. Radial nerve.
2. Brachial muscle.

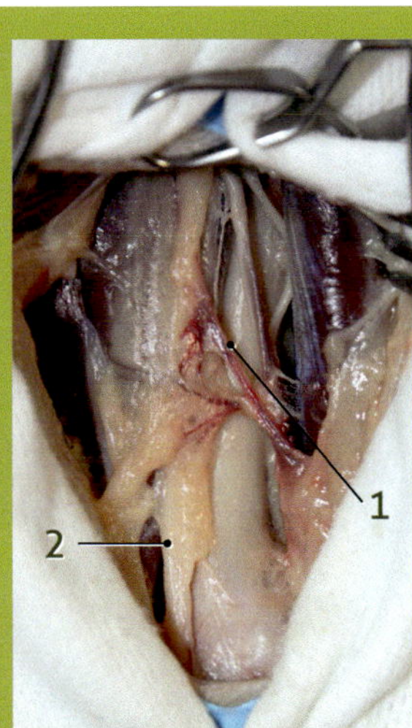

FIGURE 30. Medial approach of the distal third.
1. Ulnar nerve.
2. Median nerve.

Approaches depending on the location of the fracture

Approaches depend on the location of the fracture:

- Lateral access:
  - Intramedullary pins or external fixation systems.
  - Plates in fractures of the proximal and middle thirds.
- Medial access:
  - Plates in fractures of the distal and middle thirds.

avoid this problem, the median nerve pathway can be used as a reference as it can be palpated when it passes over the caudal area of the medial epicondyle following it until the ulnar nerve branches.

Treatment of the most frequent fractures

In this section, the most frequent humerus fractures are briefly described with the principal aspects to be taken into account to select the optimal stabilisation system, as well as their particularities.

Epiphysiolysis of the humeral head

This fracture is very infrequent. It affects more cats than dogs and is almost always a type I Salter fracture.

Firstly, it is important to not confuse the growth line with a fracture. Unfortunately, it is not that infrequent that forelimb limps are justified in young dogs of fast-growing breeds with a persistence of the opening of the proximal line of growth of the humerus. In these breeds, the cranial portion of the growth line is visible in X-rays until nearly one year of age (Fig. 31).

A growth line should not be confused with a fracture, which is possible in young dogs of fast-growing breeds.

The treatment of choice for all Salter-Harris fractures is Rush pins. These can be inserted from the greater tubercle towards the metaphysis, or from the metaphysis in a divergent manner, towards the epiphysis, avoiding their introduction in the joint cavity (Fig. 32). This is the only system that does not produce the premature healing of the growth plates.

In animals that have reached their full size, this fracture can also take place in the time it takes for the growth plate to ossify completely. In these patients, intramedullary pins can be substituted with compression screws or pins with tension-bands. Once the patient has stopped growing, these systems will not produce any bone alterations. In these cases, the osteosynthesis material is always inserted through a greater tubercle of the humerus.

Diaphyseal fractures

This type of fracture represents half of the fractures produced in the humerus.

As mentioned previously, few can be treated using intramedullary pins. This treatment should only be used in simple fractures in young animals in which movements of rotation can be neutralised. This can easily be achieved by using cerclages (Fig. 33).

In multiple fractures, aside from the rotational instability, the possibility that the fracture site could collapse must be taken into account. In these cases, although the ideal treatment would be stabilisation using plates, if the benefits of the different osteosynthesis systems are taken advantage of and they are adequately combined, they could neutralise all forces (Fig. 34).

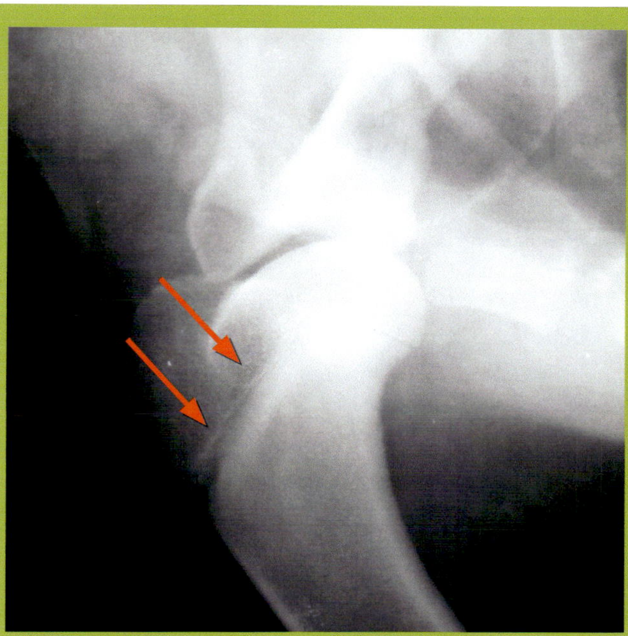

FIGURE 31. In this image of the proximal metaphysis of the humerus, the growth line can be observed (arrows). It should not be confused with a fracture.

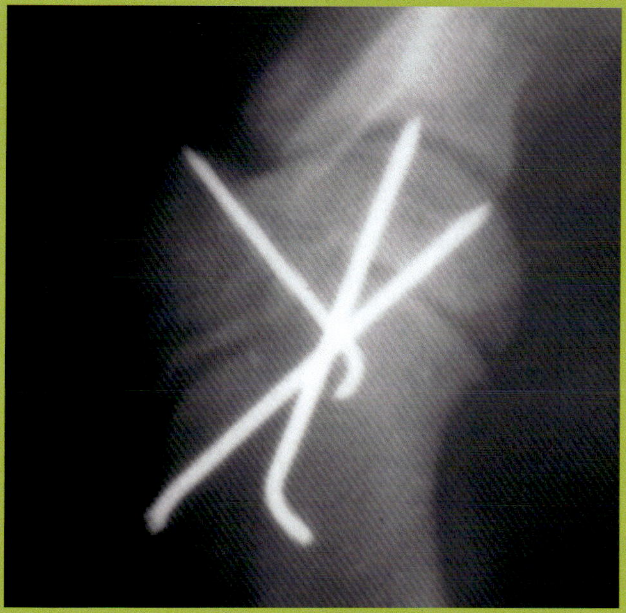

FIGURE 32. Treatment of a Salter I fracture of the proximal epiphysis of the humerus stabilised using three divergent pins inserted from the metaphysis.

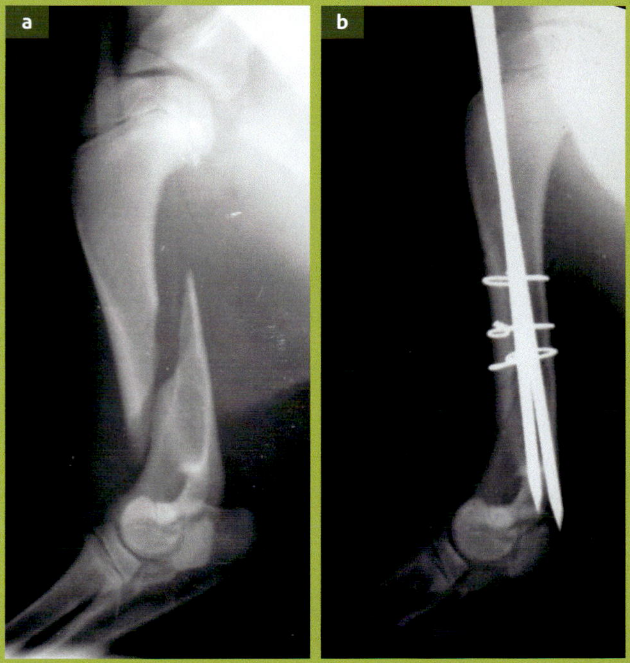

FIGURE 33. Diaphyseal humerus fracture (a), resolved with intramedullary pins associated with cerclages that impede movements of rotation (b).

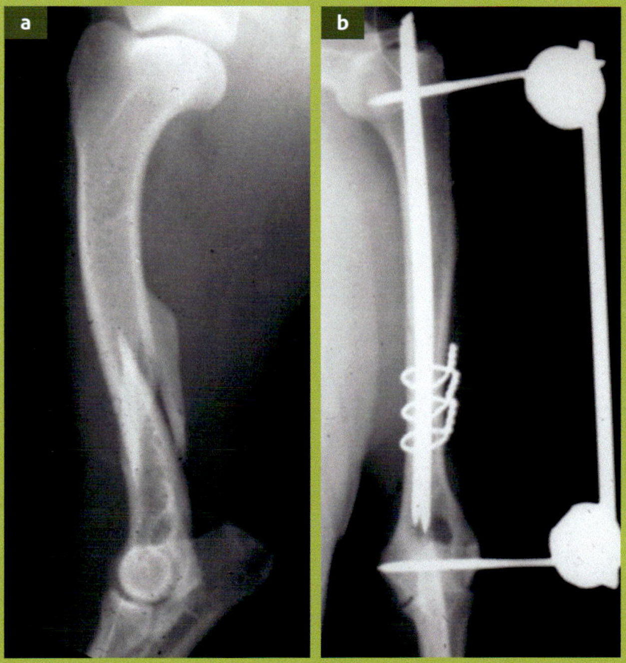

FIGURE 34. Multiple fracture of the humerus diaphysis (a). In this case, the instability of the intramedullary pins has been resolved by using an external partial fixation system (b).

Stabilisation by means of external fixation of humerus fractures should not be a first choice. However, it can be applied as a complementary system to increase the stability of other fixation apparatuses.

In multiple diaphyseal fractures of the humerus, all forces can easily be neutralised by combining different osteosynthesis systems.

It is possible that there are no other alternatives than this osteosynthesis system in certain fractures. In these cases, given the fact that due to anatomical conditioning only partial fixation can be used, the best option is to choose tie-in configurations or hybrids of this system with others (Fig. 35).

In fractures in adult animals, osteosynthesis plates are the ideal system. Logically, the type of plate used depends on the type of fracture as well as the surgeon's preferences. In most cases, diaphyseal fractures are oblique and located in the distal middle third, at the level of the isthmus. Given its location, the plate must be placed on the medial surface of the bone (Fig. 36).

If possible, it may be beneficial to associate compressive systems to the plate to increase the stability of the fracture. However, this possibility depends not only on the type of fracture but also on the surgeon's preferences (Fig. 37).

In the humerus, the greatest problem of the plates is likely the moulding of the implant, due to the shape of the bone and the great variability that exists between species and breeds.

When plates are placed on the humerus, the primary disadvantage is the moulding of the implant, due to the shape of the bone and the great variability found between species. This problem is minimised by applying locking plates in which, as previously mentioned, when the screw is tightened, the fragments are not tractioned towards the implant.

Fractures of the distal epiphysis

Among the fractures that affect the distal epiphysis of the humerus, there are two large groups: those that affect the joint surface, and those that are produced in the distal metaphyseal area.

Fractures of the distal metaphysis

The problem of metaphyseal fractures is the lack of space available in the distal fragment to place a sufficient number of screws. The stabilisation system must be selected depending on specific characteristics of each case. Many times, and primarily in small-sized patients, Rush pins may be enough with the possible association to other types of stabilisation systems (Fig. 38).

Of course, in the case of fractures that affect the growth plates, "bridge" systems cannot be used between both fragments as growth would thus be interrupted. In these

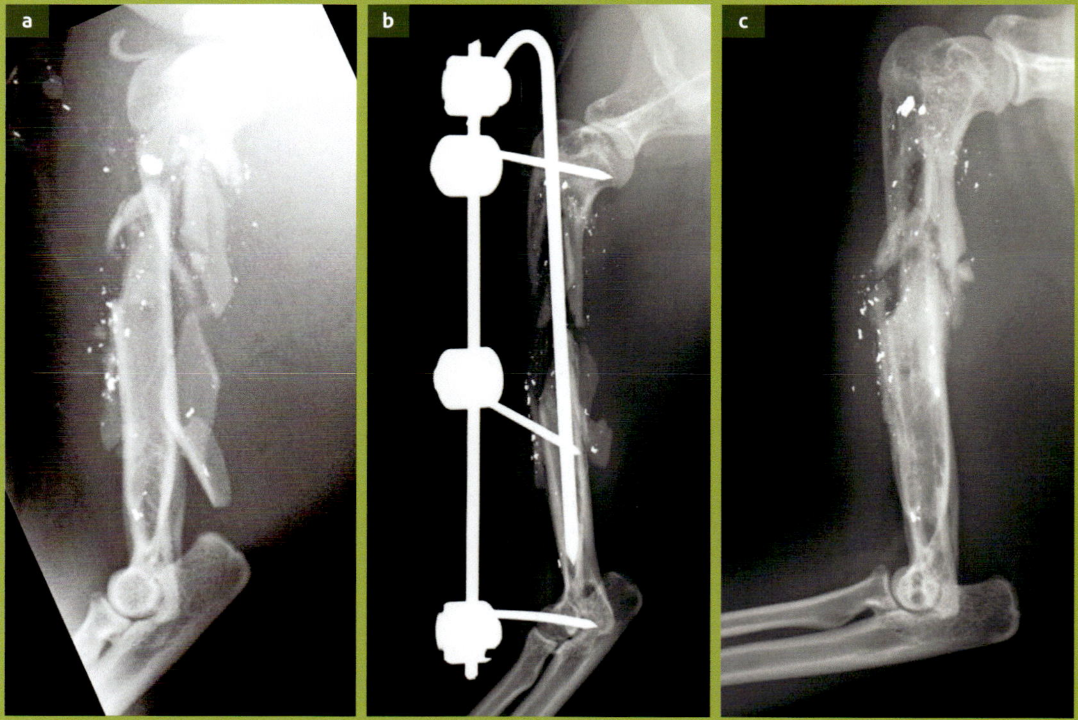

FIGURE 35. These images show how a fracture from a firearm has been resolved (a), using a tie-in configuration (b) and its progress (c).

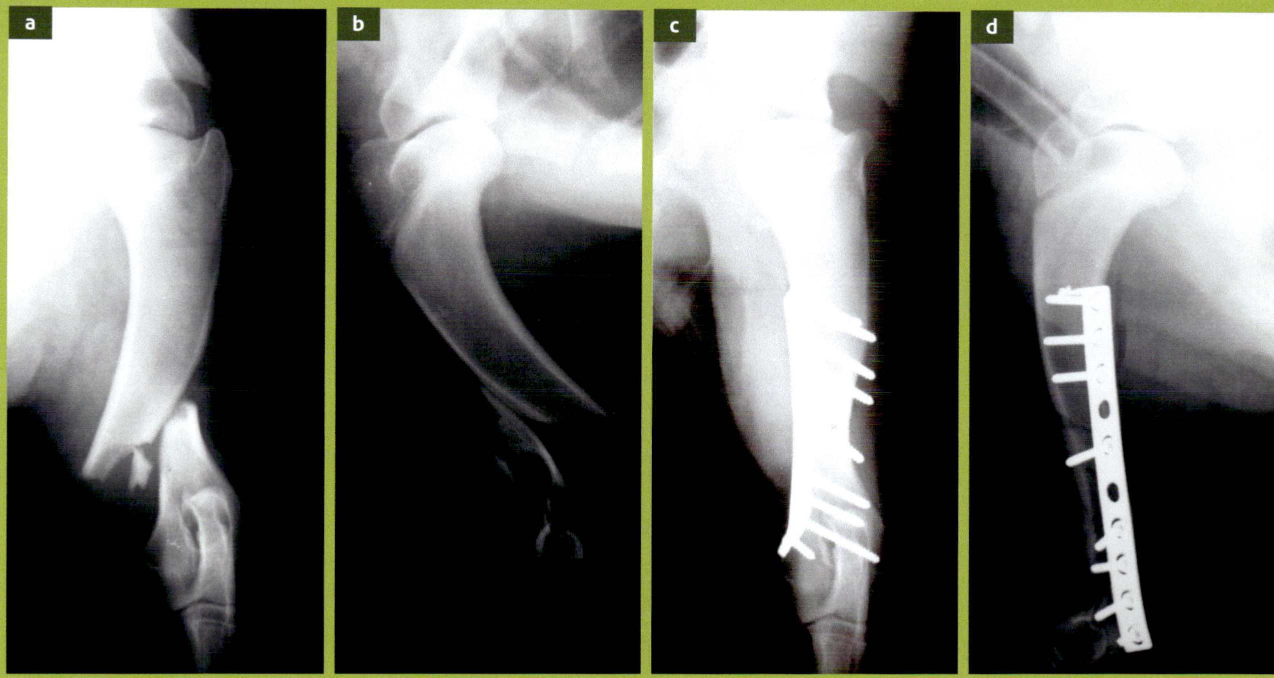

FIGURE 36. Image of a multiple fracture of the distal diaphysis of the humerus (a and b), resolved with a neutralisation plate with compression screws (c and d).

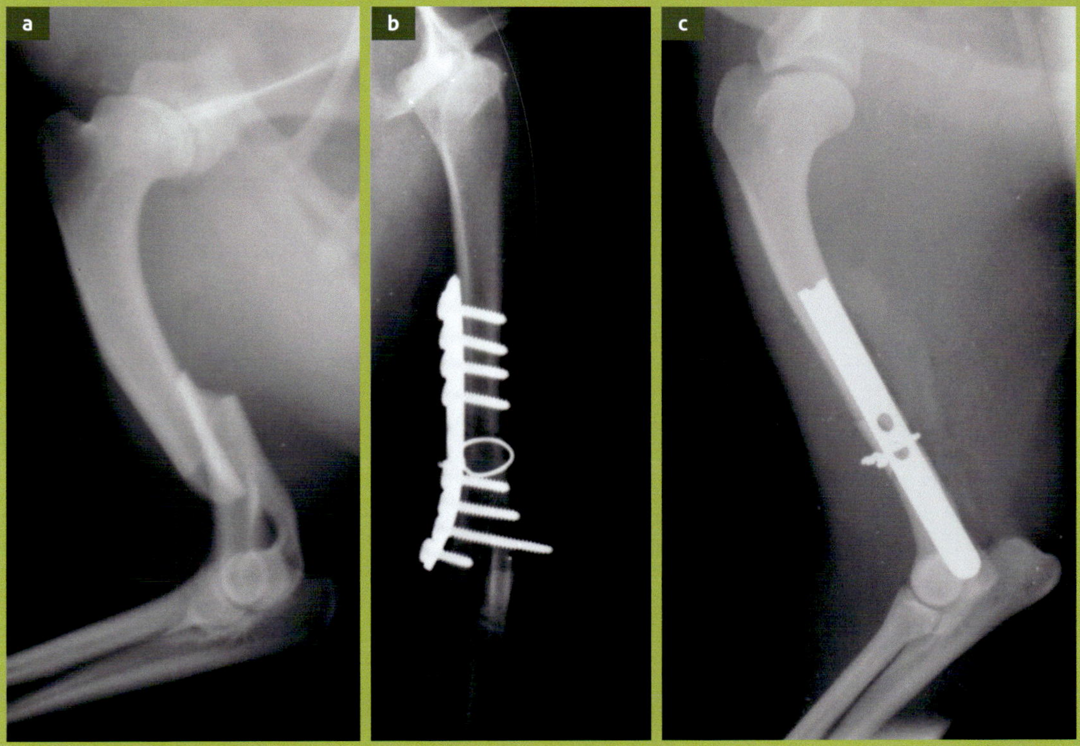

FIGURE 37. Distal fracture of the humerus (a), which is resolved with an adjustable neutralisation plate associated with wires (b and c).

cases, as in all Salter-Harris fractures, the only treatment is stabilisation using pins perpendicular to said plate (Fig. 39). In some cases, if the characteristics of the fracture require a more rigid stabilisation, pins may need to be substituted with screws. In these cases, if there is not enough space to insert three screws, two may be sufficient. If they are fasted to the condylar area, they will be more firmly anchored than if they were screwed into the compact bone area. Also, metaphyseal fractures have a greater healing capacity (Fig. 40).

> *"Bridge" systems cannot be used between the fragments of the fractures that affect the growth plates as growth would be interrupted.*

Fractures of the joint surface

The other large group of fractures that affect the distal epiphysis of the humerus are those that involve the joint. These fractures have a much less favourable prognosis and must be treated as quickly as possible. In this case, the joint surface must be reconstructed as perfectly as possible to minimise the appearance of secondary joint degeneration. Another essential condition for the correct recovery of joint function is that the patient start using said joint as soon as possible, for which the most stable osteosynthesis possible must be achieved.

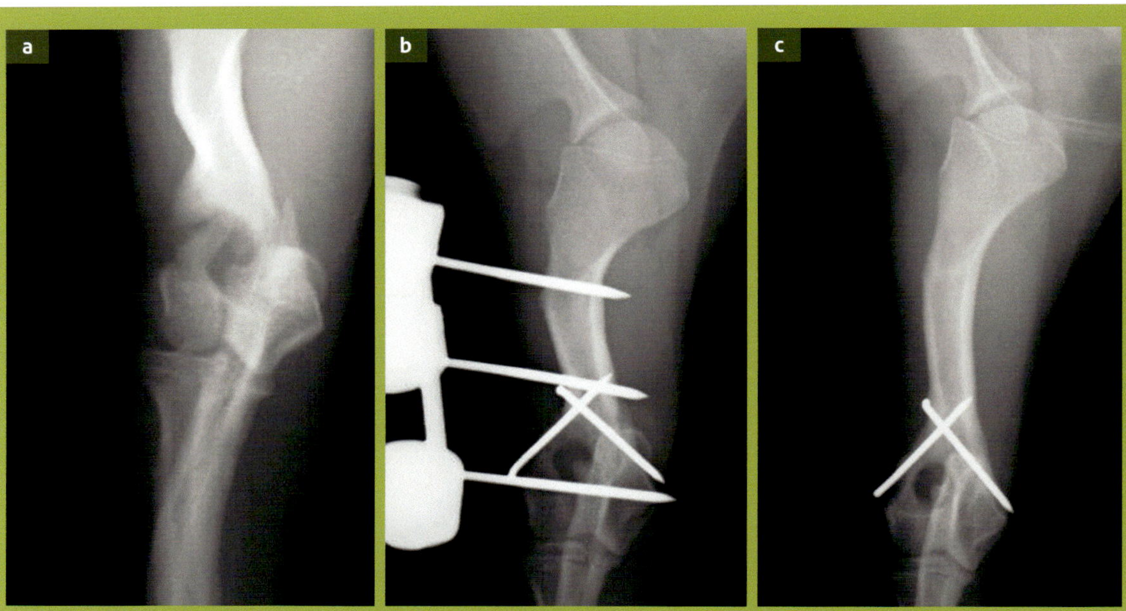

FIGURE 38. Fracture in the distal epiphysis of the humerus (a), which is resolved with Rush pins associated with a temporary external fixation system (b). X-ray of the fracture after removing the unilateral external fixator (c).

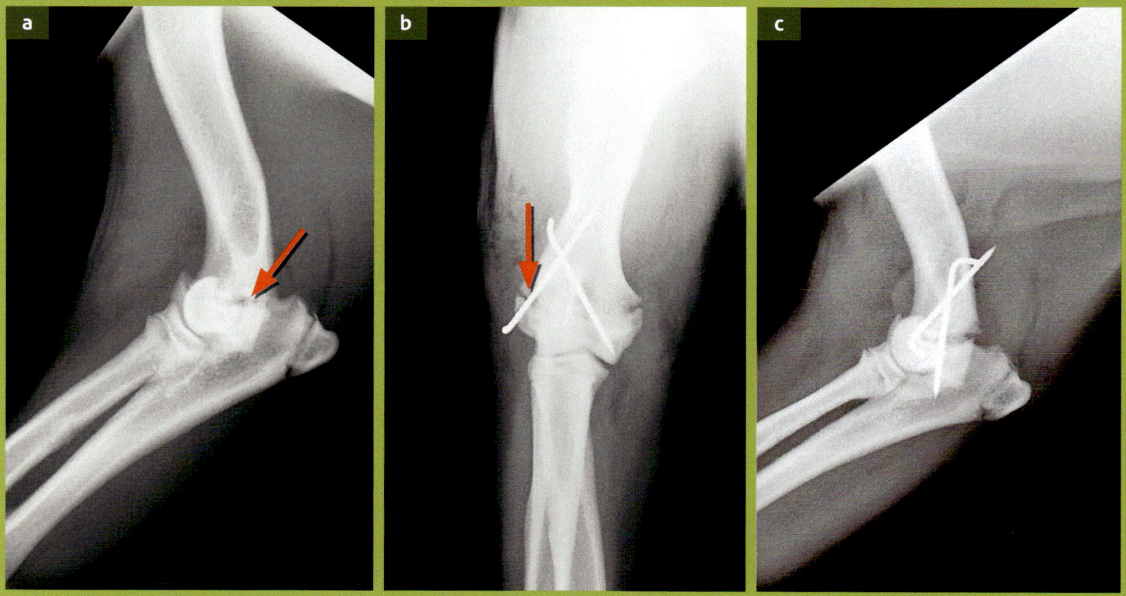

FIGURE 39. Type I Salter-Harris fracture of the distal metaphysis of the humerus (a). It can be observed here how this fracture (arrow) was resolved by inserting two pins perpendicular to the growth plate, caudo-cranial view (b). Latero-lateral view (c).

Type IV Salter-Harris fractures

In growing patients, the most frequent fracture in the distal epiphysis of the humerus is the type IV Salter-Harris fracture. The lateral condyle is the most frequently affected portion, as it is the primary weight-bearer on the proximal head of the radio (Fig. 41).

Treatment consists of placing an intercondylar compression screw after reducing the joint surface as correctly as possible using an anti-rotational pin inserted through the fractured condyle. The best procedure to perform osteosynthesis is to perforate the sliding hole from the fractured surface of the affected condyle and, once reduced, proceed with the perforation of the traction hole by means of the first hole.

In adult patients, this fracture is not very frequent, and in a large number of cases, it is produced as a consequence of a lack of ossification in both condyles. It is recommended that an in-depth study of the unaffected humerus be performed to discard said pathology.

Bicondylar fractures

The other fracture that is produced in the distal epiphysis of the humerus is the bicondylar fracture. It has an uncertain prognosis, and to achieve proper recovery of the patient, an osteosynthesis that is as stable as possible within the limitations of the space available to insert the implants should be performed.

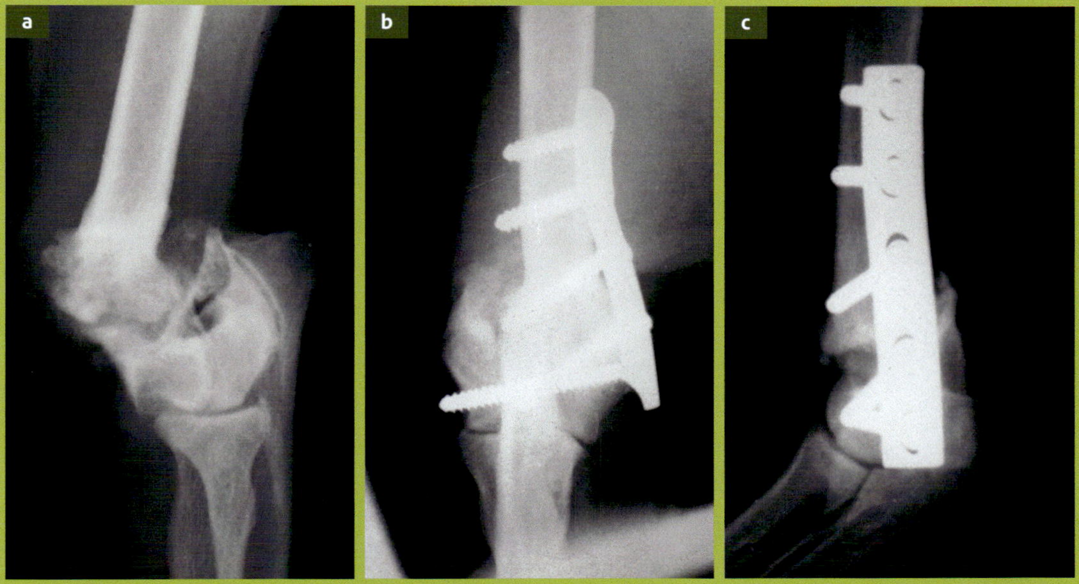

FIGURE 40. Image of the resolution of a epiphyseal fracture of the humerus through pseudoarthrosis.

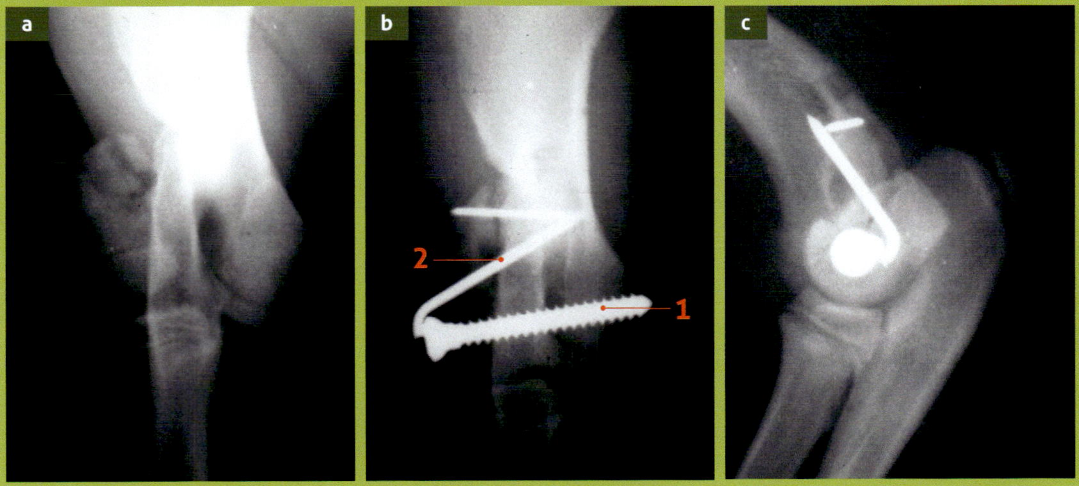

FIGURE 41. Salter IV type fracture in the lateral condyle of the humerus (a). Here, the orientation of the intercondylar screw (1) and the anti-rotational pin (2), can be observed in the caudo-cranial (b) and latero-lateral (c) views.

Once again, the ideal technique is the placement of an intercondylar compression screw associated with two plates, one a stronger medial plate, and the other a lateral plate (Fig. 42). This apparatus stabilises both condyles with the humerus diaphysis. In order for the joint to recover its function as soon as possible and avoid complications in the ossification of the olecranon, it is better to perform a double surgical approach before carrying out an osteotomy of the olecranon.

In the case of patients that are still maturing, the clinician will find him/herself faced with the disadvantage of not being able to lock the growth plates. Consequently, the osteosynthesis plates must be substituted with Rush pins, which are much less stable (Fig. 43).

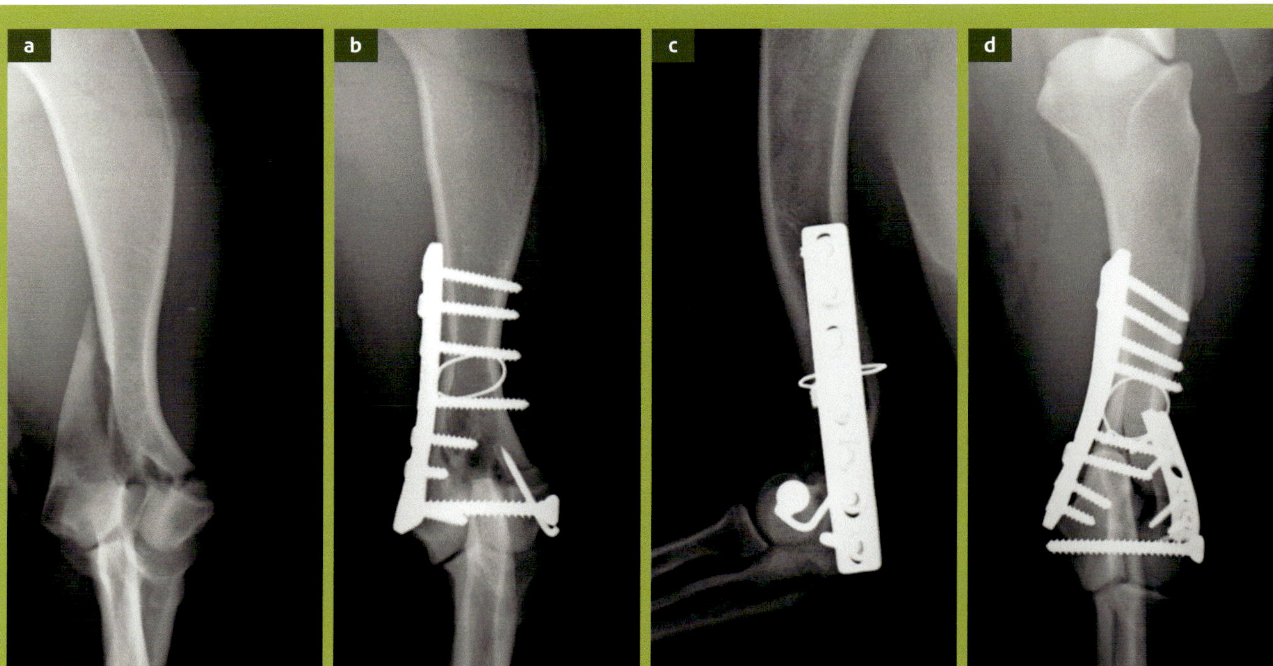

FIGURE 42. Bicondylar fracture in an adult patient (a). The fracture is resolved by placing an intercondylar compression screw, a medial plate (b) and a lateral plate (c). Latero-lateral view where the arrangement of the medial and lateral plates can be observed (d).

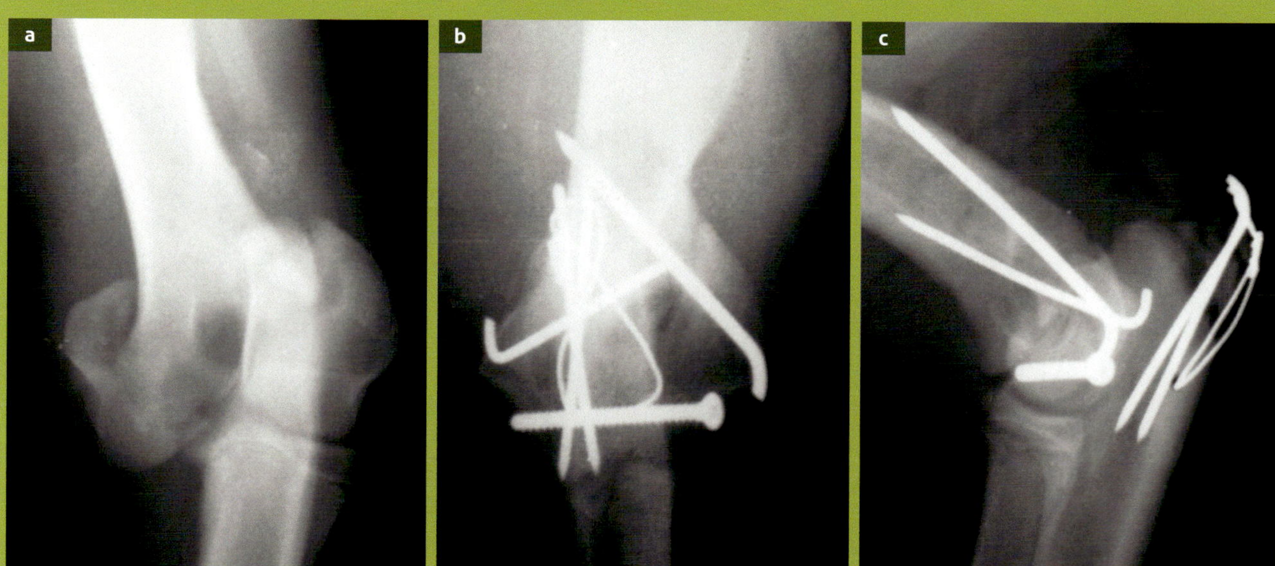

FIGURE 43. Bicondylar fracture in a young patient (a). Observe, in this case, the application of pins instead of plates to allow for bone growth. Caudo-cranial view (b) and latero-lateral view (c).

FRACTURES OF THE RADIUS AND ULNA

From a statistical perspective, the radius is the second most fractured bone after the femur. Normally, the radius and ulna are affected at the same time given their close anatomical location. However, there are certain types of fractures that only affect the ulna and that, due to their specific characteristics, will be discussed at the end of this chapter.

Anatomically, the radius is a flat bone in a straight, cranio-caudal direction (except for its distal third) in most breeds (Fig. 44). In chondrodystrophic breeds, the radius presents a slight curvature that must be taken into account due to its clinical significance when treatments are chosen.

The epiphysis of the radius is locked in on both sides: proximally by the joint surface of the humerus, and distally by the joint surfaces of the radial carpal and ulnar carpal bones. Due to this peculiarity, together with the small diameter of the medullary cavity, intramedullary fixation is completely contraindicated to stabilise fractures at this level (Fig. 45). On the other hand, the tension-bearing surface of the radius is found on the dorsal side along its entire length. In chondrodystrophic animals, due to the previously mentioned curvature, the tension-bearing surface is located slightly towards the medial side in the distal third. On the contrary, the ulna accepts intramedullary pinning perfectly as its epiphyseal extremes have no direct contact with other bones (Fig. 46).

In most cases, although both bones are usually fractured at the same time, stabilising the radius is sufficient as practically 100 % of the axial load is transmitted through this bone. The ulna heals without needing fixation, given that the fracture site, after stabilising the radius, hardly moves. In some cases, when a radius fracture cannot be perfectly stabilised, it may be useful to fixate the ulna also to provide greater stability to both bones.

Also, it should be highlighted that the entire ulna-radial area is surrounded by a muscle mass that is not especially strong. This lack of muscular mass, principally in the distal third of the forearm, causes healing to be slower than usual, which also makes the consolidation of fractures in this area more difficult. For this reason, when a simple fracture in the distal third of the radius must be stabilised, osteosynthesis systems that provide great stability should always be chosen, especially in adult dogs of miniature breeds.

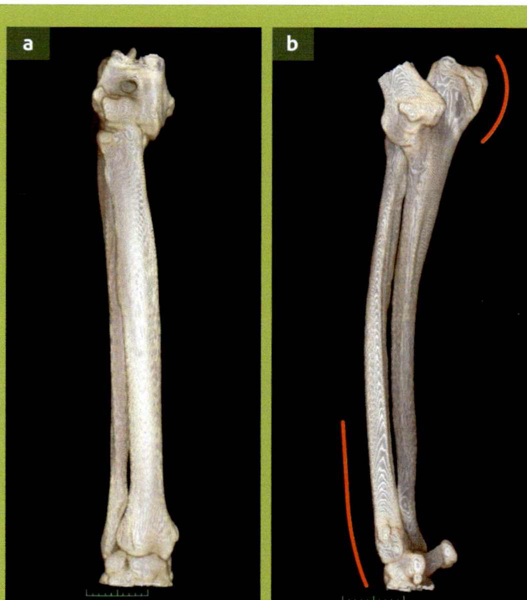

FIGURE 44. Three dimensional reconstruction of the radius and ulna using CT. The red lines represent the tension-bearing faces.

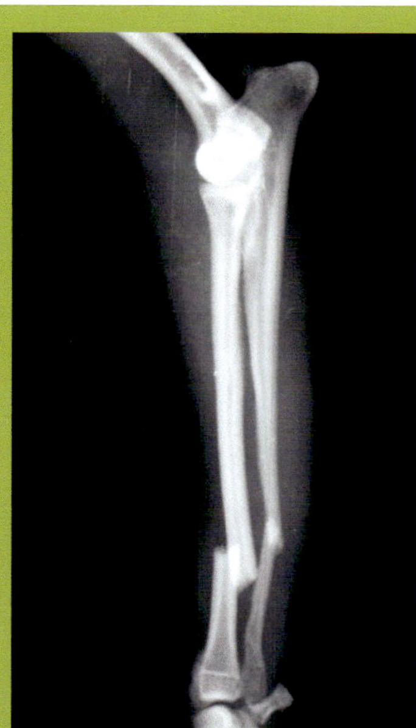

FIGURE 45. Transversal fracture of the radius and ulna. Observe the reduced diameter of the medullary cavity of the radius that makes intramedullary fixation a poor option.

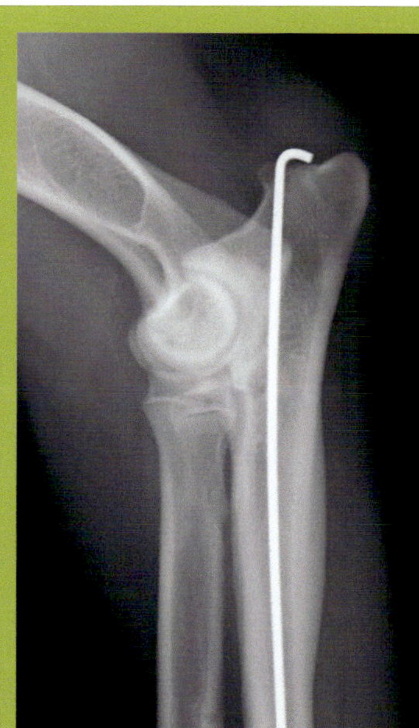

FIGURE 46. Intramedullary pin overlapping the proximal epiphysis of the ulna. The ulna has a wider medullary cavity that allows for the use of intramedullary implants.

Most of the non-unions that are observed in veterinary bone surgery are produced in fractures of the radius.

Stabilisation techniques

As previously mentioned, the diameter of the medullary cavity is one of the factors that determine which stabilisation technique to use. This way, the radius accepts all fixation systems except for intramedullary pins. Just the contrary takes place in the ulna, intramedullary pinning is the most used system for the few times that its stabilisation is needed.

Also, due to the lack of muscle mass and the possibility to effectively immobilise both joints in which the radius participates, external immobilisation using cast-type rigid bandages can be used occasionally to treat certain ulnar and radial fractures.

Fixation using intramedullary pins is not the best technique for radial fractures, however, it is ideal when a fractured ulna needs to be fixed.

External coaptation

In reality, radial and ulnar fractures that can be treated conservatively are scarce. To be able to consider this option, they must be highly stable fractures that affect young patients, in which fast healing processes compensate for the lack of stability of the fracture (Fig. 47).

Although infrequent, fractures can occur in the radius without affecting the ulna (Fig. 48), and vice versa. The fractures that only affect the ulnar diaphysis can be adequately treated using external immobilisation. In fractures that only affect the radius, the integrity of the ulna serves as an internal splint, which greatly decreases the movements of the fracture site in the radius, especially the collapsing during axial weight-bearing. If the ulna is not fractured, the possibilities for conservative treatment are greatly increased.

External coaptation is feasible in young patients that present highly stable fractures.

Conservative treatment should be carried out using bandages. There are many types of rigid bandages that are capable of stabilising the radius. Basically, all are based on the application of a light Robert-Jones bandage that covers from the distal portion of the forearm to above the elbow joint. The step to apply padding under the bandage is critical as an excess of material will allow for slight movements of the fracture site that can be counter-productive to the formation of the bone callus. After the padding, a rigid component must be applied, such as a splint, that will provide greater

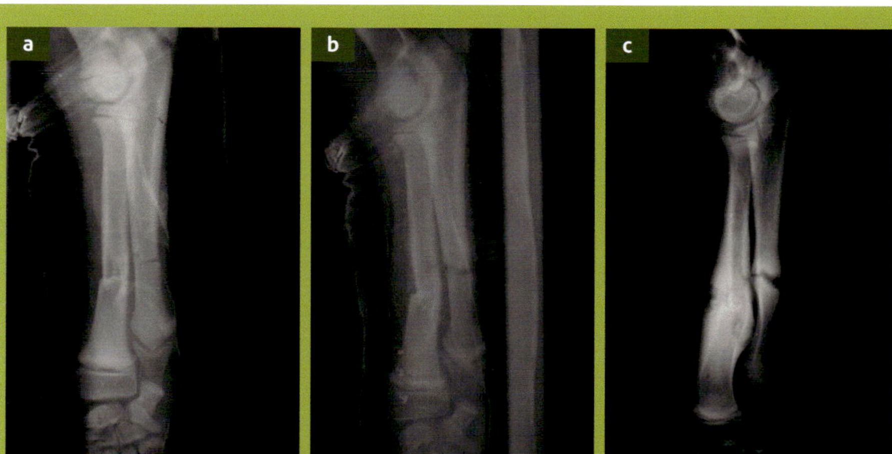

FIGURE 47. Fracture of the radius and ulna in a young patient without displacement (a), stabilised using a cast (b). Consolidated fracture after three months of treatment (c).

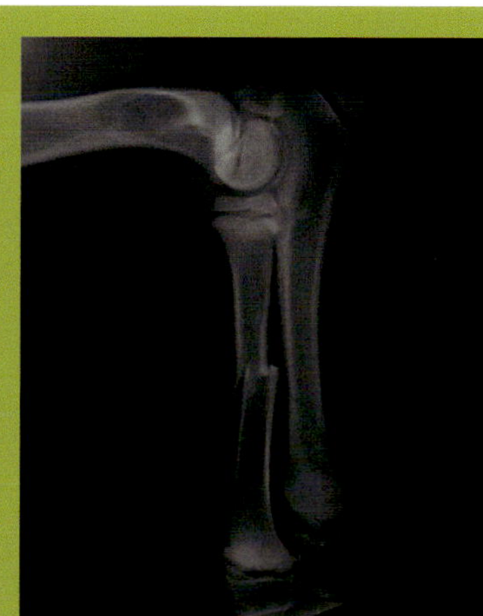

FIGURE 48. Fracture of the radius without affectation of the ulna.

Choice of treatment (surgical or conservative) in fractures of the radius depends on:

- Type of fracture.
- Location.
- Age of animal.
- Another series of factors (such as the affectation or lack thereof of both bones or habitat).

stability to the system. There are many types of splints, but the best are fibreglass casting tapes. This material is easy to use and adapts well to each patient. If great stability is needed, a complete bandage similar to traditional casts is ideal, while protecting the edges well using padding to avoid cutaneous lesions caused by rubbing.

In other cases, the application of a fibreglass splint is sufficient, preferably on the cranial portion of the radius to avoid possible rubbing with the carpal torus (padding of the accessory carpal bone). This option is much more comfortable for the patient (Fig. 49).

Intramedullary pinning

Intramedullary pinning in forearm fractures should preferably be used in those fractures that affect the ulna. The stabilisation of radial fractures using this system is not the best option due to the narrowness of the medullary cavity and because it does not completely stabilise the radius, a bone that is prone to suffering pseudoarthrosis. Also, as the fixation has to pass over one of the epiphyses, joint damage can easily be caused (Fig. 50).

In the ulnar fractures, the insertion of this type of implant is easily carried out starting at the olecranon in a normograde manner. Through a small incision in the caudal portion of the ulna, the fracture can be reduced perfectly to continue inserting the pin until anchoring it in the styloid process of the ulna once the pin has been introduced through the medullary cavity of the distal fragment. In small patients, in chondrodystrophic breeds and felines that have olecranons that are not as straight, it may be easier to introduce the pins in a retrograde manner.

External fixation

Almost all fractures that affect the radius can be treated using external fixation. The choice between this system and osteosynthesis plates is frequently the mere preference of the surgeon. That said, it must be taken into account that this external fixation system is not indicated in distal fractures in miniature breeds due to the high risk of non-union (Fig. 51). The principal advantage of external fixation compared to stabilisation using plates is the possibility to implant the fixators without opening the fracture site. No soft tissue is damaged in this process and thus the healing process is much faster. Due to the fact that no material is introduced in the fracture site, this system can be used in open fractures and those in which a great amount of soft tissue has been damaged or lost.

The radius accepts all possible configurations of external skeletal fixation, except for tie-in configurations.

As previously mentioned in the Osteosynthesis and Biomechanics chapter (page 34), the percutaneous pins must be introduced into the safe corridors, avoiding the areas with strong muscle masses. The most proximal reference point to insert the percutaneous pin is the lateral surface of the head of the radius. This point is easily identifiable as it can be palpated in a distal direction just beyond the lateral epicondyle of the humerus. In the case of having to insert the pin in a

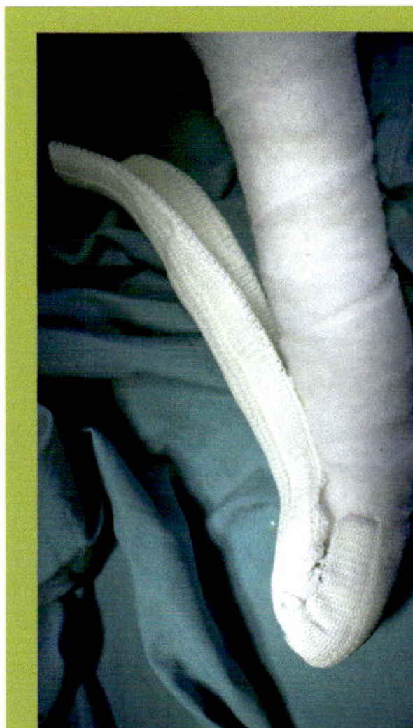

FIGURE 49. Fibreglass cast applied on the cranial surface of the radius.

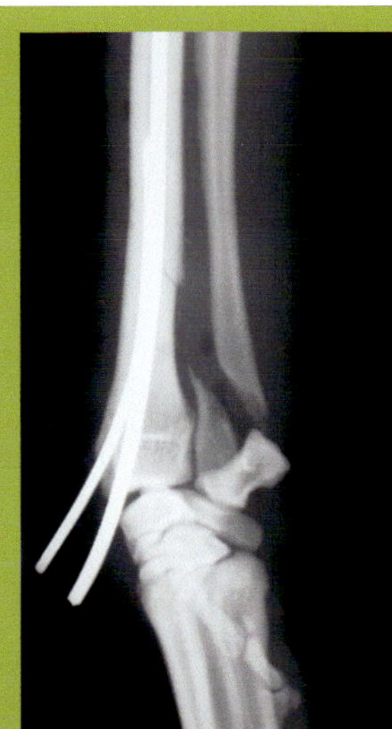

FIGURE 50. Intramedullary pins invading the carpal joint.

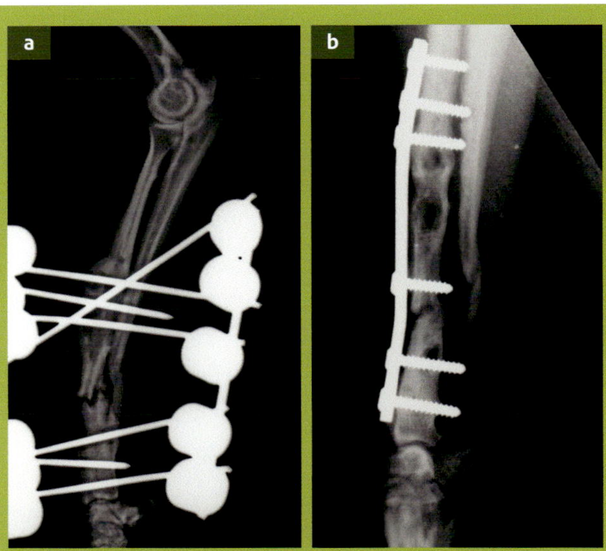

FIGURE 51. Non-union of a distal fracture in the radius due to inadequate implantation of external fixators (a).
The fracture was finally reduced through the implantation of an osteosynthesis plate (b).

more proximal location, it should be slightly oriented in a cranial direction to avoid contact with the proximal epiphysis of the ulna, which would cause pain to the animal when bearing weight on that limb. The distal screw, in turn, is inserted in a medial to lateral direction. Its insertion point is located by palpating the styloid apophysis which is found in a medial direction from the distal epiphysis of the radius. The direction of this pin depends basically on the type of fixator used. In the case of a one-plane or two-plane unilateral fixator, the direction is not important. On the contrary, if a type II or III fixation configuration is used, the same direction as the previously inserted percutaneous pin should be followed. The rest of the pins should be placed in the best position possible while working to insert them as close as possible to the fracture site (Fig. 52).

Osteosynthesis plates

Osteosynthesis plates are, for almost all surgeons specialised in bone surgery in small animals, the most adequate system to treat most radius fractures. Almost all plates that are applied to this zone can easily be applied through a dorsal approach that is made even easier with the cranial location of its tension-bearing surface (Fig. 53).

In distal fractures, they can also be placed on the medial surface of the bone (Fig. 54). With this placement, three effects are achieved:

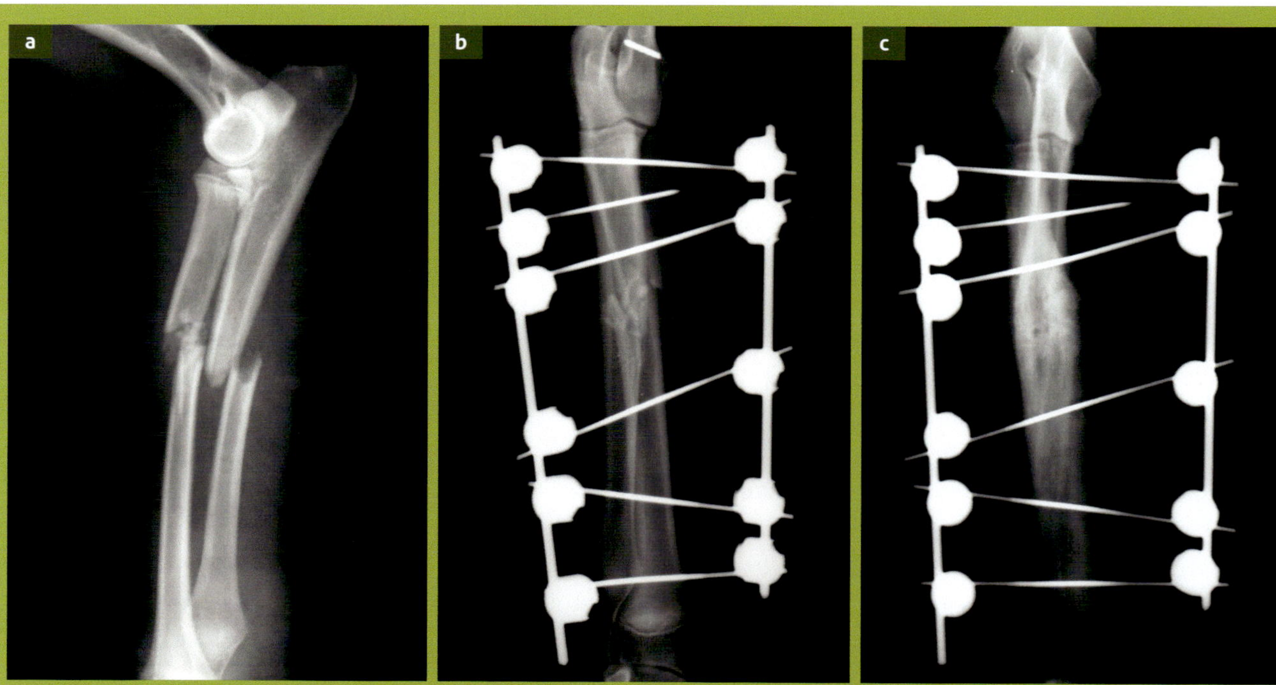

FIGURE 52. Transversal fracture of the ulna and radius (a) to which type II external fixation has been implanted (b). The fixator covers the entire length of the bone (c).

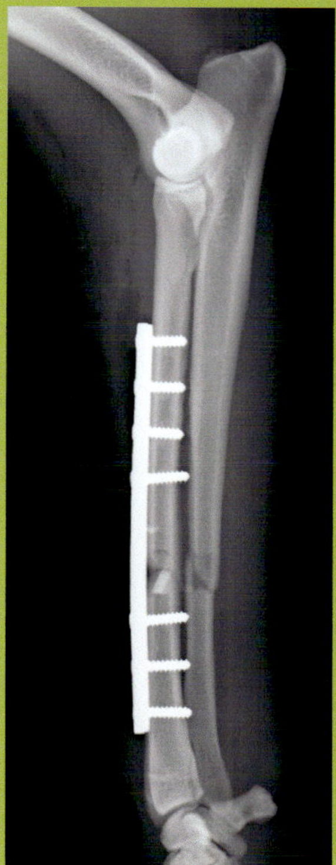

FIGURE 53. Osteosynthesis plate placed on the dorsal surface of the radius. Practically no moulding was necessary.

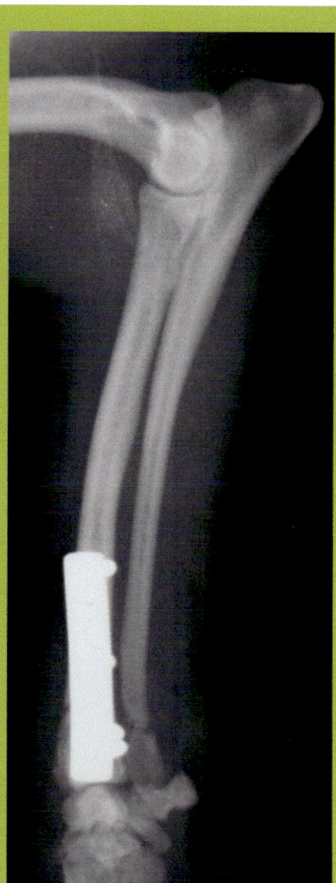

FIGURE 54. Osteosynthesis plate placed on the medial surface of the radius for the fixation of a distal fracture of the bone.

- Constant rubbing of the implant with the tendon of the extensor carpi radialis muscle is avoided, primarily in very distal fractures. This can be of great significance in working dogs (hunting or racing dogs).
- It allows more space for the screws due to the asymmetrical shape of the distal epiphysis of the radius.
- Smaller plates are used due to the location of the angled implant regarding the direction of the forces of flexion, which provides greater resistance against them. Also, as the holes are closer together, the plates need less bone length to be fastened with an adequate number of screws.

Chondrodystrophic breeds present certain cranial curvature of the distal third of the radius, which may complicate the placement of the osteosynthesis plate in the medial surface of the bone.

Due to the shape of the radius - practically straight in non-chondrodystrophic breeds -, the plate needs hardly any moulding (Fig. 53). Moulding it with a slight curve is only needed when the plate needs to be placed close to the epiphysis, or in a medial location.

Lastly, one of the intraoperative difficulties with this type of distal radius fractures is the scarcity of soft tissues for suturing; although it is important to avoid direct contact of the plate with the skin, sometimes there is no other option.

Surgical approach

Without doubt, the dorsal or dorso-medial approach is the most frequent to access the radius. First, due to the involvement of the skin, precaution must be taken to not go too deep to avoid sectioning the superficial cephalic vein. After moving the vein in a medial or lateral direction (according to the surgeon's preferences and the location of the fracture), the tendinous portion of the extensor carpi radialis muscle is moved to access the diaphysis of the radius. After this point, the approach is prolonged in a proximal or distal direction, depending on where the fracture is located (Fig. 55). Given the greater incidence of distal fractures, broadening the approach to the carpus is almost always necessary, that is, in a distal direction.

In some cases, it may be necessary to section the long abductor muscle of the first toe to facilitate treatment of the fracture as well as placement of the plate. This muscle has no important role in the functionality of the extremity and it can therefore be left without being sutured. However, whenever possible, it should be left intact to provide greater coverage to the plate after surgery.

On the few occasions when the proximal head of the radius must be reached, the approach is performed from the lateral side, being careful not to damage the radial nerve, that courses from the flexor carpi radialis muscle and is adhered to the supinator muscle (Fig. 56).

Regarding the ulna, the approach is performed in a caudal direction by palpating the edge of the bone that is covered only by skin and subcutaneous tissue. Using a periostotome, the extensor carpi ulnaris muscle is separated in a lateral direction and the digital flexor muscles in a medial direction, being careful not to damage the ulnar nerve (Fig. 56).

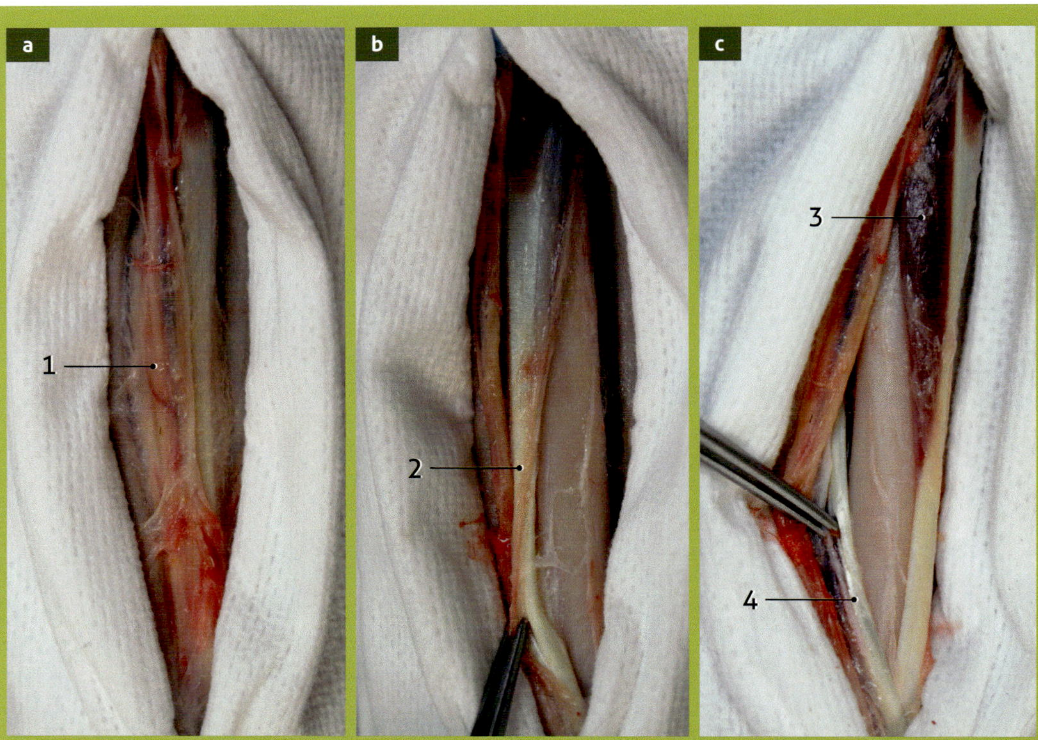

FIGURE 55. Medial and lateral approaches of the diaphysis of the radius. Dorsal incision (a), medial approach (b) and lateral approach (c).

1. Cephalic vein.
2. Extensor carpi radialis tendon.
3. Extensor carpi radialis muscle.
4. Tendon of the abductor of the first toe.

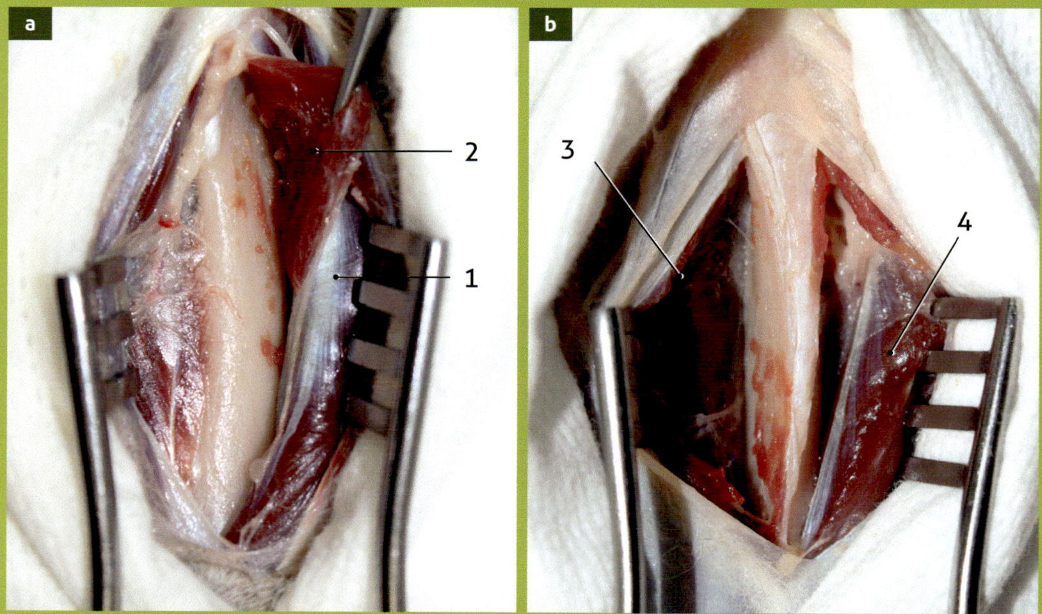

FIGURE 56. Lateral approach of the proximal head of the radius.

1. Extensor carpi radialis muscle.
2. Supinator muscle.
3. Flexor muscles.
4. Extensor carpi ulnaris muscle.

Treatment of the most frequent fractures of the radius

Fractures of the proximal epiphysis of the radius

Radius fractures in the proximal epiphysis and multiple fractures are infrequent in dogs and cats. When they occur, they are usually comminuted fractures of the proximal third of the bone.

> *Most fractures that affect the radius take place in the middle or distal third of the bone.*

In simple fractures, the best option for treatment is stabilisation using osteosynthesis plates applied to the craniolateral surface of the radius (Fig. 57).

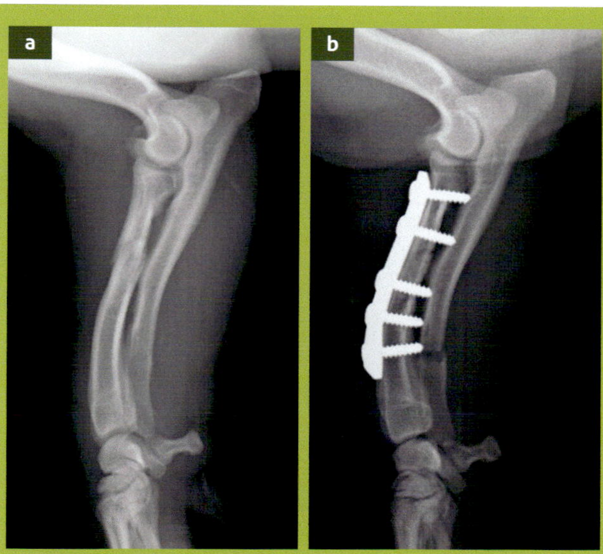

FIGURE 57. Proximal fracture of the radius in a chondrodystrophic dog (a) that has been fixated using an osteosynthesis plate on the cranio-lateral surface (b). Correctly moulding the plate is essential in these breeds.

In comminuted fractures, there are two possibilities: stabilisation using osteosynthesis plates, or by means of external fixation. The decision between one option or the other depends on various factors, but the most significant, aside from the patient's age, is the length of the proximal fragment. In this type of fractures, where there is no capacity of transmission of forces between the proximal and distal fragments, the lever forces applied by the plate on the fragments in which it will be anchored, increase considerably. For this reason, if the proximal fragment is short, there is a risk that the screws will loosen.

In the radius, unlike the humerus and the femur, any type of external fixation can be applied, and adequate stability can be achieved even in heavier patients and in fractures with a high degree of comminution (Fig. 58). In extreme cases in which the proximal fragment is not wide enough to place a minimum of two percutaneous pins, the possibility of creating a mixed configuration has been described using the fixator anchor in the proximal area of the ulna.

The union between the radius and the ulna near the elbow joint is very firm, thanks to the existence of the annular ligament. As the ulna cannot move in relation with the distal fragment of the radio, the fracture site suffers no significant excessive displacement.

On the other hand, and unlike the distal third, there is sufficient muscle mass in the proximal third of the radius that surrounds the bone, and thus the vascularisation provided allows for a vital contribution of cells responsible for the healing process during the first few days. For this reason, delays in healing are infrequent in fractures of the proximal third of the radius. Also, as external fixation can be applied without opening the fracture site, the iatrogenic damage to soft tissues is practically nonexistent, which aids in the further avoidance of problems with healing.

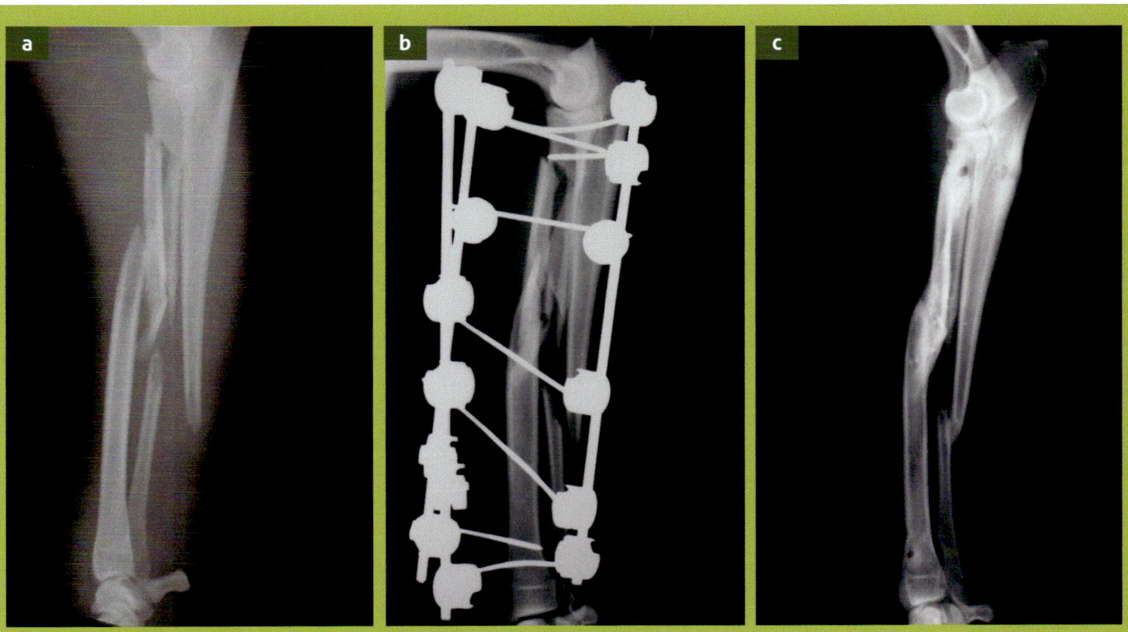

FIGURE 58. Extremely proximal comminuted fracture of the radius and ulna (a) treated with type III external fixators (b). The result obtained is acceptable (c).

One risk when percutaneous pins are placed in an extremely proximal location is the appearance of profuse bleeding a few days after surgery. This happens as a consequence of placing one of the pins too close to a vein due to the rubbing of the pin on the tunica adventitia. When the patient bears weight on the extremity, an aneurysm is formed that ruptures spontaneously after a few days. The bleeding is easily controlled by compression but, if the origin of the problem is not eliminated, it will happen again. In these cases, the percutaneous pin causing the bleeding must be removed and substituted by another pin, slightly modifying the entry point.

> *External fixation in a closed site reduces the risk of infection and avoids delays in the healing process.*

Fractures of the diaphysis of the radius

All fractures that affect this area can be treated both externally through external skeletal fixation, or internally, with osteosynthesis plates. The decision depends on the type of fracture as well as the surgeon's preferences. Normally, there are no problems of having enough space in this location to place an adequate number of screws in both of the primary fragments, and thus fixation using plates is usually the most indicated option (Figs. 59 and 60).

The surgical approach of the diaphysis of the radius is not difficult. However, the correct positioning of the patient is key to be able to easily manipulate the fractured limb. There are two options:

- Place the patient in a supine position with the extremity extended towards the posterior third.
- Place the patient in a sphinx position with the front paws resting on the table. To keep the anaesthetised animal in this position, its head must be held using a bar at a height that keeps its humerus bones in a vertical position (Fig. 61). This position allows for greater precision and comfort when perforating the holes as the animal's forearms are firmly resting on the table.

Logically, the function of the implant depends basically on the type of fracture being treated. Rigid osteosynthesis systems are not recommended for multiple fractures of the radius as the use of cerclages presents difficulty due to the flat shape of the bone, which can also complicate the tightening of the wires.

> *The flat shape of the radius makes the tightening of the wires in rigid osteosynthesis systems difficult, and therefore, the use of cerclages is not recommended.*

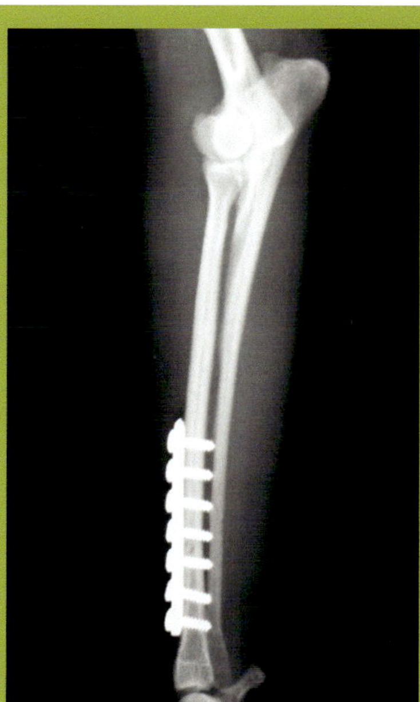

FIGURE 59. Compression plate in a transversal radius fracture.

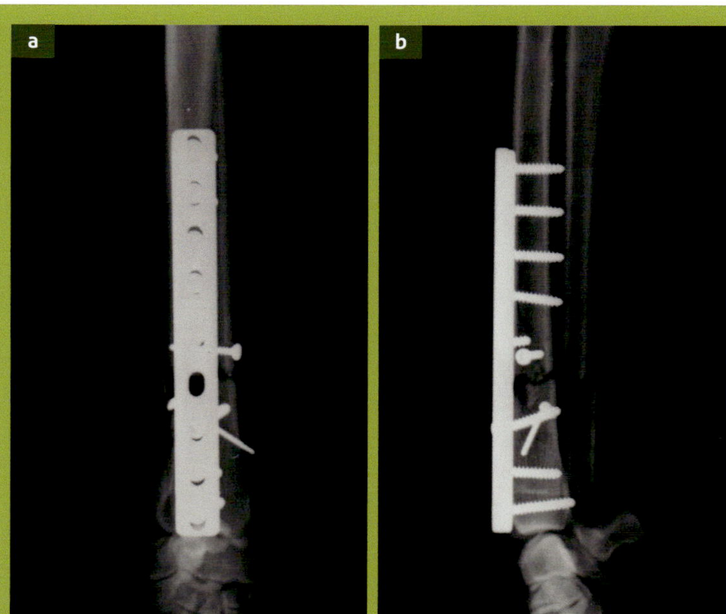

FIGURE 60. Neutralisation plate in a multiple radius fracture. Dorso-palmar view (a) and latero-lateral view (b).

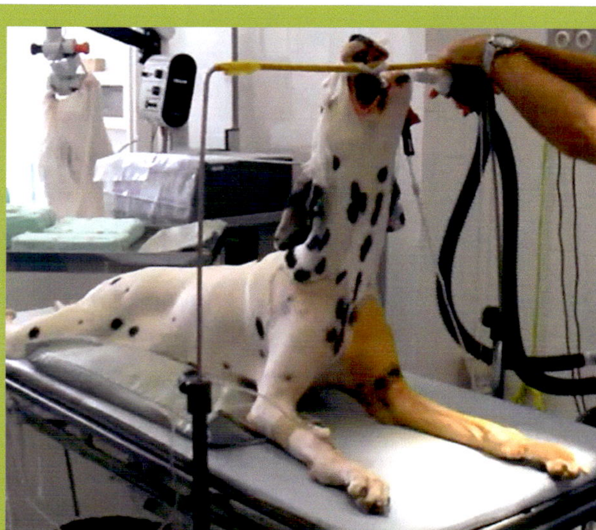

FIGURE 61. Patient in sphinx position to operate in a comfortable position on a radius fracture.

In miniature breeds, one of the problems when treating fractures of the distal third of the radius is the appearance of "protection stress". Due to deficient vascularisation and a decrease in the weight-bearing on the radius - as this is absorbed by the implant -, the bone suffers a process of halisteresis, that is, the progressive loss of bone mass (Fig. 62). This loss of mass can lead to bone reabsorption and posterior disappearance of bone tissue. If this is detected, the implant must be removed as soon as possible. To do so, the screws must be removed progressively, eventually leaving the plate with no screws. The plate is left as an internal splint given that the simultaneous extraction of the plate and the screws would leave the bone unprepared for physiological weight-bearing, with its respective risk of new fractures. Once the bone has recovered its normal density, the implant can be completely removed (Fig. 63).

Fractures of the distal epiphysis

The fractures of the distal epiphysis of the radio are more frequent in cats, after falls from great heights, and in dogs of miniature breeds.

As a general rule, whenever a young animal with a distal fracture in the forearm is attended to, the owners should be informed about the possibility of alterations of the bone growth.

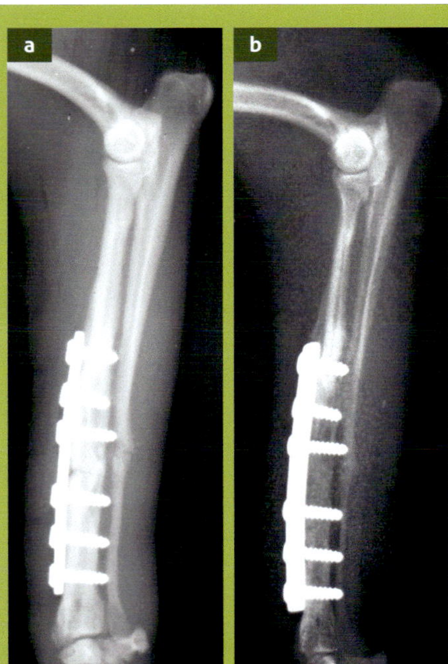

FIGURE 62. Loss of bone mass (halisteresis) due to protection stress.
Progressive bone density lose is visible between (a) and (b).

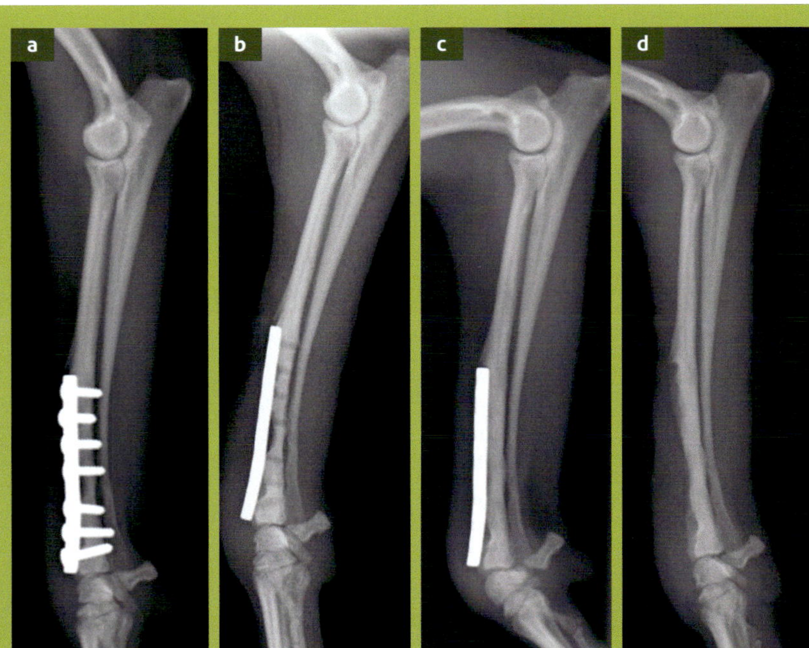

FIGURE 63. Progressive dynamisation of an osteosynthesis plate to avoid repeated fractures. First the screws are removed (a) and the plate is left as an internal splint to stimulate osteosynthesis (b and c). Later, the plate is removed (d).

This typology of fractures of the distal third should be treated under the same precepts as diaphyseal fractures, as long as they are not excessively distal, in which case the surgeon will find the same disadvantages as those in fractures of the proximal third.

Unlike the case with proximal fractures, the implantation of external fixators is not recommended in this type of fractures, especially in small breeds. As previously mentioned, the reason is the precariousness regarding its vascularisation due to the lack of well-irrigated muscle mass, where complications could arise with processes of bone halisteresis. Also, most distal fractures at this level are simple, and thus stability should be maximum, which is harder to achieve through external fixation. This does not mean that correct healing of the bone cannot be achieved if structures such as type III fixators that provide great stability are used (Fig. 64).

In the case of very distal fractures, in which there is not enough space to place three screws as recommended by the AO technique, there are various options:

- Place only two screws in the distal fragment. This option is only recommended in cases of fractures that are sufficiently transversal to apply static compression using a plate. When compressing the fracture, the stability needed is achieved so that all forces of flexion can be supported by just two screws (Fig. 65).
- Place only two screws in the distal plate with a locking osteosynthesis plate. As previously explained in the corresponding chapter (page 94), this is a safer option as when the screw is fastened not only to the bone but also to the plate, only two screws are needed to achieve adequate stability (Fig. 66).
- Place the plate on the medial surface of the radius, where a small amount of space is gained, not only due to the location, but to the possibility to use an implant with screws with a smaller diameter (Fig. 67).
- Place one plate on the radius, and another on the ulna. The combination of both plates provides magnificent stability to the bones together, where two screws placed on the distal portion of the radius are enough to correctly neutralise the forces (Fig. 68).

There are plates on the market that are designed to fit a greater number of screws in a smaller bone space. To achieve this objective, the plates are symmetrical and they have one end that is wider than the other, this way the holes are parallel to each other (Fig. 69). The most common are called T plates due to their shape. These implants are located under the extensor tendons and their horizontal edge levels with the most distal portion of the radius, where three screws can fit in

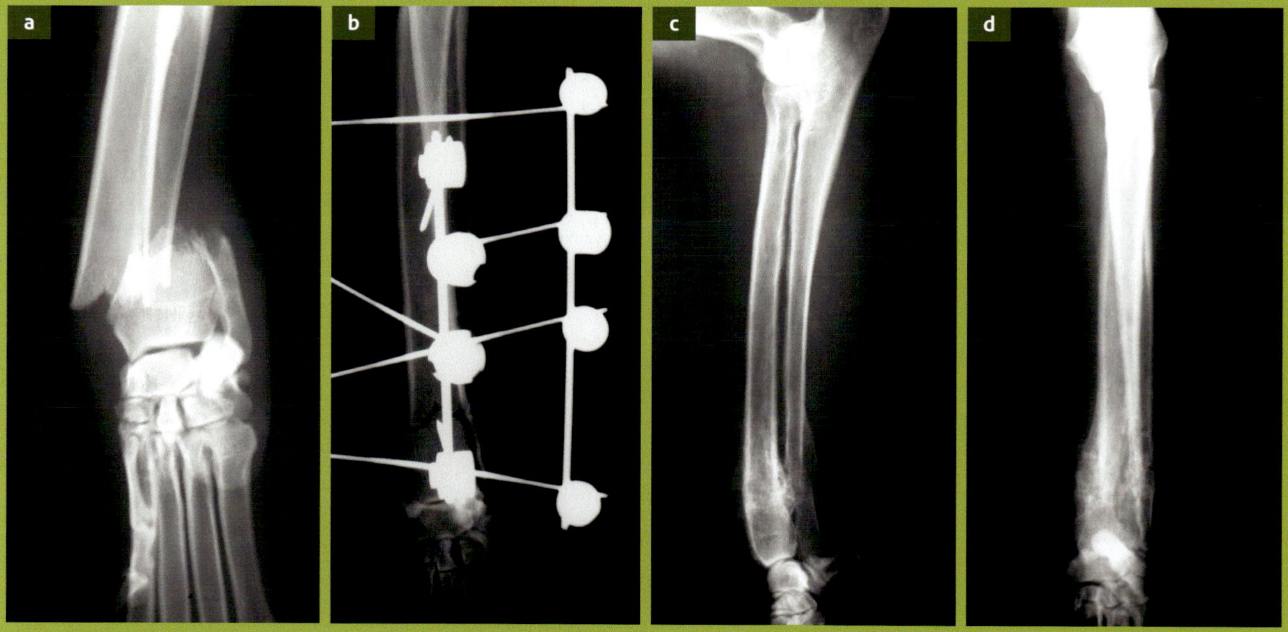

FIGURE 64. Distal transversal fracture of the radius (a) treated with three-dimensional external fixation (b). If good stability is achieved, the postoperative results are good (c and d).

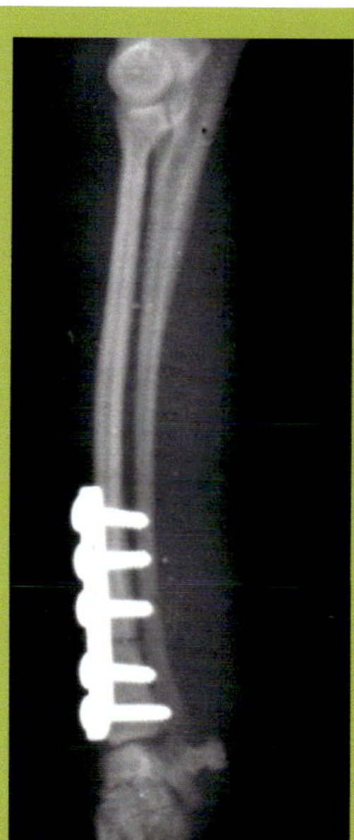

FIGURE 65. Transversal radius fracture stabilised using two screws in the distal fragment.

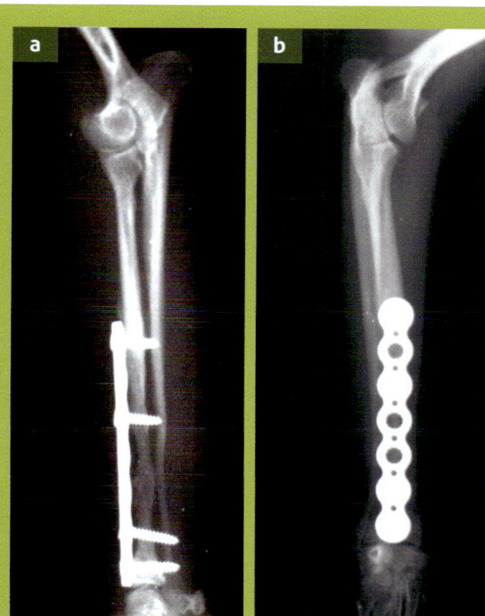

FIGURE 66. Medio-lateral view (a) and dorso-medial view (b) of a locking plate stabilised using two screws on each side.

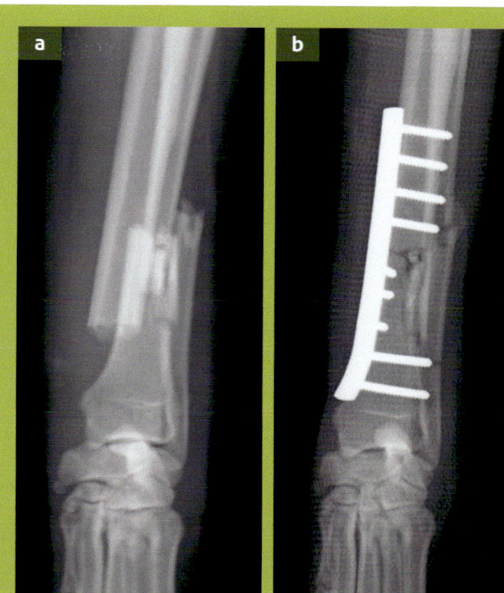

FIGURE 67. Distal radius fracture (a) stabilised using a plate placed on the medial surface of the radius (b), which allows for the use of screws with a smaller diameter.

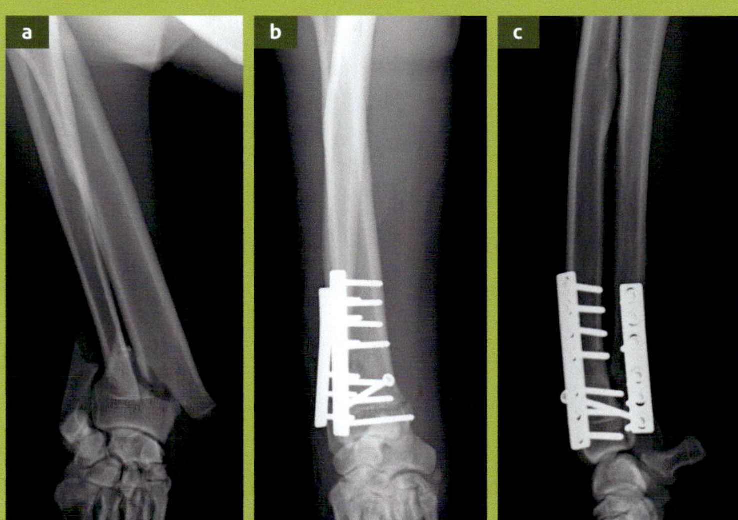

FIGURE 68. Extremely distal radius fracture (a) stabilised using small plates applied to the radius and ulna. Caudo-cranial view (b) and latero-lateral view (c).

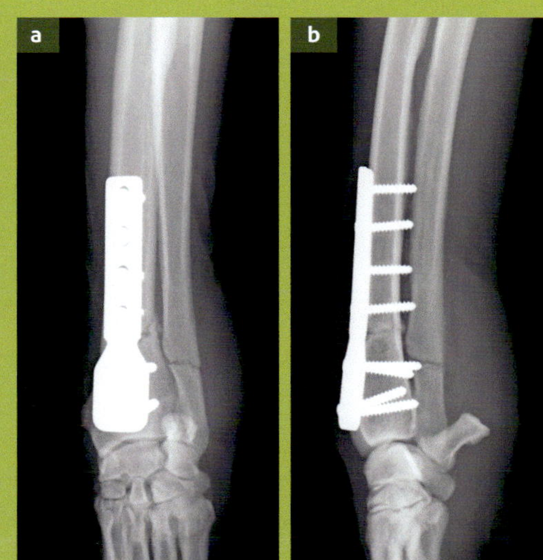

FIGURE 69. Cobra-type plate to stabilise a distal radius fracture.

one smaller bone fragment. Traditionally, human bone plates have been used that were meant for hand surgeries, but these implants have a very thin profile and sometimes break (Fig. 70). Currently, there are T plates designed specifically for veterinary purposes with a thicker profile and a slightly triangular shape, instead of a strict T shape, which provides greater resistance (Fig. 71).

Salter-Harris fracture of the distal epiphysis of the radius

Type I Salter Harris fractures are more frequent in felines. The fracture is produced at the level of the distal growth plate of the radius (Fig. 72). These fractures should be treated as soon as possible to achieve a correct reduction, especially if the fracture affects the distal growth plate of the radius.

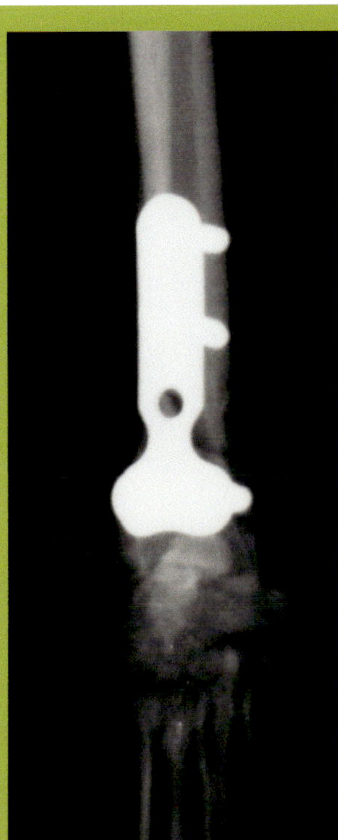

FIGURE 70.
T plate for bone surgery in humans.

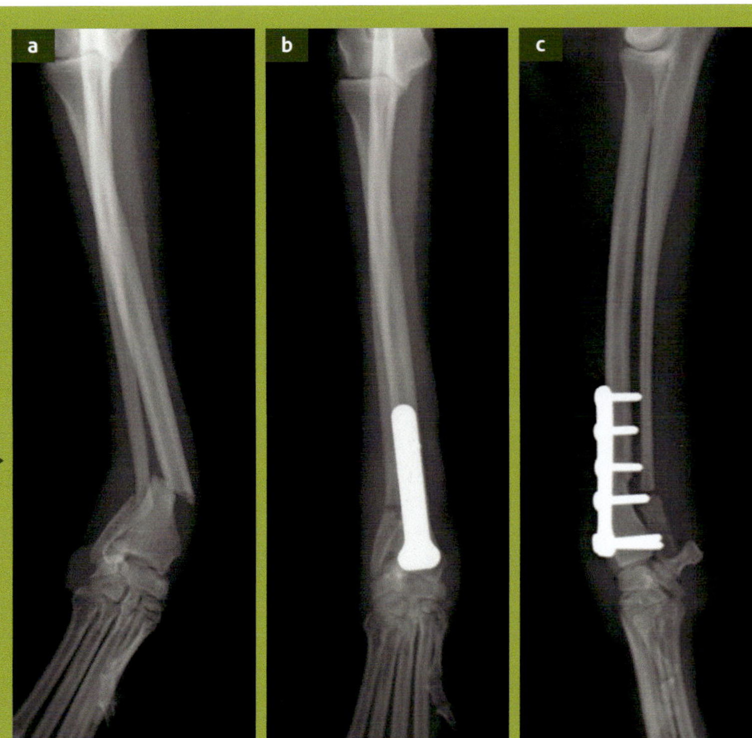

FIGURE 71.
T plate specifically made for veterinary bone surgery, which is thicker and presents a more triangular profile.

If various days have passed since the fracture, the tendons of the extensor muscles, the frequently associated ulnar fracture and the small size of the distal fragment make its reduction considerably complicated and the correct implantation of the implants complex.

Treatment consists of the insertion of two pins on both sides of the distal epiphysis of the radius oriented towards the diaphysis of the radius, once the fracture is reduced (Fig. 73). Due to the small size of the medullary cavity of this bone, which is practically nonexistent in the distal portion in small breeds, the pins function like Rush pins. That is, the growth of this plate and, therefore, of the bone at this level, will be neutralised. Normally, this does not impede any functionality of the limb thanks to the vicarious growth of the proximal plate of the radius and to the possibility to extend the angle of flexion of the elbow and shoulder when bearing weight. When dealing with patients that are still growing, it must be taken into account that the growth plate of the ulna may be damaged as a result of the trauma, which causes the premature closing of the distal epiphysis and consequent appearance of radius curvus. In the case of patients with a great growing potential - young animals or large breeds -, it may be helpful to perform a preventive ulnar ostectomy (Fig. 74).

Treatment of the most frequent fractures of the ulna

When either the radius or the ulna are fractured, the latter does not usually need treatment as long as the radius can be adequately stabilised. Surgery is not normally needed when only the diaphysis of the ulna has been fractured, however, intramedullary fixation helps to stabilise the fracture (Fig. 75). There are, nonetheless, certain fractures that always require treatment due to their location.

Fractures of the olecranon

The fractures of the olecranon are usually due to avulsion and thus require correct stabilisation. Tension band systems are the most frequently used systems to treat this type of fractures. They allow for the transformation of forces of traction into compressive forces that accelerate the healing process.

For a correct surgical approach, the patient should be placed in a supine position with the elbow flexed 90°. In this position, the surgical approach is very simple as the proximal epiphysis of the ulna can easily be palpated. Also, both the reduction of the fracture and the placement of the implants are more easier.

Once the fracture is identified, it is then reduced while being careful to cause the minimal amount of damage to soft

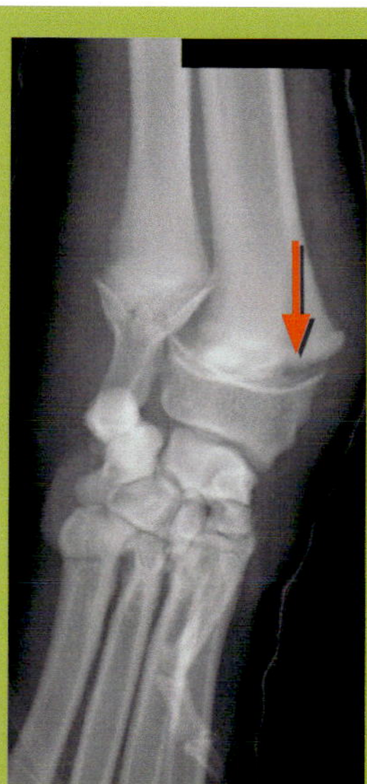

FIGURE 72. Type I Salter-Harris fracture of the distal epiphysis of the radius. The arrow points at the fracture line in the growth plate.

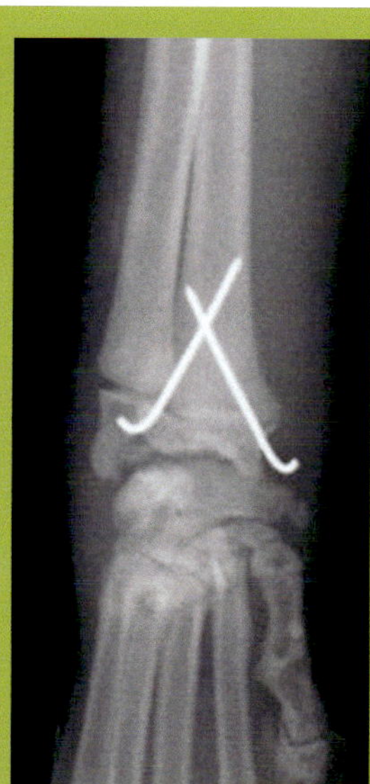

FIGURE 73. Stabilisation of a type I Salter Harris fracture using Rush pins.

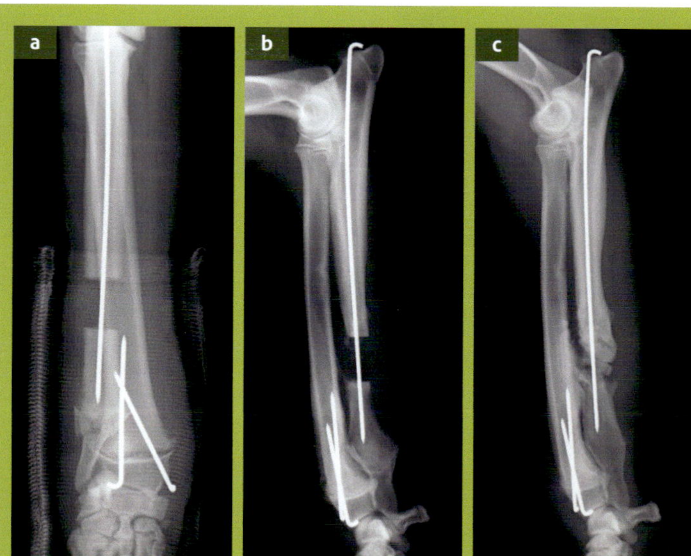

FIGURE 74. Preventive ostectomy of the ulna to avoid radius curvus (a and b) and its postoperative progress (c).

tissues and avoid over-manipulation. If the surgeon decides to insert the pins in a retrograde manner, they should be inserted through the fracture site. Once the fracture is reduced, the pins are inserted towards the medullary cavity (Fig. 76). The pins do not need to be inserted excessively given that their function is to avoid the rotation and lateral displacement of the fragments, as well as acting as an anchor for the wire. Next, a hole is made in the distal fragment close to the fracture line, being careful to leave a margin towards the edge of the fracture as well as the caudal compact bone of the ulna. The wire should not break the bone tissue near the fracture plane when the contraction of the triceps muscle tractions the wire. Later, the cerclage is passed through the hole and both ends are crossed over the caudal compact bone of the ulna. One of the ends is then placed in front of the part that overlaps the pins and the tension band is tightened by tying one end with the other under traction (Fig. 77). Lastly, the pins are bent and cut, and the "hooks" created are oriented in a cranial direction to hold the wire (Fig. 78). To finalise, the wound is sutured by layers.

In fractures of the olecranon with more than two fragments, and primarily in those in which one or more of the fragments are located in the cranial area of the ulna, stabilisation using pins with tension bands may be insufficient. By transforming the forces of traction into forces of compression, the pins with tension bands cause the forces to be concentrated principally in the cranial area of the ulna. Any loose fragments in this area would move, causing the fracture site to become unstable. In these specific cases, it is better to apply a treatment using osteosynthesis plates placed on the caudal surface of the ulna (tension-bearing surface of the bone). Depending on the position in which the fracture is found, the plate should be placed in a more or less proximal position (Fig. 79). In the case of very proximal fractures, it is helpful to fold the implant to accommodate the olecranon and insert the screws in different directions to avoid their ends coming into contact with each other (Fig. 80).

Another possible option is to place the plate on the lateral or medial surface of the ulna. This way, with the angled plate, the implant acts in a stable manner against the forces of traction produced by the triceps muscle (Fig. 81).

Monteggia fracture

The Monteggia fracture is a combination of a fracture of the middle or proximal third of the ulna associated with a cranial dislocation of the head of the radius (Fig. 82).

Treatment consists of stabilising the ulnar fracture using intramedullary pinning or plates, depending on the type of fracture. If the radius is not fractured, the osteosynthesis system applied in the ulna does not need to be especially powerful. Its function is basically to keep the fracture site from collapsing and to place the radius back in its place.

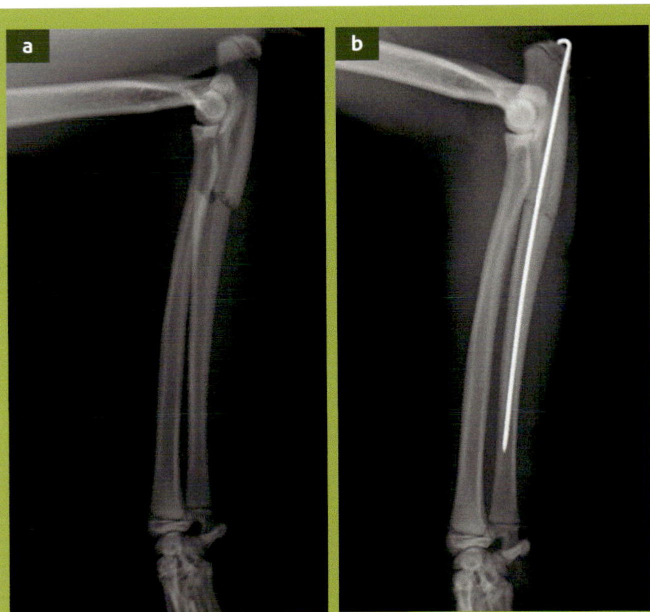

FIGURE 75. Proximal fracture of the ulna (a) treated with intramedullary fixation (b).

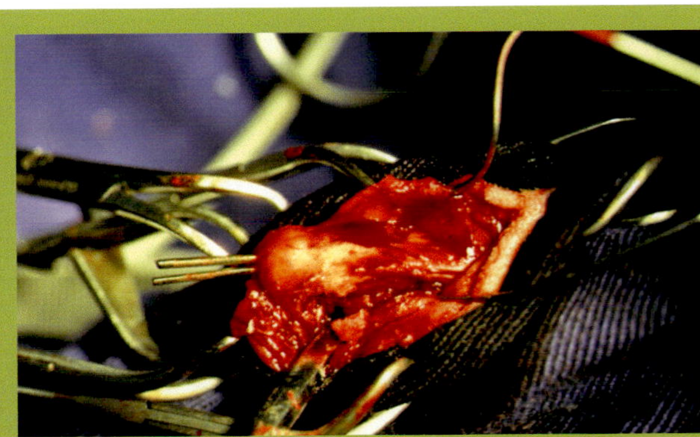

FIGURE 76. Pins inserted with the elbow flexed towards the medullary cavity in the surgical resolution of an ulnar fracture.

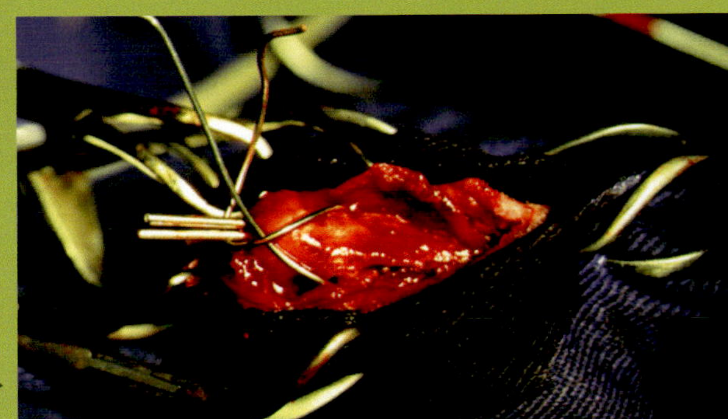

FIGURE 77. Cerclage applied around the pins in the ulnar fracture of Fig. 76.

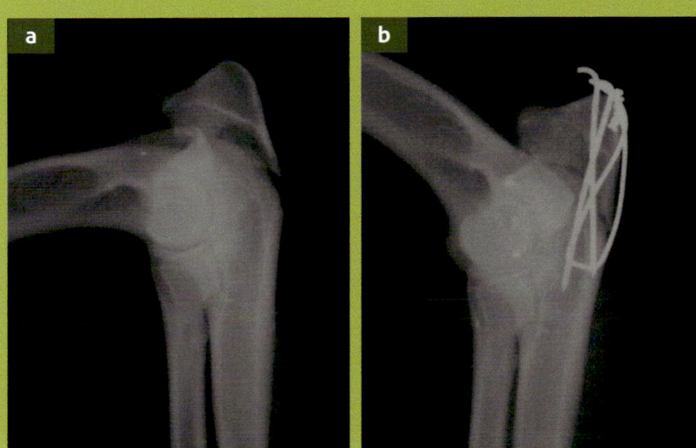

FIGURE 78. Application of pins with a tension band to stabilise a fracture of the olecranon..

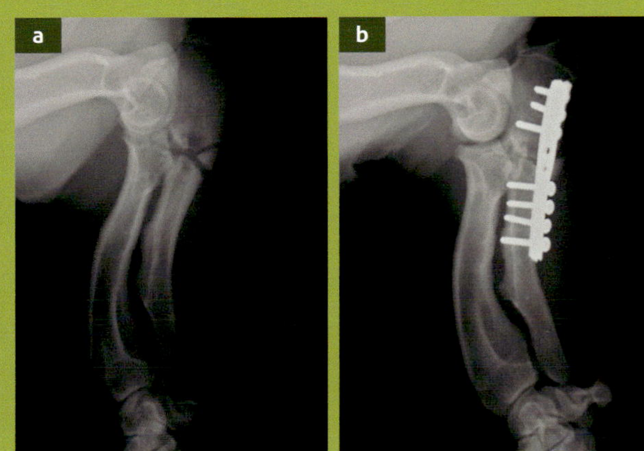

FIGURE 79. Ulnar fracture (a) stabilised using a plate in a proximal and caudal position (b).

In order to stabilise the cranial dislocation of the radius, after stabilisation, the function of the annular ligament must be substituted artificially. This ligament hugs the head of the radius in a cranial direction and it inserts into both sides of the proximal portion of the ulna, allowing for slight movements of both bones.

There are two options to substitute the function of the annular ligament:

- The first consists of applying a screw from the ulna to the radius, anchoring both bones. This avoids displacement of the radius in a cranial direction. This system is not recommended in cats as firmly fastening the radius with the ulna impedes the physiological movements of displacement between the two bones which are inherent to felines, which would make movements of pronation and supination that are necessary to this species

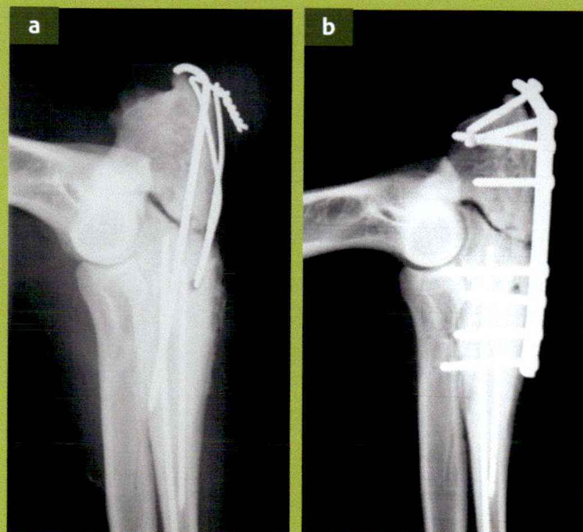

FIGURE 80. Erroneous implantation of pins with tension bands (a) stabilised with a caudal plate in an excessively proximal position (b).

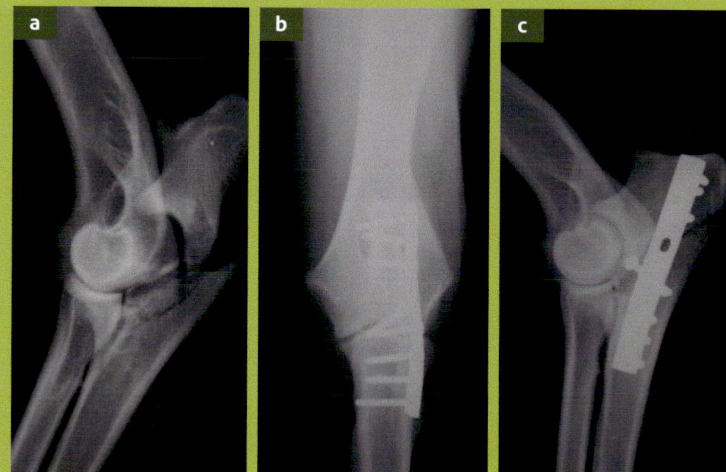

FIGURE 81. Multiple fracture in the joint portion of the ulna (a). Anterior fracture stabilised using a medial neutralisation plate associated with a compression screw to stabilise the articular fragment (b and c).

very difficult. Dogs, however, better tolerate this system as their forearms have more limited movement between the ulna and the radius, although the screws implanted always end up breaking due to wear.

- The second option, which is more recommended, is to place a cerclage that surrounds the radius and the ulna from the metaphyseal area, right where the ligament is located. To do so, a cerclage wire or another nonmetallic synthetic material can be used, making sure that the medial or radial nerves are not trapped between the radius and the cerclage. If it is trapped, when tightening the cerclage, the nerve could be badly damaged. It must be taken into account that the objective is not to perform compression of one bone on the other as if it were a fracture, but that the cerclage should be adjusted to allow the physiological movements of one bone over the other, but without allowing for the radius to move in a cranial direction (Fig. 83).

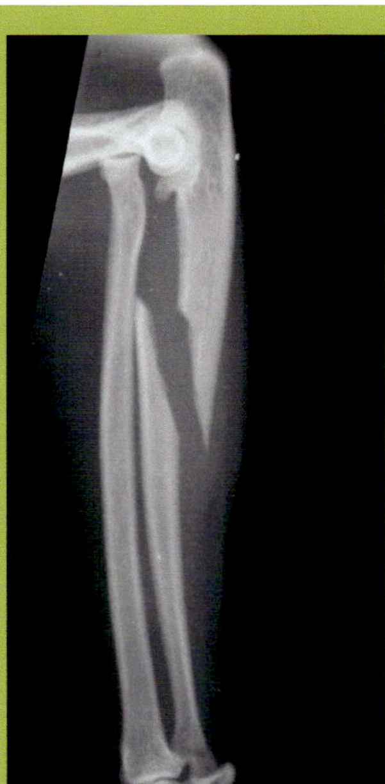

FIGURE 82. Monteggia fracture (fracture of the proximal third of the ulna associated with the cranial dislocation of the head of the radius).

FIGURE 83. X-rays that show the treatment applied to the fracture in Fig. 82. Cerclage implanted around the radius and ulna associated with another cerclage and intramedullary pinning. Caudo-cranial view (a) and latero-lateral view (b).

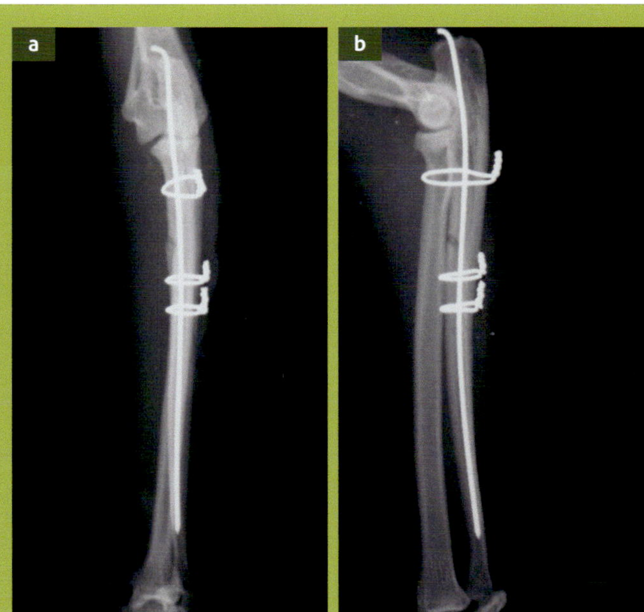

CARPAL FRACTURES

Fortunately, the lesions of the bones of carpal joint are not frequent. This joint, as is the case with the tarsus, tolerates secondary joint degeneration poorly that usually derives from these types of lesions. For this reason, the definitive solution of carpal injuries is performing a pancarpal or carpometacarpal arthrodesis. If the surgeon believes that the radiocarpal joint, which is responsible for the 90° joint movement of the carpus, can be saved, the best option is to perform only a carpometacarpal arthrodesis (Fig. 84). Pancarpal arthrodesis basically consists of fusing the radius, the carpal bones and the metacarpal bones to form one single bone, in order to impede movement capacity of the joint to eliminate the pain caused by the arthrosis.

It must be taken into account that the carpus is the joint that presents the best prognosis when immobilised through arthrodesis as it maintains an angle similar to that used when the extremity is placed on the ground (close to 180°), allowing for ideal weight bearing (Fig. 85). When walking, the patient flexes the elbow and the shoulder slightly more to compensate for the lack of flexion of the carpus, but this posture allows for the patient to carry out a completely normal life at all times, showing hardly any signs of it while moving. An assessment should be made regarding whether it is worth it or not to perform a pancarpal arthrodesis as a first option depending on the possibilities of recovery with reconstructive surgical techniques. The best option is to perform surgical techniques that, if they fail, can be resolved through arthrodesis of the joint, but this will depend greatly on the owner's preferences.

> *A large number of fractures that affect the carpus can be corrected through surgery.*

Carpal injuries can be divided into three large groups:

- Fractures of the distal head of the radius.
- Fractures of the radial carpal bone.
- Dislocation of the radial carpal bone.

Fractures of the distal head of the radius

This type of injuries are infrequent in pets. Generally, they are caused by a strong impact to the distal portion of the extremity which is transmitted through the metacarpal bones producing a sharp blow from the radial carpal bone on the joint surface of the radius. This type of lesions are almost always caused from falls from great heights.

The diagnosis is very simple. The patient presents a limp without bearing weight, that appears suddenly, with prior trauma. The definitive diagnosis is made through an X-ray

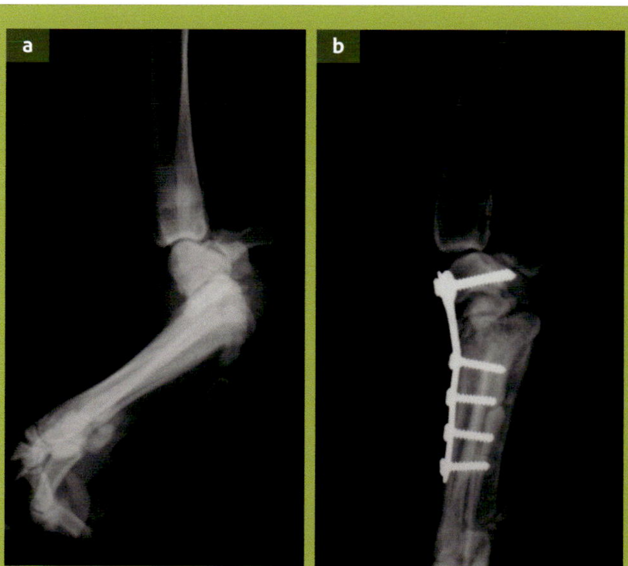

FIGURE 84. Carpometacarpal arthrodesis. Image of the fracture (a) and its treatment by means of arthrodesis (b).

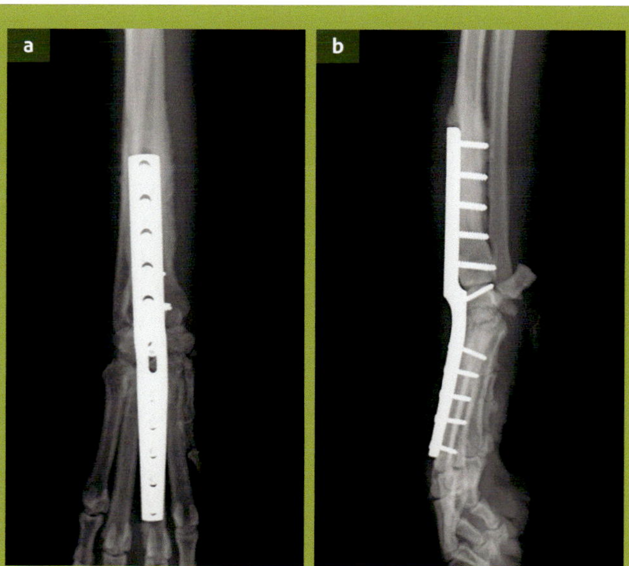

FIGURE 85. Pancarpal arthrodesis. Caudo-cranial view (a) and latero-lateral view (b).

exam (Fig. 86). It is important that the study be performed with the animal under general anaesthesia to be able to carry out stress X-rays. This way, along with being able to evaluate the severity of the bone lesions, the integrity of the joint ligaments can also be confirmed (Fig. 87). Joint ligament lesions will require modifications to treatment and determine whether arthrodesis can be considered as an option or not.

When the surgeon plans treatment for a fracture of the distal head of the radius, he or she must consider the possibilities of recovery of the extremity. When faced with a joint fracture, he/she must take into account that these are frequently associated with lesions of the interosseous ligaments that are difficult to assess and worsen the prognosis.

The treatment of fractures of the distal head of the radius is the same as that implemented for any joint fracture. First of all, the fragments must be perfectly reduced to obtain a continuous joint surface with no defects. Otherwise, the possibilities of secondary joint degenerative processes are very high. The fragments are stabilised using traction screws, or in the case of very small fragments, with pins.

The biggest problem of stabilisation with Kirschner pins is that they can break when the patient begins to bear weight on the extremity.

Once the joint surface is repaired, the metaphyseal fracture is reduced and stabilised. In these cases, the surgeon is faced with the additional problem of lack of space to place the osteosynthesis plates; frequently, the only option is to stabilise using pins.

Once the bone is reconstructed, and given that minimal osteosynthesis has been performed, a system to reinforce the stabilisation systems used must be applied. For this purpose, there are rigid bandage systems or temporary transarticular external fixation systems (Fig. 88). The choice of which system to use depends, primarily, on the stability achieved and the size of the patient. In the case of insufficient stability and in large breeds, the use of a transarticular external fixator for two to three weeks is a better choice given that the external stability achieved using bandages is always less and may cause *débricolage* of the fracture.

As previously mentioned, if the intervention fails or if the prognosis is poor, the joint should be permanently immobilised by means of pancarpal arthrodesis.

Fractures of the radial carpal bone

This type of fracture is primarily produced in animals subjected to high physical stress, such as dogs used for sledding, competitions or hunting, as a consequence of jumping or specific overstrain. The fracture is caused by the combination of sudden pressure and shear strain.

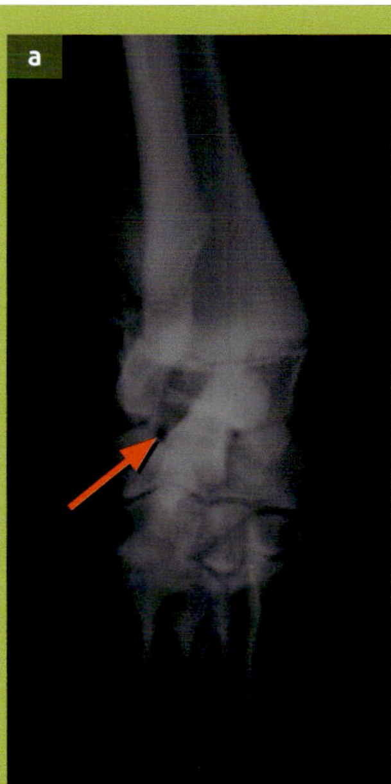

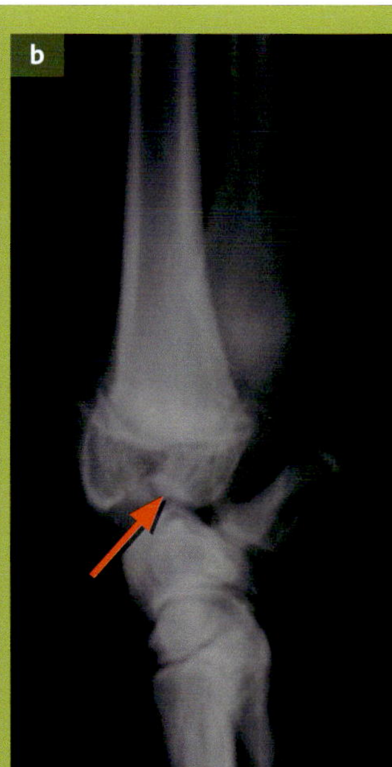

FIGURE 86. Cranio-caudal view (a) and latero-lateral view (b) where a fracture of the distal epiphysis of the radius is observed.

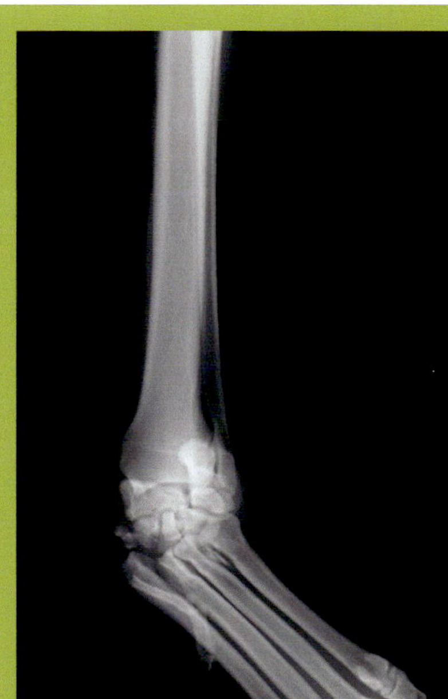

FIGURE 87. Stress X-ray to confirm the possible rupture associated with medial collateral ligaments.

The typical fractures are usually detachment of small fragments in the cranial area of the radial carpal bone, caused by the impact that said bone suffers against the radius or the bones of the second line of the carpus. Another typical fracture is that produced in the middle of the bone, just underneath the styloid process of the distal head of the radius (Fig. 89).

Frequently, these fractures are not easily identified if little time has passed since the trauma due to the structures that surround this bone and keep it under pressure. However, a few days later, as a result of the processes of reabsorption that take place along the edges of the fracture, it becomes more visible. For this reason, when there are suspicions of a fracture of the radial carpal bone and it cannot be identified by X-ray, an X-ray should be repeated a few days later. A CT scan can be performed on the first day to clear up any doubts the surgeon may have.

Treatment of the fractures of the radial carpal bone must always be surgical.

Once the cranio-medial approach of the joint is performed, the size of the fragments should be confirmed. If they are small, they should be removed as long as they do not directly affect the weight-bearing areas; if their size is adequate, treatment consists of fixating them using compression screws. For these interventions, 1.5 to 2 mm screws are usually used.

In the case of transversal fractures of the radial carpal bone, the surgical approach is similar to that used for fractures of the humerus condyle. That is, a sliding hole must be made from the fracture plane. Later, the fracture should be reduced and the compression screw inserted (Fig. 90). Achieving proper reduction of the fracture to avoid irregularities in the joint surface is of great importance. Sometimes, it is impossible to recognise by X-ray all of the lesions that have been produced (Fig. 91).

Once the intervention has been completed, the joint should be temporarily immobilised. For this type of fracture, the application of a rigid bandage is preferable to the use of a transarticular external fixator. As this is a joint fracture, excessively rigid stabilisation is not ideal, as long as proper stability has been achieved through the use of osteosynthesis systems.

In cases in which the radial carpal fracture is too comminuted, or in those in which the desired results are not obtained through surgery, a pancarpal arthrodesis should be performed.

Dislocation of the radial carpal bone

This lesion, caused by falls from height in which the patient lands on its front limbs, is infrequent. The trauma is similar to that produced in cases of carpal dislocations and fractures,

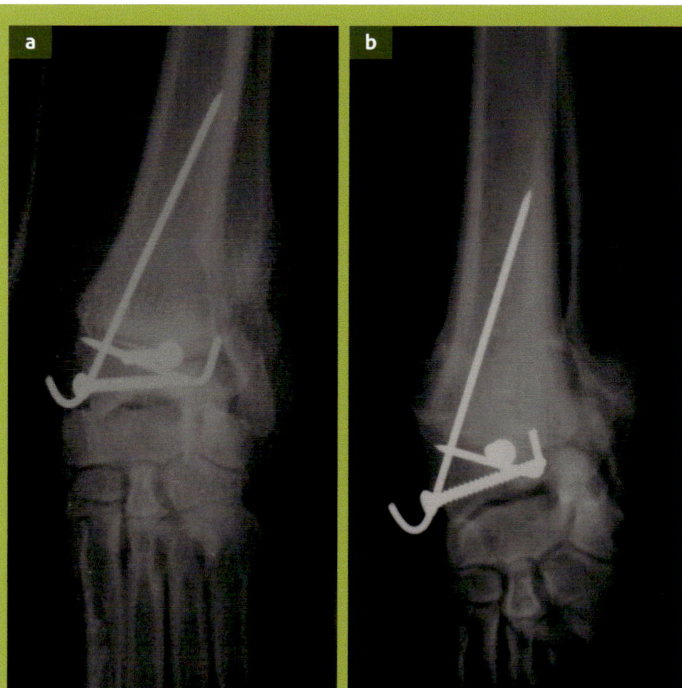

FIGURE 88. Minimal osteosynthesis with external coaptation. Cranio-caudal view that shows the fracture (a) and its progress (b).

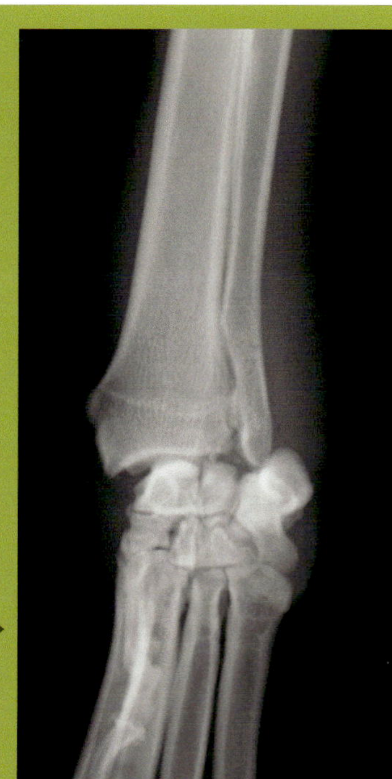

FIGURE 89. Fracture of the radial carpal bone. Oblique X-ray for better viewing of the fracture.

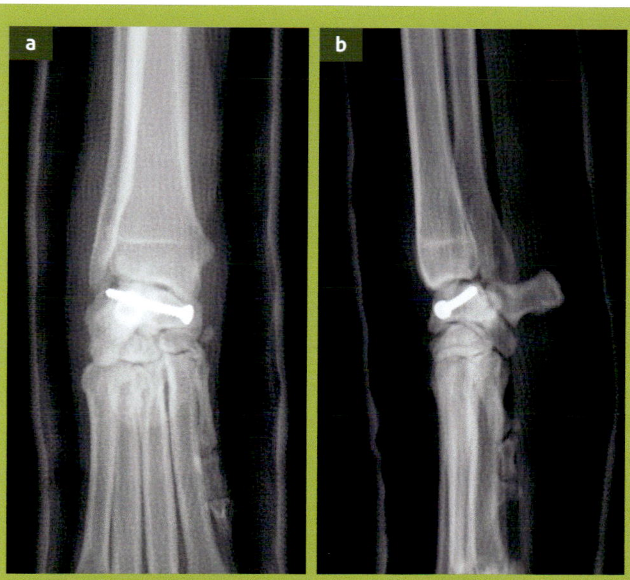

FIGURE 90. Compression screw in a radial carpal fracture. Caudo-cranial view (a) and latero-lateral view (b).

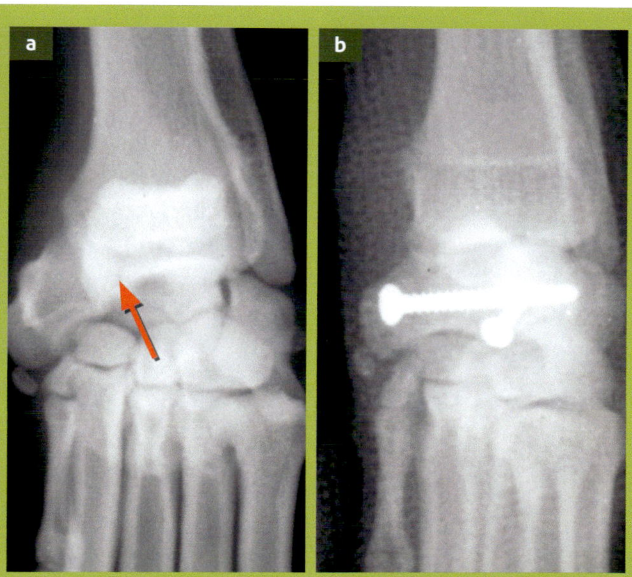

FIGURE 91. Double fracture of the radial carpal bone. One of the fractures is not recognisable in the X-ray (a). Compression screws are used for stabilisation (b).

however, in these cases, the collateral ligaments resist the impact. The radial carpal bone breaks the joint capsule and moves out of the joint space, rotating 90° in a medial and dorsal-palmar direction.

The X-ray diagnosis is very simple as the displacement of the wound is easily detected (Fig. 92).

Manually reducing the closed fracture dislocation may be possible in recent cases, but in practice and primarily in large-sized animals, performing an open reduction is preferable. In this case, after performing a cranio-medial approach to the carpus, the radial carpal bone is located and moved into its correct anatomical position within the joint space. It is important to take into consideration the existence of possible fractures of said bone, as well as small fragments that are attached to the ulnar carpal bone due to a fracture from avulsion produced by the ligament that connects both bones (if the fragment is small, it is better to remove it as it cannot be fixated).

Once the dislocation is reduced, the joint capsule is then closed. The radial carpal bone must be stabilised in its position to allow for healing of the damaged soft tissues. In this context, the Kirschner pin or a screw can be introduced that goes through this bone and is anchored to the ulnar carpal bone. This avoids another dislocation of the same bone. This system impedes certain physiological movements between the radial carpal bone and the ulnar carpal bone (Fig. 93). Another possibility that is less

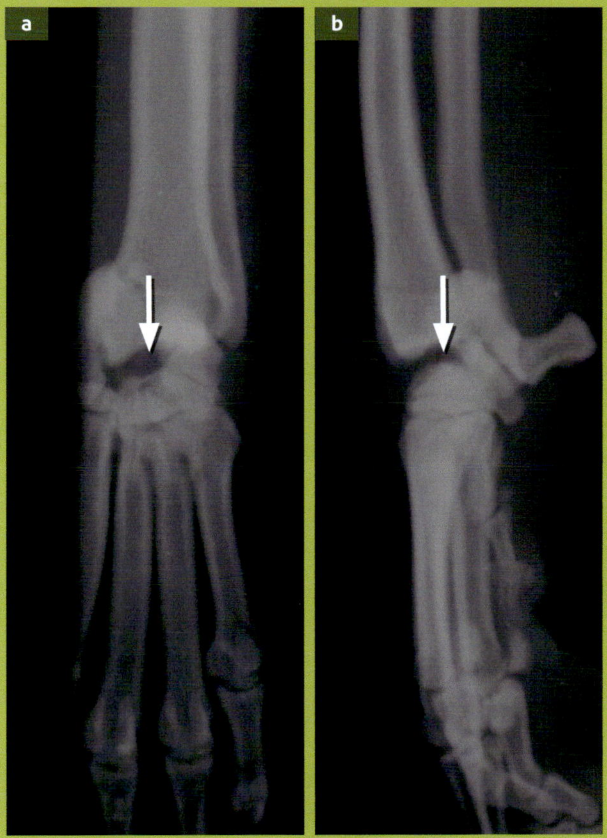

FIGURE 92. Dislocation of the radial carpal bone that is detected by an increase in the joint space of the bone (arrows). Caudo-cranial view (a) and latero-lateral view (b).

traumatic and with a better prognosis, is to temporarily immobilise the joint using a rigid bandage system or a transarticular fixator (Fig. 94). This system is more reliable, given that it provides a more rigid stabilisation to the joint, compared with the external coaptation systems that allow for certain movements and lose their effectiveness as the days go by.

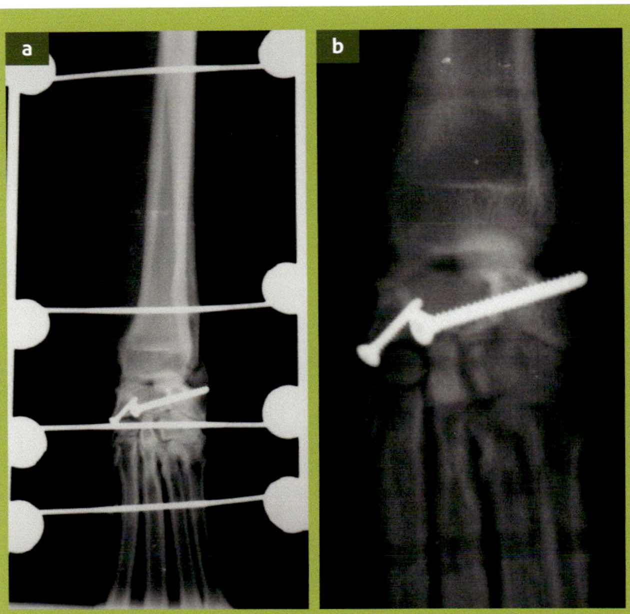

FIGURE 93. Screw between the radial carpal bone and the ulnar carpal bone (a). Also, a radial carpal fracture is observed that has been treated with a compression screw (b).

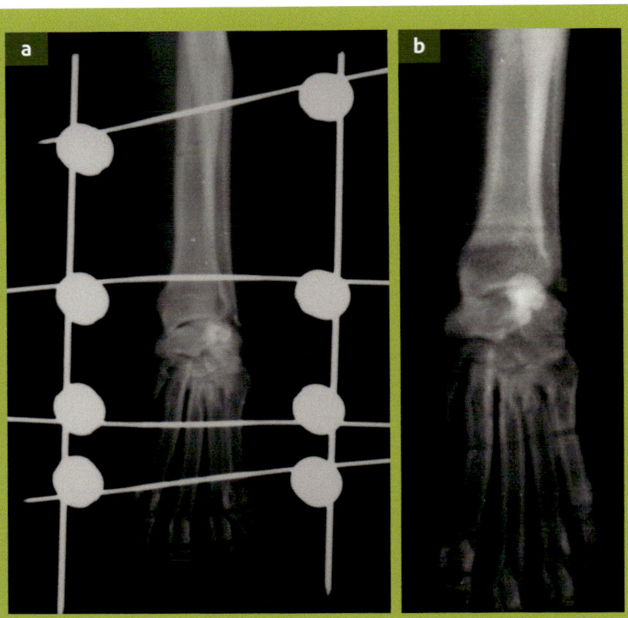

FIGURE 94. Temporary transarticular fixation without internal fixation. Fracture similar to that shown in Fig.92, without applying internal fixation.

FRACTURES OF THE METACARPUS AND THE METATARSUS

Due to the common characteristics of these two anatomical regions, their orthopaedic problems will be covered together in this chapter.

Both regions compose of four fine long bones whose epiphyses are blocked by other bones that they articulate with. The proximal epiphyses are in close contact with the carpal and tarsal bones, while the distal epiphyses articulate with the first phalanx of each toe (Fig. 95). The distal joints, although they are blocked, allow for intramedullary pins to project out of them if they are placed in their dorsal portion.

As the four bones are parallel to each other and in close contact with each other, they each serve as an internal splint to the other bones. In the proximal portion, movement between the bones is much less and, moving towards the distal portion, the two middle bones are slightly displaced in a dorsal direction, increasing the possibility for movement between them.

On the plantar surface of the joint with the first phalanx, there are two sesamoid bones that are calcifications of the flexor tendons. There is also a dorsal sesamoid bone in some large breeds of dogs that should not be confused with a bone fragment (Fig. 96).

The metacarpal fractures are generally produced from falls from height. Metatarsal fractures, which are much less frequent, are usually produced by trauma caused by objects falling onto them or from when the animal has gotten its foot trapped in a hole/cavity when trying to jump (this is frequent in cats that jump off of radiators, getting their limb stuck between the segments).

Fractures of these bones are usually produced in the distal middle third, where there is greater mobility. However, if the impact takes place on the proximal portion, a dislocation is produced.

Within the metacarpal fractures there is, however, a proximal epiphyseal fracture that has its own entity and treatment, it is a fracture of the proximal epiphysis of the V metacarpus that is described below.

Fracture of the proximal epiphysis of the V metacarpus

This lesion is relatively frequent in middle and large breed dogs, primarily as a consequence of jumping from considerable heights. Normally, an oblique fracture occurs from the proximo-lateral portion to the medial portion, resulting from the traction carried out by the lateral collateral ligament (Fig. 97). Although at first sight it may seem like an insignificant fracture, given its location, it is a fracture caused by avulsion that, if not treated correctly, causes

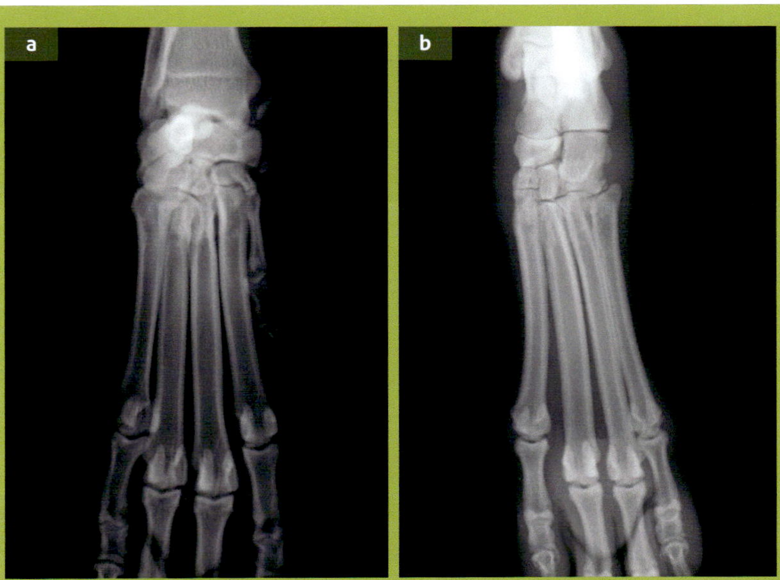

FIGURE 95. Metacarpal (a) and metatarsal (b) region. Observe the anatomical similarity between them.

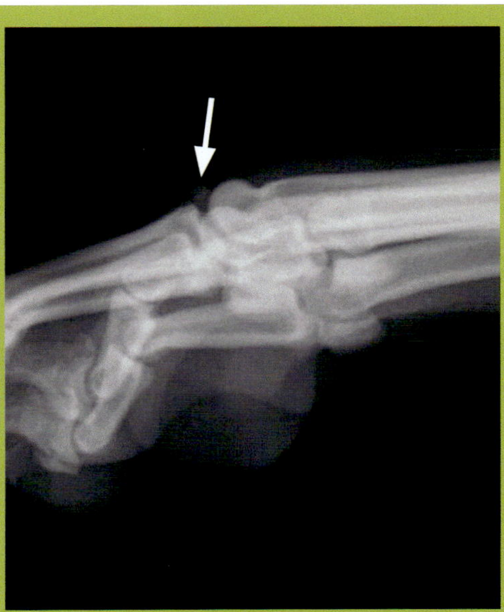

FIGURE 96. Dorsal sesamoid bone of the metatarsophalangeal joint (arrow). It should not be confused with a fracture.

instability of the carpal joint; secondary joint degeneration takes place progressively that can possibly derive in an arthrodesis of the joint.

Treatment is based on stabilisation using a fixation system that counteracts the forces of traction. The most used system consists of placing a pin with a tension band or a cerclage that compresses the oblique fracture. The insertion of two pins is not necessary as this type of fracture does not tend to rotate.

If the patient is large or subjected to physical stress, treatment using an osteosynthesis miniplate is the best option (Fig. 98). In these cases, the insertion of three screws per fragment is not strictly necessary as the fracture is relatively stable.

Fractures of the diaphysis of the metacarpal and metatarsal bones

As previously explained at the beginning of this chapter, the fractures that affect both areas will be explained together, given their biomechanical similarities.

When the surgeon is faced with this type of fracture, he or she must first analyse if surgical treatment is indispensable or, if conservative treatment is required that provides sufficient stability as needed for correct consolidation (Fig. 99).

To determine which treatment is better, different aspects must be taken into consideration. The most important aspect is the number of fractured bones. Taking into account that, as previously mentioned, each bone acts as an internal splint for the rest, it is logical to deduce that fewer injured bones means that the joint fractures are more stable. There is no fixed standard about when surgical treatment should be implemented or not, or regarding how many bones should be stabilised, it is the surgeon's choice. In general, more than two fractured bones should never be left untreated, and of course, surgical treatment is always safer. The age of the patient must also be taken into account as healing processes in young animals are produced in a more active manner.

More than two metacarpal or metatarsal fractures should never be left without stabilisation.

To stabilise fractures of the metacarpal and metatarsal bones, there are various options: intramedullary pinning, application of osteosynthesis plates and, in certain cases, external fixation.

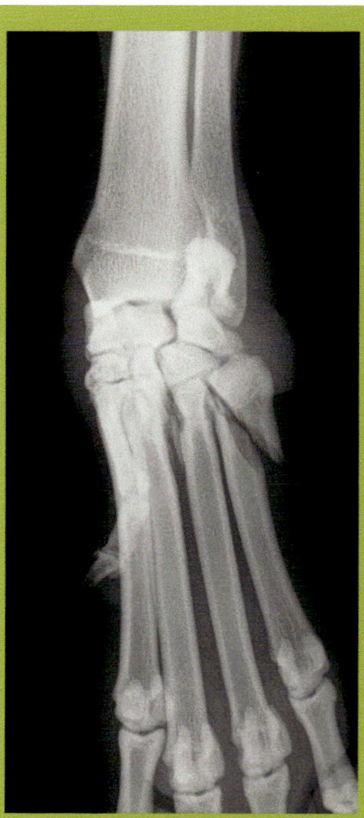

FIGURE 97. Fracture of the V metacarpal bone.

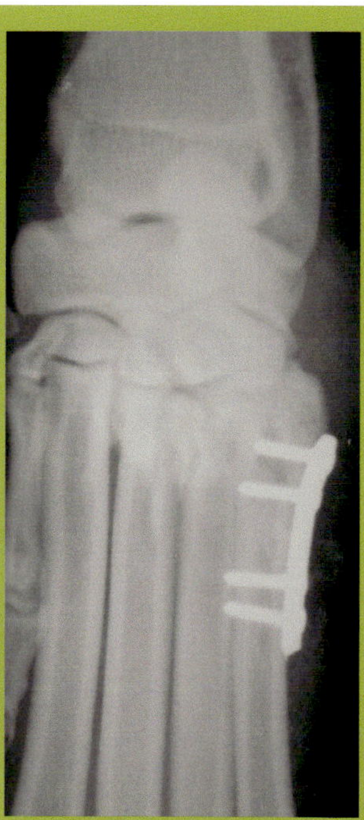

FIGURE 98. Previous fracture stabilised using a miniplate.

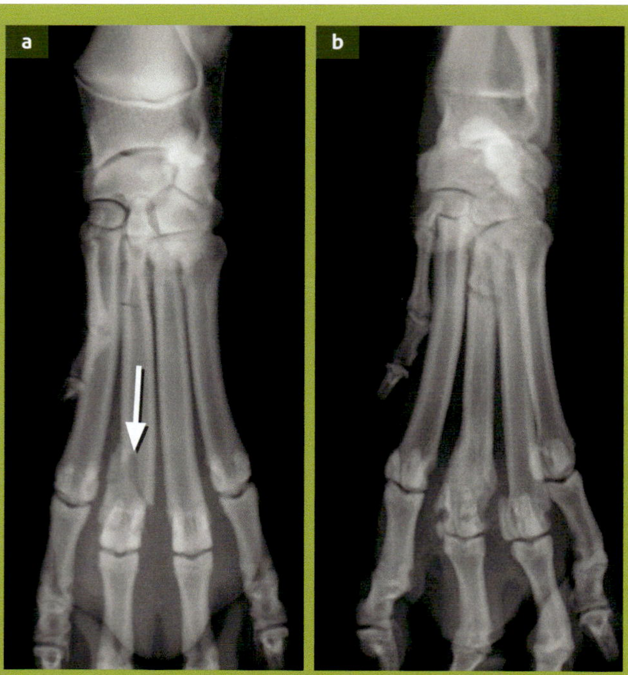

FIGURE 99. Conservative treatment of a double fracture of the III metacarpal bone (a). Progress of the fracture (b).

Intramedullary pinning

Intramedullary pins can be applied two ways: leaving an end out of the distal epiphysis without damaging the joints with the first phalanx, or leaving the entire pin inside of the medullary cavity.

There are two alternatives to insert the pin according to the first technique. In the first, it is introduced in a retrograde manner forcing it to exit through the dorsal portion of the joint, and once the fracture is reduced, it is introduced into the medullary cavity of the proximal fragment. Next, the end is bent and cut, adapting the pin so that it causes as little damage as possible to the joint (Fig. 100). This way, before bending the end, it is a good idea to pull it slightly out, and once bent, reintroduce it to the previous position and thus move the curved portion as close as possible to the epiphysis. Regarding the second alternative, it consists of creating a small hole in the metaphyseal area to introduce the pin in a normograde manner. This option is more laborious, but it does not cause damage the joint with the phalanx.

Whenever this system is used, the implants should be removed when the bones have healed. This way, damage to the flexor tendons and the appearance of secondary joint degeneration are avoided.

The second technique consists of stabilising the fracture using pins that are left completely inside of the medullary cavity. This system can be applied to fractures that are not in an excessively distal location. First, the pin is introduced in a retrograde manner in the medullary cavity of the longer fragment (normally the proximal fragment). Once it is introduced as far as possible, the pin is cut close to the fragment, leaving a few millimetres outside of the fragment. The fracture must then be reduced, introducing the part that remains outside into the cavity of the other fragment. Using a haemostat clamp introduced between both fragments, the pin is clamped and pushed until it is centred (Fig. 101).

This system does not damage the joint nor does the compact bone have to be filed, however, it is less stable in non-transversal fractures. In the case of infection, removing the implant is laborious and complicated.

Plates

In large patients, or in the case of comminuted fractures, intramedullary fixation may not solve the problem entirely. In these cases, it is recommended that plates be used for stabilisation.

As in the case with intramedullary fixation, stabilising the bones is not always necessary. On many occasions, maintaining half of the bones aligned is enough to achieve adequate stabilisation of the group of bones.

The approach for metacarpal and metatarsal bones is simple. The incision area of the skin depends primarily on how many bones need to be stabilised. Two bones can

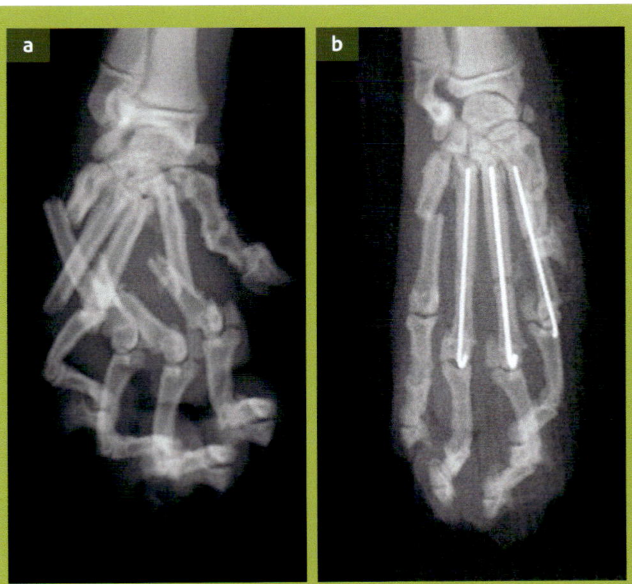

FIGURE 100. Fracture of the four metacarpal bones (a) treated using intramedullary pins bent at the distal metaphysis (b).

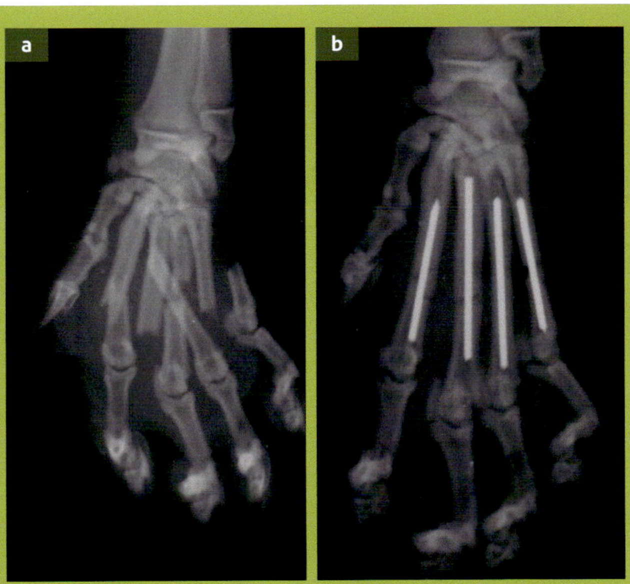

FIGURE 101. Fracture of the four metacarpal bones (a) treated using intramedullary fixation without overlapping from the distal area (b).

easily be stabilised through one incision. If three implants or more are needed, it is recommended that two parallel approaches be carried out between the I and II and the III and IV metacarpal/metatarsal bones. Excessive manipulation of the soft tissues while trying to access three bones from one single incision may lead to the appearance of serious licking problems.

Attention must be paid to not damage the tendons of the digital extensor muscles, which are found in an oblique direction in a fan shape on top of the bones, from lateral to medial.

Due to the shape of both the metacarpal bones as well as the metatarsal bones, there is almost no need to bend the plates. Taking into account the stability that each bone provides in cases of very proximal or distal fractures, inserting three screws into each primary fragment is not indispensable (Fig. 102).

Depending on the stability achieved, it is usually helpful to apply some type of external coaptation for a few weeks.

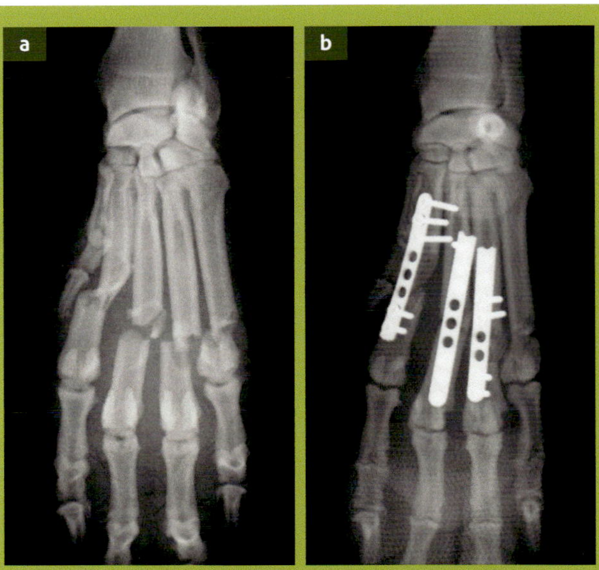

FIGURE 102. X-ray image of a fracture of the four metacarpal bones (a). The fracture is treated using adjustable plates (b).

External fixation

Although this system can be applied to almost all metacarpal and metatarsal fractures, it is recommended that they only be used in fractures where there has been a significant loss of soft tissues; that said, said loss does not necessarily imply that other stabilisation systems such as plates be discarded (Fig. 103). However, the use of cerclages or intramedullary fixation are not recommended due to the poor tolerance of these implants against infection.

These bones, as they are not anatomically located on one single plane, especially in their distal portion, do not accept single plane structures well. Given the peculiar position and the need, on many occasions, to apply percutaneous pins with different diameters, the connecting rods should be substituted with structures made of

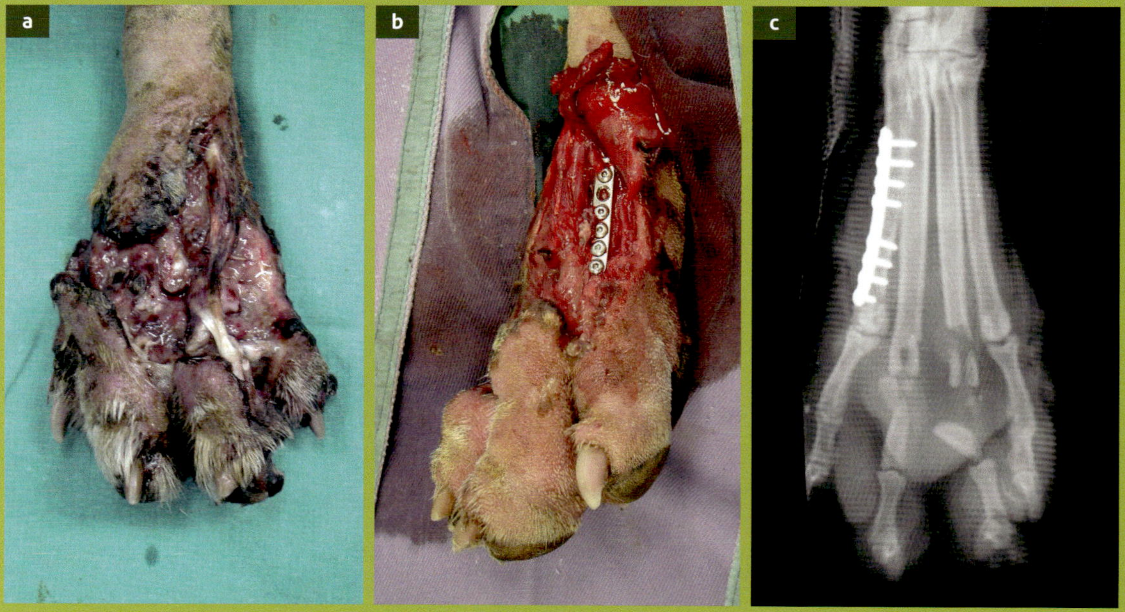

FIGURE 103. Open fracture (a). It is stabilised using an osteosynthesis plate (b). X-ray image where the treatment applied is visible (c).

methyl methacrylate. Acrylic cements allow for the initial insertion of the pins in the most adequate position and direction to later stabilise them without needing to keep them in one single plane and, also, they offer the possibility of combining percutaneous pins of different diameters (Fig. 104).

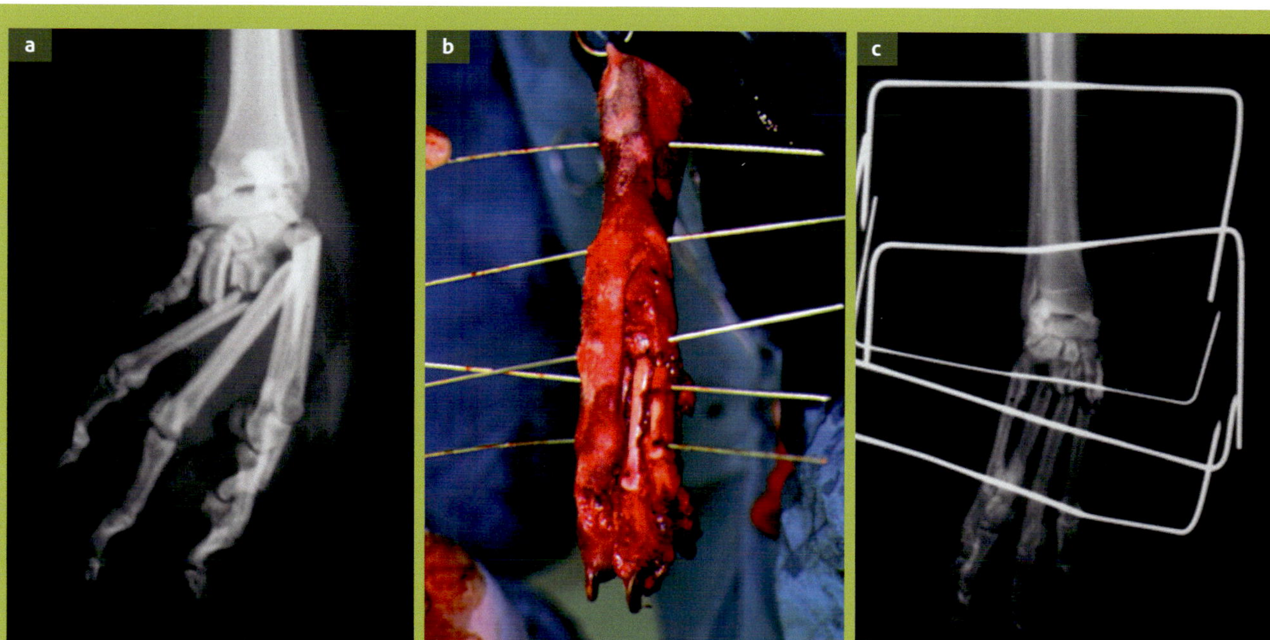

FIGURE 104. Open fracture of the four metacarpal bones with significant loss of soft tissues (a and b). Stabilisation has been carried out using type II external fixation with methyl methacrylates and a skin flap. Observe the different diameters and orientation of the percutaneous pins (c).

9 Hindlimb fractures

HIP FRACTURES

Introduction

Hip fractures are relatively frequent in small animals. According to certain authors, they may reach 20 to 30 % of all fractures. This joint supports and transmits forces towards the vertebral column that the coxofemoral joint is subjected to when walking or running.

Anatomically, the hip is made of the union of three bones: the ilium, the ischium and the pubis (Fig. 1). The three bones converge in the acetabulum. In a cranial direction, the hip articulates with the sacrum by means of a synarthrosis located on the iliac wings.

Due to its anatomical configuration, fractures that only affect one of the hip bones are rare. This characteristic is easy to understand if the pelvis is considered as a frame formed by the sacrum, the two ilium and ischium, and the pubis. When a fracture is produced, this frame is deformed, which may cause at least two different situations:

- Fracture of at least two of the bones that form the joint.
- Fracture of one bone and dislocation of the ilium in relation with the sacrum on one of its sides.

On the other hand, the fractures that affect the hip are rarely open due to the great muscle mass that surrounds the joint. However, given that these bones form a "bone ring" round the pelvic canal, attention must be paid to other types of concomitant lesions that can occur. In fact, hip fractures are frequently a consequence of major trauma, and thus a physical examination should be performed with special emphasis on discarding other lesions such as possible injury to the bladder or urethra, as well as rupture of a tendon at its point of insertion or a rectus abdominis muscle tear that may lead to the appearance of abdominal hernias (Fig. 2).

Other lesions that must be discarded are spinal fractures due to the intimate anatomical relation that the spine has with the bones that form the sacroiliac joint. Whenever a patient is received with a hip fracture, a basic examination of the sensitivity of the hindlimb must be performed with an X-ray study of at least the lumbar portion of the vertebral column (Fig. 3).

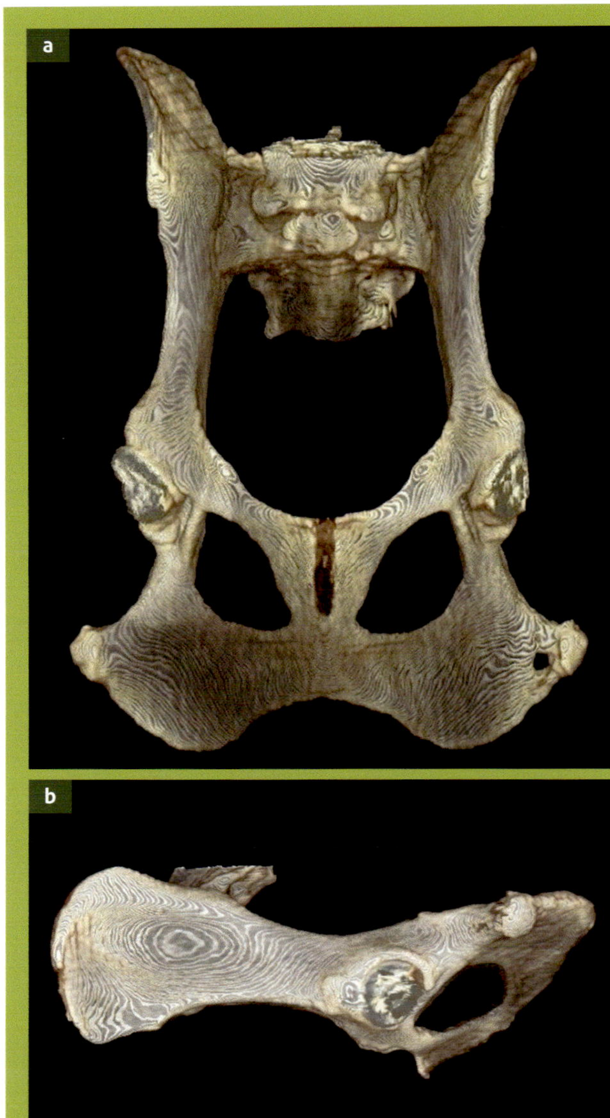

FIGURE 1. Three dimensional reconstruction of the pelvis using CT.

For the correct diagnosis of hip fractures, an X-ray study must be performed that includes X-rays of the pelvis, taking both ventrodorsal views (which provide more information), as well as lateral views. Oblique views of the acetabular area may be necessary in some cases to correctly

Characteristics of hip fractures:

- These fractures are usually produced in various points, at times combined with sacroiliac dislocation.
- Open fractures are not frequent due to the great muscle mass surrounding the pelvis.

It is important to assess the following when faced with a diagnosis of a hip fracture:

- Existence of organ damage (ruptured bladder or urethra).
- Appearance of abdominal hernias (muscular tears or detachment of insertions).
- Existence of neurological damage (associated spinal fractures).

evaluate if the coxofemoral joint is affected or not (Fig. 4). The X-ray view in a "frog" position enables a complementary assessment of the integrity of the pelvis and it also avoids unnecessary traction of the femurs, which in turn decreases the patient's pain during manipulation (Fig. 5).

That said, the need for a complete X-ray study sometimes requires general anaesthesia for the correct positioning of the patient. Lastly, assessment using computerised tomography (CT) obviously provides more precise images of all of the concomitant lesions present, but this test is not normally necessary.

Treatment of the most frequent hip fractures

As a general rule, any fracture located in a cranial position to the caudal portion of the acetabulum should be reduced, that is, those that affect the ilium and the acetabulum, per se.

Taking into account the transmission of the previously mentioned forces, it is easy to understand that pubic fractures and caudal fractures of the acetabulum hardly suffer any displacement when the patient bears weight on the limb. Also, the elevated healing capacity of the flat bone found in the pelvic bones - rich in cancellous tissue -, together with the rich blood supply of the area and the scarce movement of the previously mentioned fragments, makes conservative treatment a good option (Fig. 6).

Fractures caudal to the acetabulum

Fractures that affect the pubis do not usually require surgical treatment, except if any of the fragments of the fracture has caused damage in the rectum or urethra, in which case they need to be surgically removed.

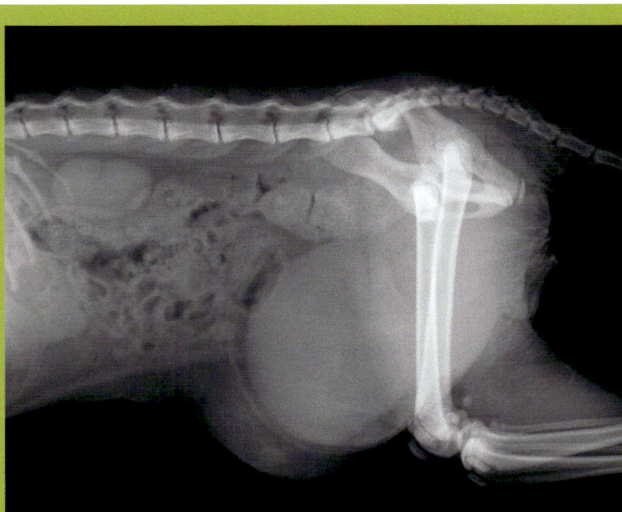

FIGURE 2. Bladder hernia as a consequence of a hip fracture.

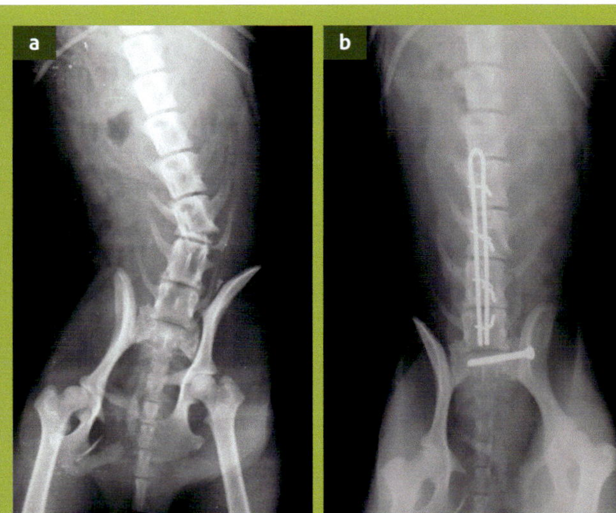

FIGURE 3. Fracture of lumbar vertebra L5 associated with a hip fracture (a) and resolution of the same fracture after surgery (b).

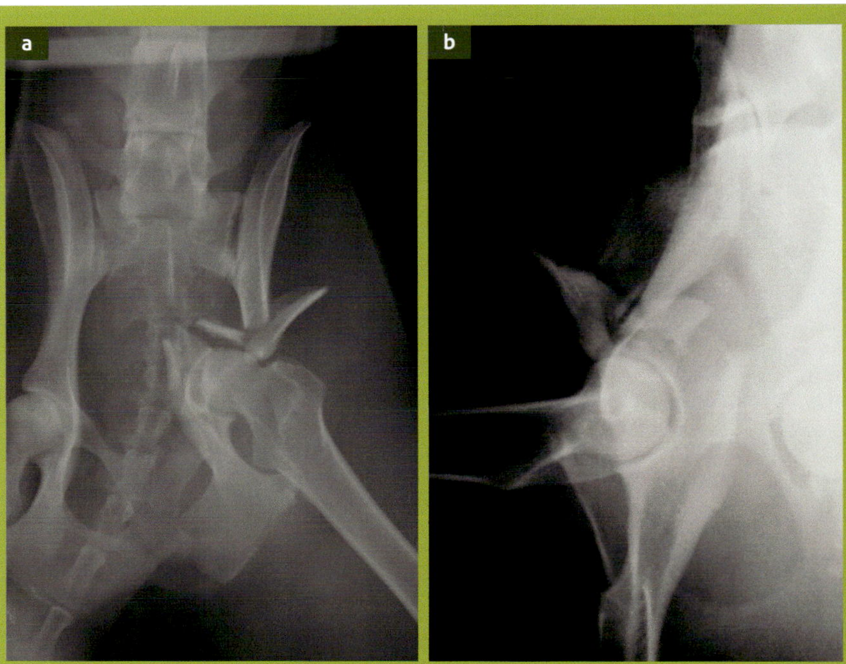

FIGURE 4. Ventrodorsal (a) and oblique (b) X-rays of the hip. Note how the acetabulum appears to be fractured in the ventrodorsal view but the oblique view shows that it is not.

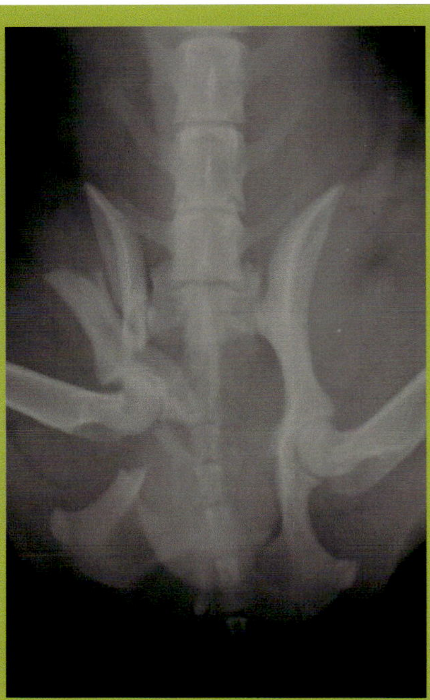

FIGURE 5. The "frog" position view is less painful for the animal and allows for complete evaluation of the pelvis.

The following factors should be taken into account when planning how to treat hip factors:

- Bones affected by the fracture.
- Displacement of the fragments.
- Integrity of the sacroiliac joint and the acetabulum, and location of the fracture if applicable.
- Age, size and body weight of the animal.

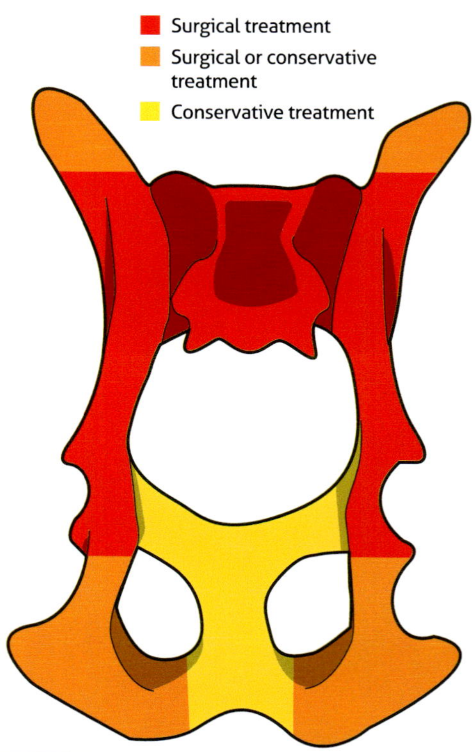

FIGURE 6. Selection of surgical or conservative treatment depending on the location of the fracture.

Fractures of the ischium

Fractures of the ischium can be treated surgically or conservatively.

If the fracture affects the ischial tuberosity - where the semitendinosus and semimembranosus muscles insert -, the ischium may suffer a delay in its ossification due to the fact that these are avulsion fractures. In these cases, the patient's age and size should be taken into consideration as well as the displacement of the fragment to select one treatment or another. In most cases, conservative treatment provides correct functional results (Fig. 7).

In most cases, conservative treatment can usually be implemented in fractures that affect the ischium with satisfactory results.

Due to the delicate approach and manipulation in this area, the convenience of carrying out conservative treatment should be considered. If surgical treatment is selected, stabilisation is usually achieved using pins. These should be inserted from the ischial tuberosity towards the body of the ischium, associated or not with cerclages depending on each fracture and the stability achieved with the pins.

The fractures that affect the sciatic notch respond well to conservative treatments. However, in some cases, the fracture callus may apply pressure to the sciatic nerve and cause temporary discomfort.

Surgical treatment of fractures that affect the sciatic notch is especially delicate due to the fact that the sciatic nerve passes through it.

If surgical treatment is chosen, performing an osteotomy of the greater trochanter is recommended to access the area without the risk of damaging the sciatic nerve. This way, a tenotomy of the superficial gluteal muscle is first performed (Fig. 8) to later mark the osteotomy line right on the limit of the insertion of the quadriceps muscle (Fig. 9). This osteotomy is performed with the help of an osteotome or an oscillating saw, with the cutting direction towards the beginning dorsal area of the femur neck (Figs. 10 and 11). This manoeuvre enables the lifting of the gluteal muscles right where they insert into the femur, providing access to nearly all of the acetabular rim. To reach the notch and simultaneously protect the sciatic nerve, a tenotomy of the gemellus muscle can be performed so that, when moved in a dorsal direction, the nerve is removed from the surgical field.

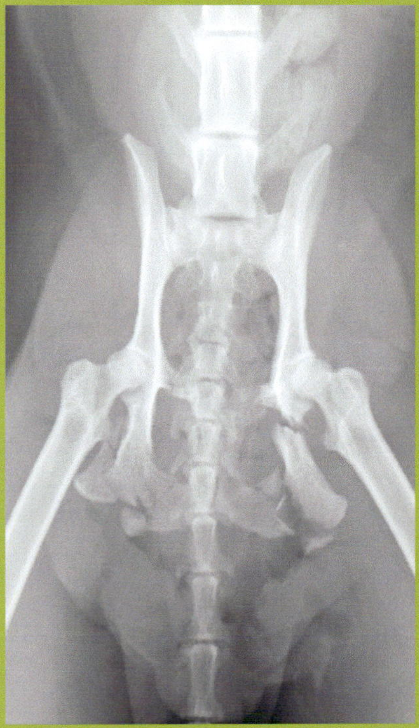

FIGURE 7. Comminuted ischium fracture. In this case, surgical treatment was not necessary.

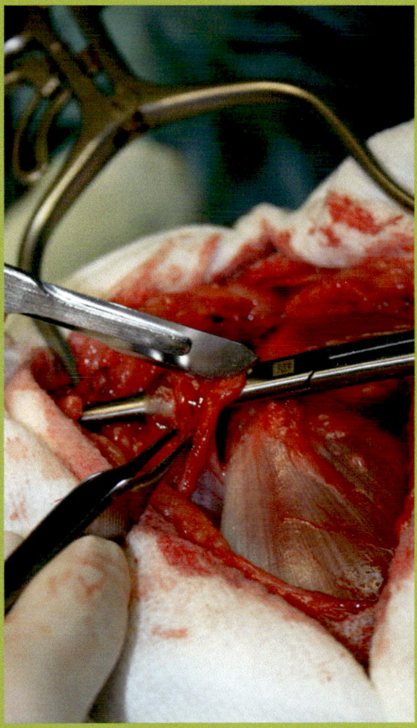

FIGURE 8. Tenotomy of the superficial gluteal muscle to access the sciatic notch.

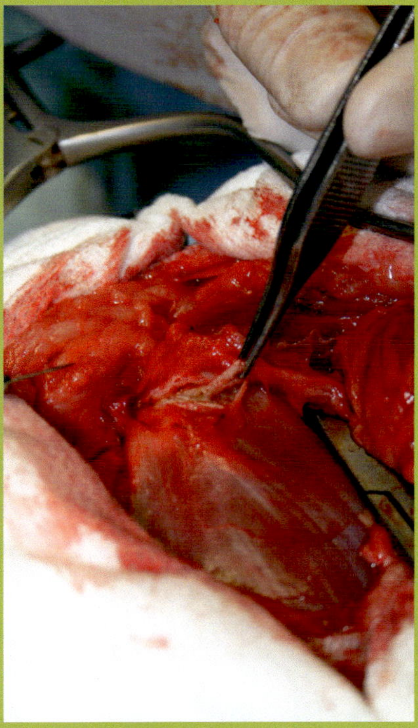

FIGURE 9. Beginning of the osteotomy at the edge of the insertion of the quadriceps to access the sciatic notch.

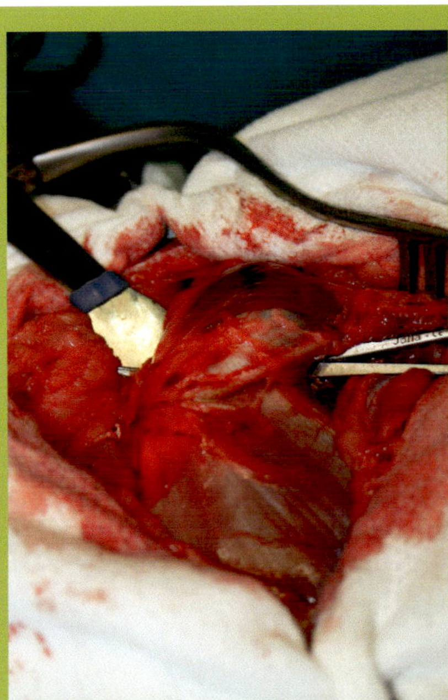

FIGURE 10. As a reference to perform the osteotomy, a curved haemostat clamp can be placed under the deep gluteal and middle gluteal muscles.

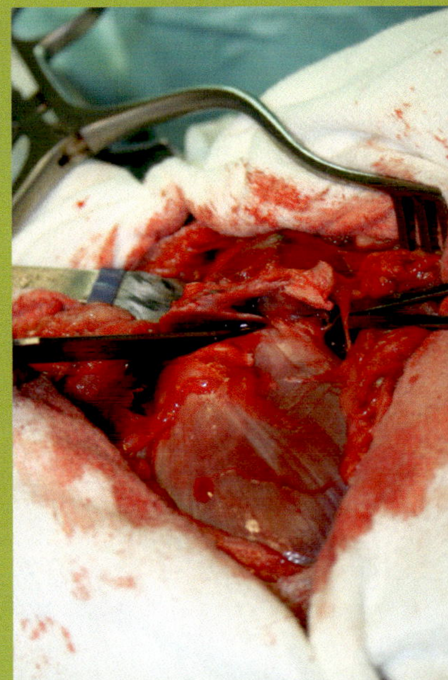

FIGURE 11. Osteotome with chisel directed at the haemostat clamp.

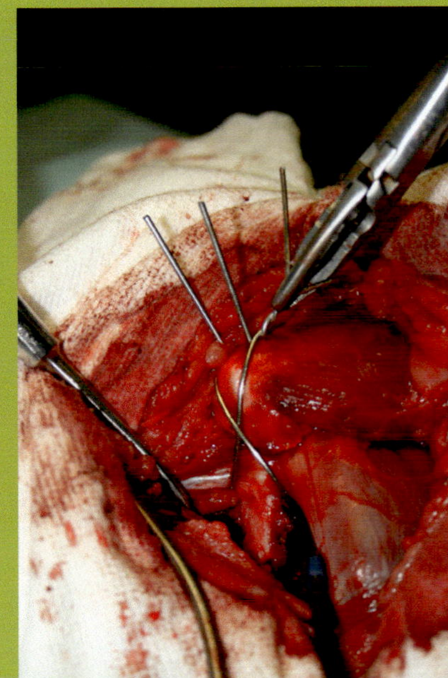

FIGURE 12. Stabilisation of the ischium fracture using pins and a tension band.

Taking into account the bone's curvature in this area, the ideal system to stabilise these fractures is the application of reconstruction or locking osteosynthesis plates. Once the fracture is stabilised, it is then reduced and the greater trochanter is fastened through the application of a tension band pin system (Fig. 12).

Fractures of the ilium

This is, without doubt, the bone that is most affected in hip fractures. The most frequent ilium fracture is an oblique fracture of the bone's body, from the dorsal area of the ilium, in a cranio-ventral direction, to just below the joint with the sacrum (Fig. 13). It has been mentioned before that this fracture, due to previously explained anatomical reasons, is associated with another pelvic lesion.

As it is a flat bone rich in cancellous tissue, the ilium has a high healing capacity. Also, as it is surrounded by a great muscle mass formed by the gluteal muscles, the movements that the bone fragments are subjected to in the case of fractures are not significant. Therefore, osteosynthesis systems used for treatment of the fracture do not need to be excessively rigid. Osteosynthesis plates are the treatment of choice for ilium fractures. Other surgical techniques have been described such as compression screws, pins and even external fixation. The latter should only be used in very specific cases due to the lack of stability and the need for more exhaustive postoperative care that this type of implant requires.

The tenotomy of the gemellus muscle permits the removal of the sciatic nerve from the surgical field.

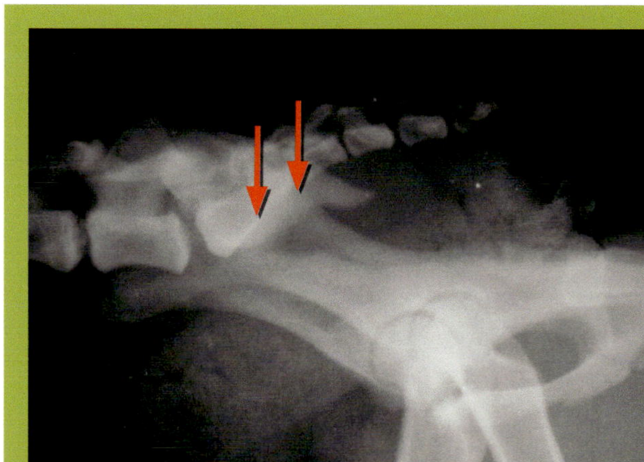

FIGURE 13. Oblique fracture of the body of the ilium. The arrows indicate the fracture line in a dorsoventral direction.

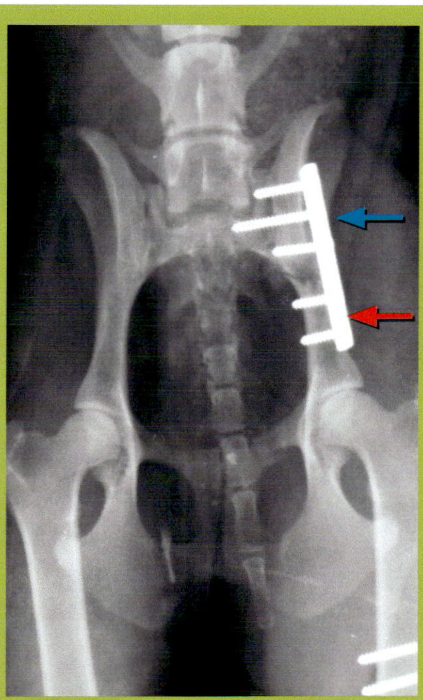

FIGURE 14. Plate stabilised with the screws in the distal fragment (red arrow, a) and a screw anchored in the sacrum in the proximal fragment (blue arrow, b).

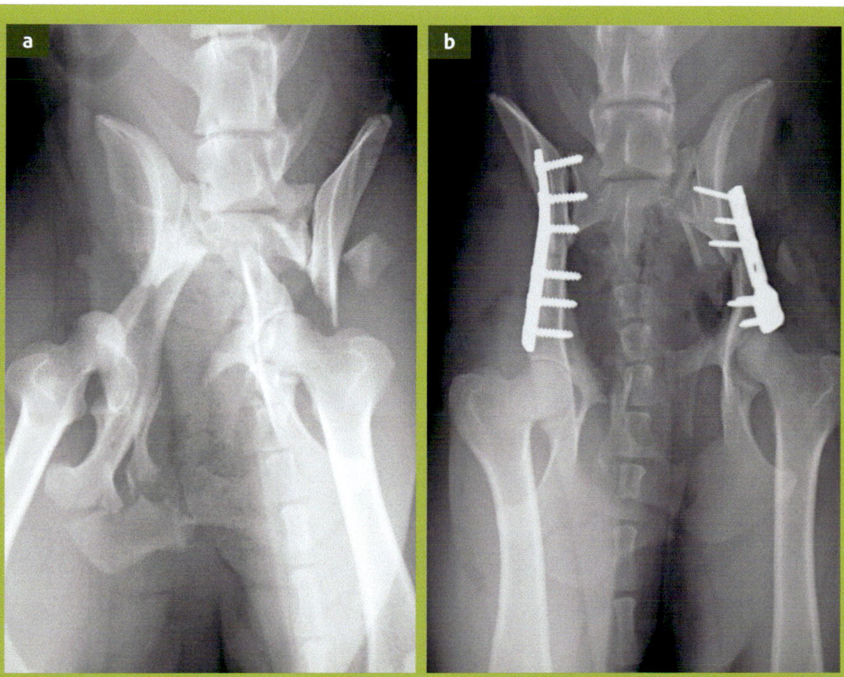

FIGURE 15. X-ray image of a bilateral iliac fracture before surgery (a). Resolution plates. A "cobra" plate is used in the right ilium due to the small size of the distal fragment (b).

As previously mentioned in the Osteosynthesis and Biomechanics chapter (page 34), the plates should always be fixated with at least three screws per fragment. However, in the case of ilium fractures, there is not always enough space. On some occasions, only two screws can be used in one of the fragments (Fig. 14, red arrow, a). More than two screws should be used in the proximal fragment as the bone is very thin and the screws loosen easily. For this reason, and to achieve a more resistant anchoring of this fragment, it is recommended that the body of the sacrum is reached by one or more of the screws (Fig. 14, blue arrow, b). In some cases, the use of special plates may be appropriate due to the lack of space (Fig. 15).

This deficit in the stability of the plate does not usually cause problems as the distal fragment in this type of fractures tends to move in a dorsal direction, and the plate is thus subjected to forces parallel to its greater plane when the animal bears weight on the limb. Therefore, plates that are smaller than those that would correspond with the patient's weight can be used. On the other hand, the predominant forces do not pull on the screws, which makes it possible to neutralise the forces of rotation in the plane of the plate and adequately stabilise the fracture with only two screws.

In the case of infrequent comminuted fractures, longer plates should be used to attempt to cover the entire length of the affected side of the pelvis. In these cases, reconstruction plates are of great use as they will have to be moulded on all planes (Fig. 16).

The surgical approach for the ilium presents no difficulties; one incision is made from the dorsal edge of the ilium wing to the area of the greater trochanter. Once the subcutaneous tissue has been separated, an incision is made through the fascia lata, extending the cut to the area above the tensor fasciae latae muscle in a cranial direction (Fig. 17).

To access the body and crest of the ilium, the middle gluteal muscle must be displaced in a dorsal direction, detaching the insertion of the ilium using a periostotome and the deep gluteal muscle must be displaced in a ventral direction, detaching the insertion from the body of the ilium. This muscle is frequently found to be partially detached as a consequence of the fracture (Fig. 18). Although this does not usually cause problems, if damaged, attempts should be made to preserve the integrity of the superior gluteal nerve.

The caudal portion of the fragment is frequently found to be displaced in a medial direction within the pelvic canal. In these

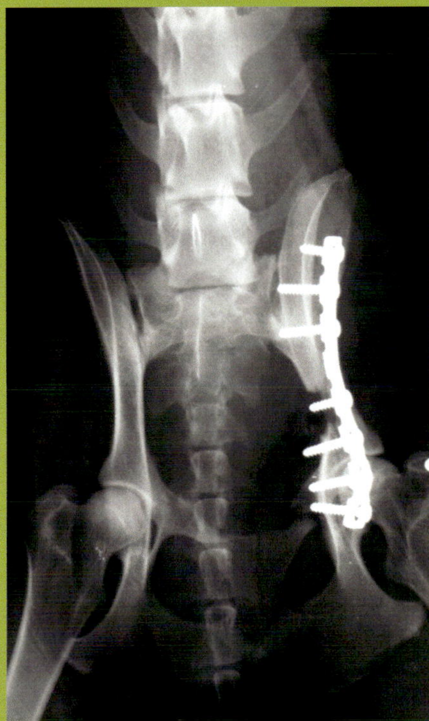

FIGURE 16. Reconstruction plate in a comminuted ilium fracture.

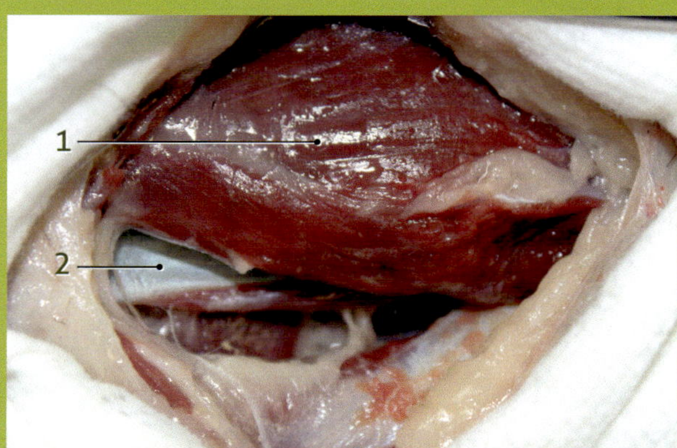

FIGURE 17. Surgical approach to the iliac wing.
1. Middle gluteal muscle.
2. Deep gluteal muscle.

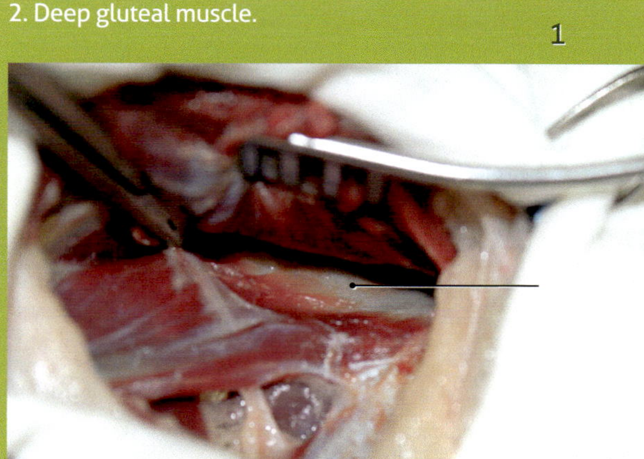

FIGURE 18. Surgical approach to the iliac wing. 1. Iliac wing.

cases, it may be useful to introduce a Hohmann elevator, hook the cranial portion of the fracture and move it to rest on the cranial fragment to act as a lever, displacing it in a lateral direction. Once the fragment found inside of the pelvic canal is placed in a lateral position, holding the ilium with a fragment reduction clamp just below the acetabulum is helpful. At the same time, if a Hohmann elevator is placed in a dorsal direction over the transition area between the crest and the body of the ilium, the middle gluteal muscle will be lifted for proper visibility of the fracture area (Fig. 19).

Once reduced, these fractures are relatively stable, while the caudal fragment usually collapses slightly in the ischial area due to the lack of support from the pubis. This deficient alignment should be taken into account to avoid any mistakes when bending the implant.

Once the plate and its position are selected, the plate is then moulded. Next, the corresponding screws are fixated. It is recommended that the screws for the caudal fragment are inserted first as their anchoring is much firmer due to the quality of the bone (Fig. 20). Later, the cranial screws are inserted which, if the moulding of the plate is correct, will lift the caudal fragment of the fracture by approximating the implant to the bone, placing it in its correct position (Fig. 21).

The flat bone that makes up the ilium, in spite of favouring ossification, is less resistant than the cortical bone. This, together with the thinness of the ilium crest, causes the screws placed in this area to loosen more easily. To strengthen their attachment, self-tapping screws should be used. If these screws are not available, another alternative is to not pass the thread insert of the screw through the entire thickness of the bone, allowing for the screw itself to finish carving the threading. This operation is possible thanks to the lack of hardness of the flat bone.

If self-tapping screws are not available, it is recommended that the thread insert not be screwed through the entire thickness of the bone. This way, the screw itself finishes carving the threading and will be better anchored.

In multiple fractures of the hip, all of the fracture lines must be carefully observed to assess which truly require surgery. When correctly stabilising a primary fracture, the rest can frequently be treated conservatively (Fig. 22).

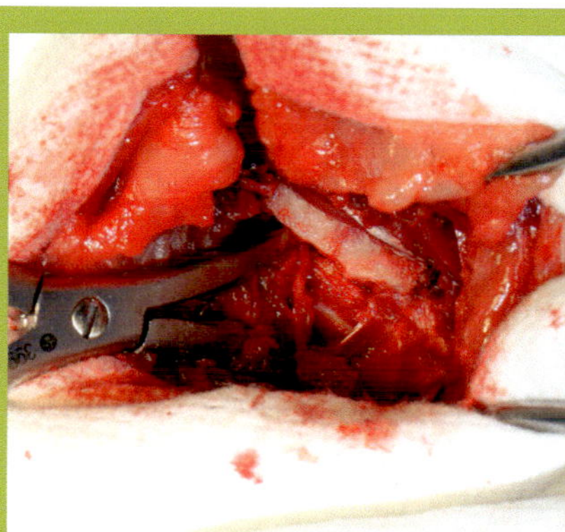

FIGURE 19. Surgical approach to an oblique fracture in the right hemipelvis.

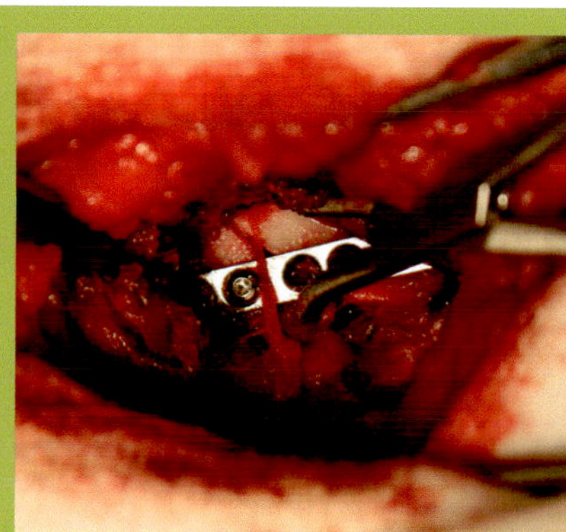

FIGURE 20. Plate screwed into the caudal fragment of the fracture. Ideally, the first screw should be inserted in the caudal part to ensure proper anchoring of the plate.

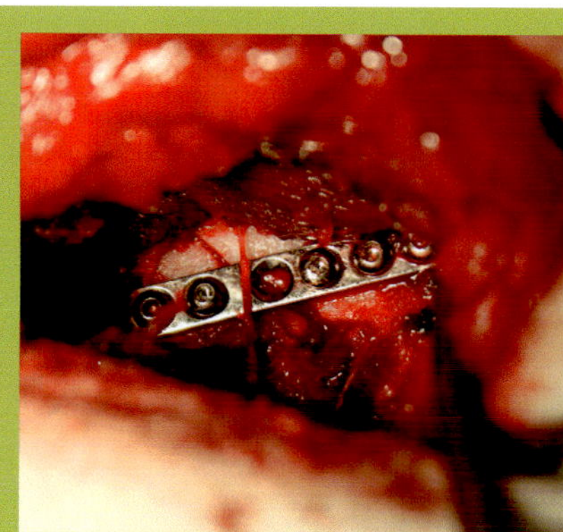

FIGURE 21. Stabilised fracture. The reduction of the fracture has improved by fixing the screws to the cranial portion.

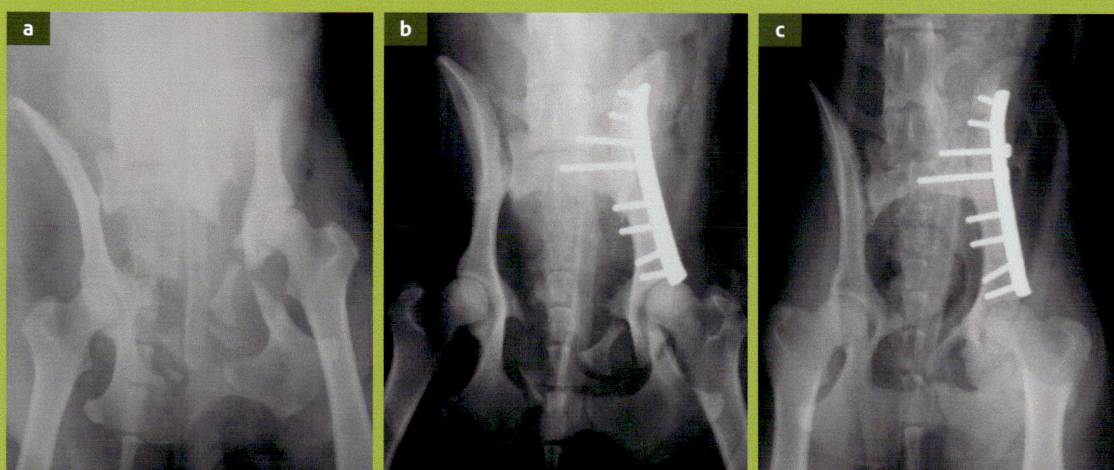

FIGURE 22. Multiple fracture of the hip (a). The stabilisation of the ilium (b) has allowed for the establishment of conservative treatment for the rest of the fractures (c).

Acetabular fractures

Like any joint fracture, acetabular fractures should be considered as surgical emergencies. Following the steps for joint surgeries previously described in Chapter 1 (Joint Fractures, page 24), attempts should be made to achieve the most perfect reduction possible of the joint surface to minimise the appearance of arthritis in the future.

The ideal osteosynthesis system for surgical treatment of acetabular fractures is the implementation of plates that will be placed in a dorsal side of the acetabular rim. For correct placement of the plates, an osteotomy of the greater trochanter will almost always be necessary, as described in this chapter (page 184).

Reduction of these types of fractures is simple, however, keeping the bones temporarily stabilised until the implant is inserted can frequently be difficult. The best system is to hold the fragments in the desired position using twin point reduction forceps, applied in cranial and caudal positions from the acetabulum.

When positioning the dorsal acetabular rim, the implant acts like a dynamic compression plate (Osteosynthesis and Biomechanics chapter, Fig. 137, page 89). This plate does not need to be very thick as the forces that it will have to neutralise - those created when bearing weight by the separation of the fracture edges of its dorsal portion - are of little importance. The primary problem with these fractures is the difficulty in achieving a perfect moulding of the implant. Any defect in the shaping will cause a loss of reduction of the joint surface that is frequently undetectable, given that the correct reduction of the fracture can only be confirmed in the acetabular labrum.

Said moulding is easier with reconstruction plates (Fig. 23). Likewise, there are acetabular plates in the shape of horse shoes that make the process easier (Fig. 24). That said, the incorporation of locking plates has shown to be the ideal treatment for this type of fractures (Fig. 25) as, with this type of plate, once the fracture is reduced, the screws do not pull on the bone excessively no matter how much they are tightened, maintaining the reduction of the fracture even if the moulding of the plate is not perfect.

> *Correct moulding of the plate is a key factor in the success of the surgical treatment of acetabular fractures.*

In small patients that tolerate arthritis much better, conservative treatment can be chosen when the acetabular fracture affects the most caudal portion as the greater amount of weight bearing of the femur against the acetabulum falls on the most cranial part.

Although infrequent, acetabular rim fractures can occur. In these cases, the size of the fragments must be confirmed to ensure they are big enough to be stabilised through surgery. If stabilisation is considered to be possible (sometimes this can only be assessed in surgery or by means of CT scans), compression screws will be applied (Fig. 26). The prognosis of this type of lesion is usually poor, especially if the cranial area is affected, given that, as previously mentioned, this is where the forces of greater intensity are produced. If the fracture cannot be stabilised or if the implants are not successful, the possibility of performing a hip replacement or an excision arthroplasty should be considered.

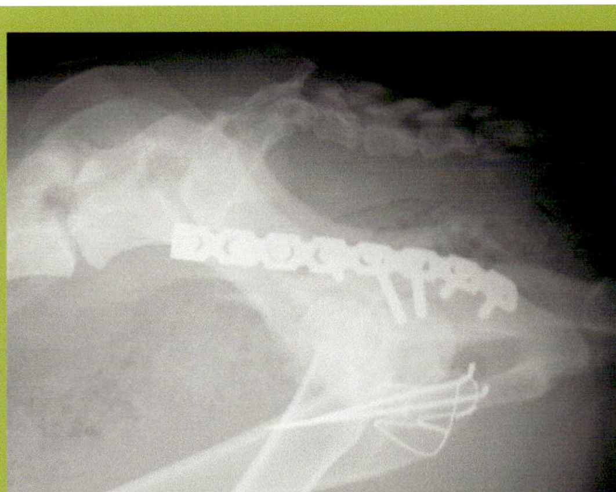

FIGURE 23. Reconstruction plate that can easily be moulded for the treatment of acetabular fractures.

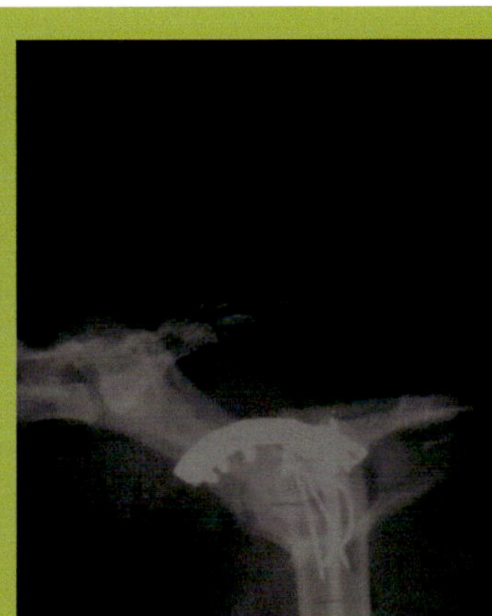

FIGURE 24. Horseshoe plate that enables the reduction of acetabular fractures.

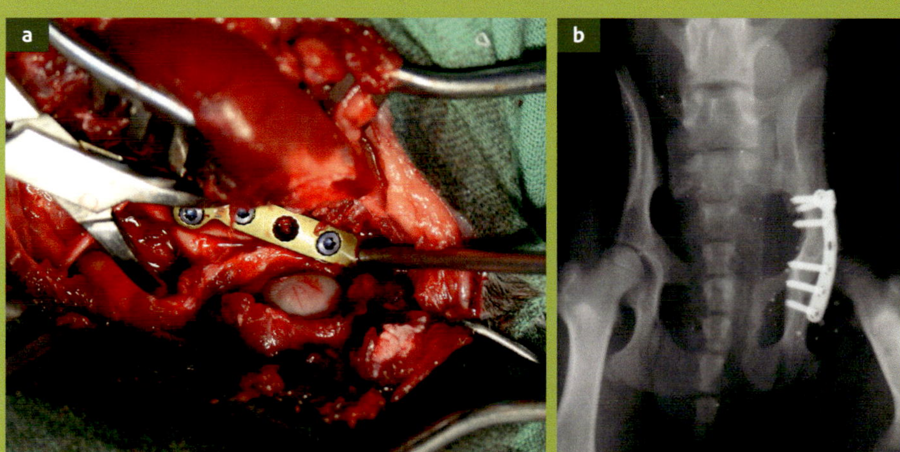

FIGURE 25. Locking plate implanted in an acetabular fracture. This type of plate is the best option for this type of fractures as the screws do not pull on the bone after reduction.

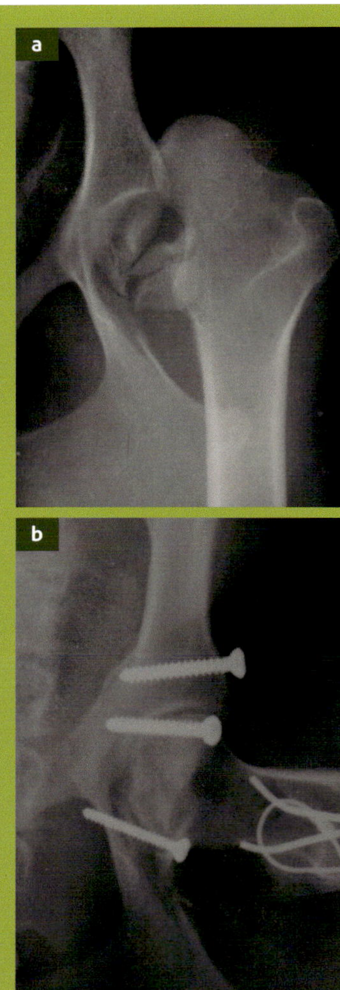

FIGURE 26. Fracture of the acetabular rim treated with a compression screw. Image before (a) and after (b) surgery.

Sacroiliac dislocation

Another problem associated with hip fractures is sacroiliac dislocation. In spite of it being a dislocation, this lesion should be treated as a fracture as it is produced in a synarthrosis, that is, in a joint with no movement.

Sacroiliac dislocations are more frequent in cats and, in some cases, it can go unnoticed if close attention is not paid. It is usually associated with ilium fractures on the other side and is rarely bilateral.

Diagnosis

The X-ray diagnosis of this dislocation is easy by means of a ventrodorsal X-ray of the hip. For correct detection, following the medial cortical bone of the body of the ilium will suffice that should follow the caudal edge of the sacrum in a smooth manner. The latter should form a horizontal arch to the contralateral joint (Fig. 27). Care should be taken to not confuse this lesion with the image of a healthy joint itself, which is radiolucent. If the positioning of the hip is not completely symmetric when the X-ray is done, one of the joints will appear much more radiolucent than the other, which may lead to mistakes by the veterinary surgeon.

For the correct diagnosis of a sacroiliac dislocation, the animal should be placed in a perfectly symmetrical position in the ventrodorsal X-ray. If not, the radiolucency of the joint itself may lead to making an erroneous diagnosis.

Treatment

Although most patients will recover with conservative treatment, this type of dislocation should be treated surgically if the displacement of the joint is greater than 50 %, or when it occurs associated with a fracture of the opposite limb. Surgical treatment is recommended for all other cases (except in young animals with little displacement) given that functional recovery will be much faster and pain-free.

Surgical procedure

Stabilisation using a compression screw from the ilium wing to the body of the sacrum is the most suitable surgical treatment, at times associated with a pin to avoid movements of rotation on the axis formed by the screw

To access the joint, an incision is made over the iliac wing with the patient in a lateral decubitus position laying on the unaffected side. The affected limb can be tied to the table for easier handling of the dislocation and to be able to pull on the limb (Fig. 28).

Once the subcutaneous tissue is separated, the insertion of the middle gluteal muscle is incised along the iliac crest, separating the muscle in a ventral direction. Subsequently, the insertions of the lateral dorsal sacrocaudal muscles and the longissimus lumbarum that insert in the medial surface of the iliac crest are incised and the muscles are retracted.

Next, the ilium is held using reduction forceps and turned 90° in a lateral direction with the help of a Hohmann elevator

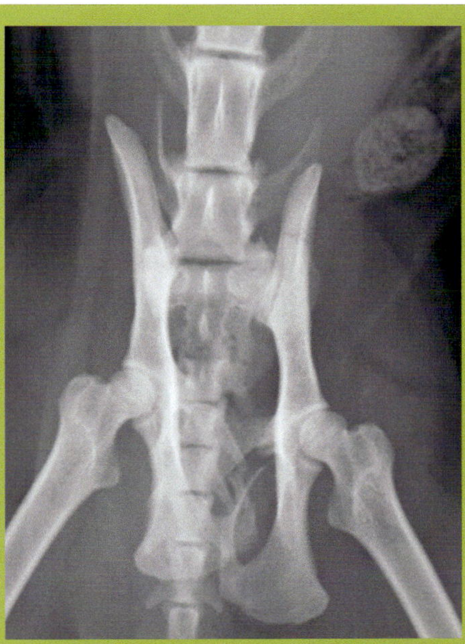

FIGURE 27. Sacroiliac dislocation in a cat.

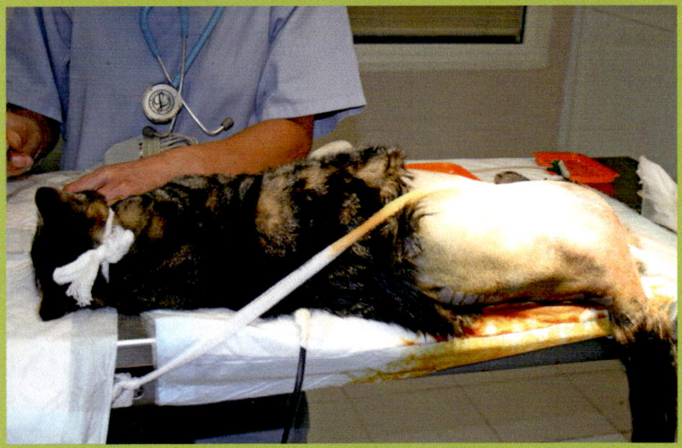

FIGURE 28. Patient prepared for surgery of a sacroiliac dislocation. The bandage below the limb allows for traction of the affected limb.

resting on the ventral part of the sacrum (Fig. 29). Great care must be taken with the tip of the Hohmann elevator to not damage the nerve endings that travel in a ventral direction to the sacrum.

This position provides access to both joint surfaces. The joint surface of the sacrum is easily identified due to its crescent-shaped cartilaginous surface. The sacroiliac ligament is found in the centre of this cartilaginous "C", where the traction hole should be made with the drill bit that corresponds with the diameter of the nucleus of the selected screw (Fig. 30).

The articular area of the iliac wing is found by palpating; it has a rough surface that is easily identified by touch. The gliding hole is perforated in the centre of said zone, medial to laterally, with a drill bit that corresponds with the diameter of the threading of the screw (Fig. 31).

After this, the length of the screw is measured in the perforated hole in the sacrum and a screw that is one or two sizes larger is selected, depending on the size of the patient, to offset the thickness of the ilium wing. The screw is inserted, medial to laterally, through the hole in the iliac wing and screwed in until the tip sticks out from the medial surface. The tip of the screw should be oriented towards the hole in the sacrum and progressively tightened (Fig. 32). This way, as the screw enters the sacrum, its head will pressure the iliac wing, forcing it into the correct position.

In young patients, or in patients that present a very soft iliac wing upon perforation, it may be useful to place a washer

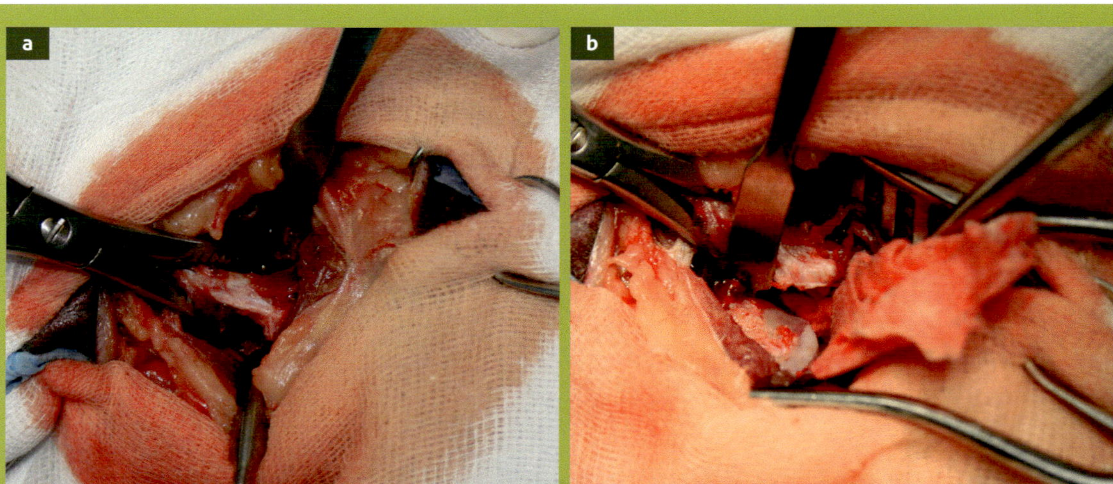

FIGURE 29. Iliac wing held in place using reduction forceps (a) and 90º turn to reveal the sacrum (b).

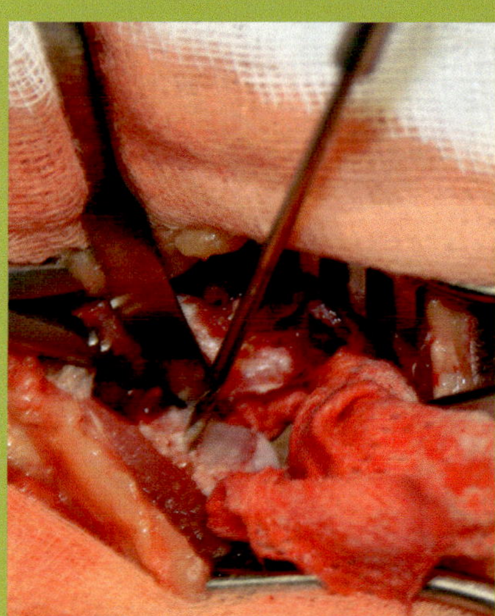

FIGURE 30. Perforation of the traction hole in the centre of the joint surface of the sacrum.

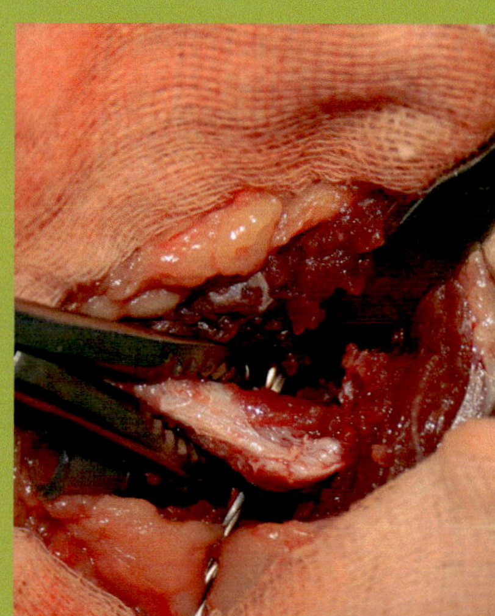

FIGURE 31. Perforation of the gliding hole in the iliac wing.

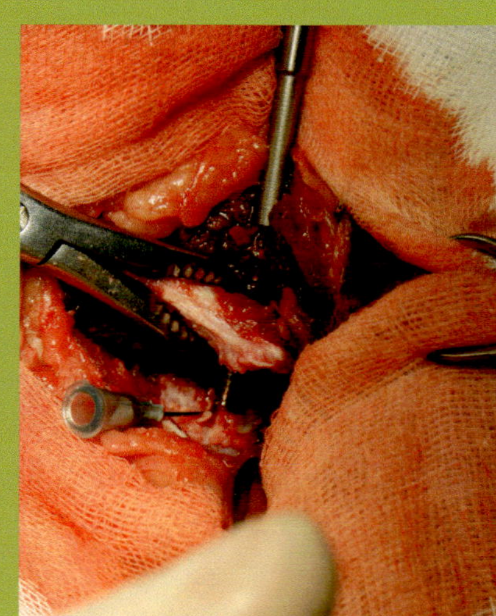

FIGURE 32. Screw tip (marked with a pin) oriented towards the sacral hole.

underneath the head of the screw. In this manner, the forces of pressure are distributed on a greater surface and the screw will not lose its effectiveness if the head is partially inserted into the ilium (Fig. 33). Depending on the surgeon's preferences, the stability of the fracture-dislocation, and of the size of the patient, a pin or even another anti-rotational screw can be inserted in a caudal direction from the screw (Fig. 34).

In cases of highly unstable dislocations, it may be useful to stabilise both iliac wings together. This can be done by perforating both iliac wings with a Kirschner pin and later bending the tips. However, the ideal technique is to implant a trans-iliac screw which consists of a threaded rod with a tip to which nuts are screwed into on each side once it is in place.

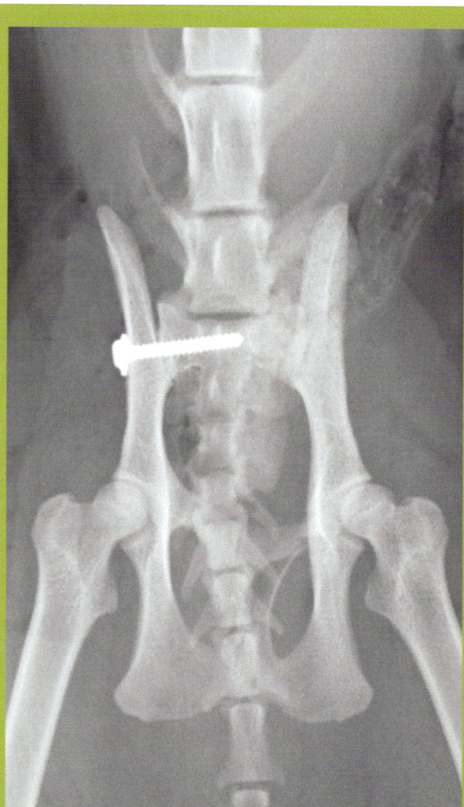

FIGURE 33. Compression screw with a nut in a patient with a sacroiliac dislocation.

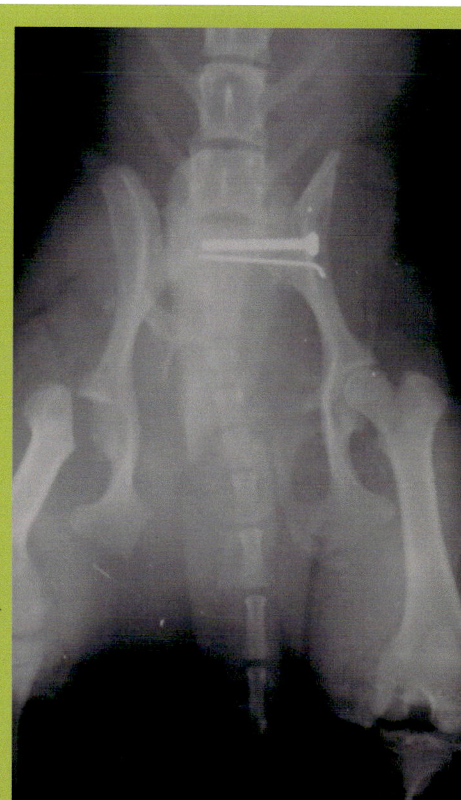

FIGURE 34. In this case, the stability of the sacroiliac joint must be increased as an arthroplasty has been performed on the other limb; an anti-rotational pin should be inserted along with the screw.

FEMUR FRACTURES

Introduction

Statistically, the femur is the bone that is most frequently fractured in pets. The fracture typically affects the middle and distal thirds of the bone. However, depending on the patient's age, the location of the fracture may vary:

- In young patients, fractures that affect the growth plate of the distal epiphysis or spiral fractures in the middle third are more frequent.
- In adult patients, the fractures are primarily located at the level of the diaphysis.

The femur has certain anatomical peculiarities that should be reviewed before explaining surgical techniques applicable to this bone.

First of all, there are differences in the femurs of dogs and cats. In dogs, the bone is slightly convex in a cranio-lateral direction (Fig. 35). The tension-bearing surface is that which bears the partial forces of distraction in the most superficial part of the compact bone in dogs (when the bone is subjected to forces of longitudinal pressure in the cranio-lateral portion). In cats, however, the diaphysis is practically straight (Fig. 36).

Secondly, the anatomical location of the femoral head, displaced in a medial direction regarding the longitudinal axis of the diaphysis, allows for fixation using intramedullary pins where one of the ends of the pin can stick out from the trochanteric fossa without invading the joint (Fig. 37).

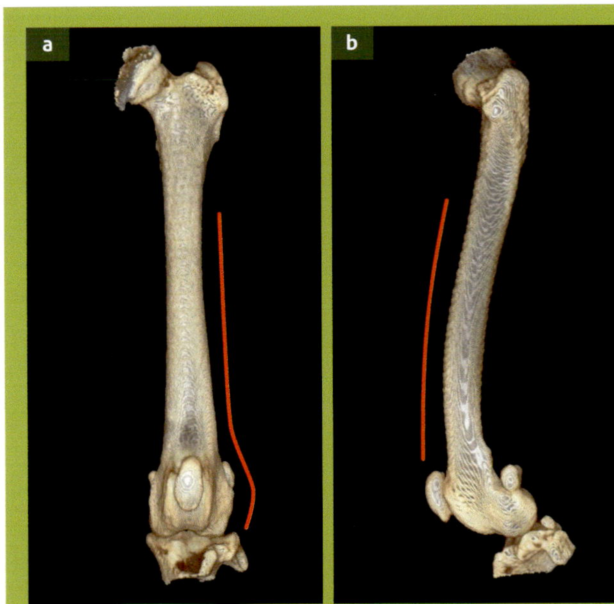

FIGURE 35. Three-dimensional reconstruction of the femur using CT.

Also, the femur is surrounded by great muscle mass, which provides excellent periosteal blood supply making delays in the healing process infrequent, provided that the right treatment is chosen.

To finish, although peripheral nerve damage is not common, a basic neurological examination should always be performed, especially if there are suspicions of concomitant hip fractures. As assessment of the reflexes cannot be

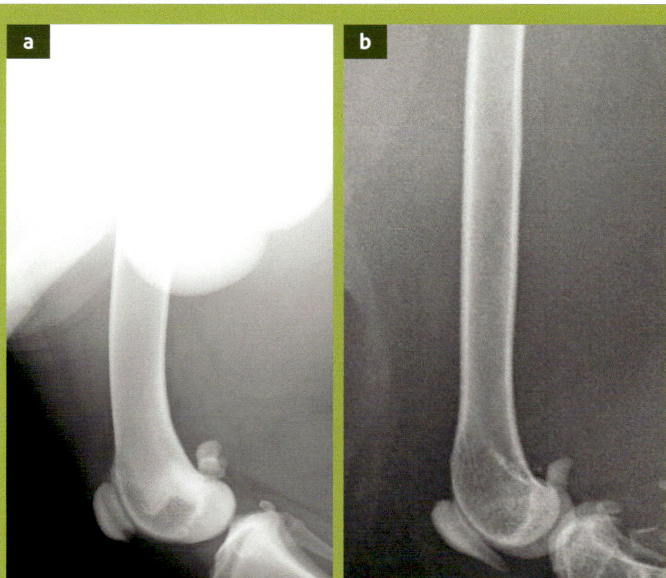

FIGURE 36. Difference between the curvature of the femur in canines (a) and felines (b).

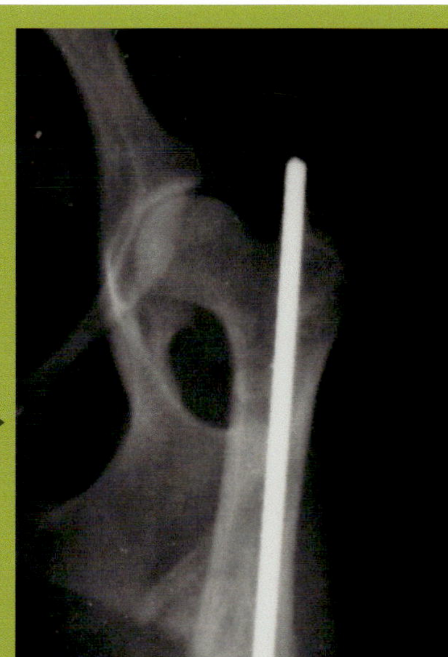

FIGURE 37. Intramedullary pin that sticks out from the subtrochanteric fossa without invading the joint.

carried out due to the loss of functionality of the extensor system of the stifle, only the sensitivity at the distal level of the limb can be tested. To do so, the last phalanx of the first and fourth toes of the limb can be pinched to determine whether the deep sensitivity is affected or not.

Almost all patients afflicted with femoral fractures present with a marked limp without bearing any weight on the limb.

Stabilisation techniques

The femur can be stabilised using most of the osteosynthesis techniques available: plates, intramedullary fixation and even external fixation when necessary. However, external immobilisation (casts or bandages) should never be used as a stabilisation system due to the fact that hip joints cannot be immobilised, also, with the great muscle mass surrounding the femur, adequate reduction of movements of the fracture site of this type is not possible. If conservative treatment is chosen, the patient should ideally be kept in a small cage instead of applying bandages.

Intramedullary pinning

As previously mentioned in the chapter on intramedullary fixation (page 34), this osteosynthesis system, with the exception of interlocking pins, is not effective in correctly stabilising the rotation or distraction-compression movements of the fracture site.

Although this osteosynthesis system is not ideal for the treatment of femoral fractures, oblique and long spiral fractures, and simple fractures without a tendency to rotate can, in some cases, be treated using intramedullary pins that are usually associated with cerclages. These fractures are more frequently produced in growing animals in which the lack of stability is partially offset by the greater speed of the mechanisms of bone healing.

Also, this osteosynthesis system may present problems derived from the curvature of the diaphysis. When attempting to stabilise a curved bone with a straight implant, a perfect reduction will never be achieved, impairing stability. This happens primarily in distal fractures, mostly in dogs, in which the curvature is greater (Fig. 38). Therefore, the greater the curvature of the femur, the greater the contraindication to use this system. Patients of chondrodystrophic breeds, with a significant curvature of the distal part of the femur, should not be treated using this system. Nonetheless, this problem is minimised in cats as the bone is much straighter.

The greater the curvature of the femur, the greater the contraindication for its stabilisation using intramedullary pins.

If intramedullary pinning is ultimately chosen, the pin must be anchored both proximally -sticking out by the subtrochanteric fossa of the femur- as well as distally -in the metaphyseal or epiphyseal cancellous bone- without, of course, invading the joint (Fig. 39). The pins should be inserted in a normograde manner so that the implant is more firmly anchored in the proximal fragment. Also, it is important to keep in mind that, if the distal fragment is extremely short, little stability will be achieved as the implant allows for slight side-to-side movements slowly pushing the pin in a proximal direction with its respective progressive loss of function.

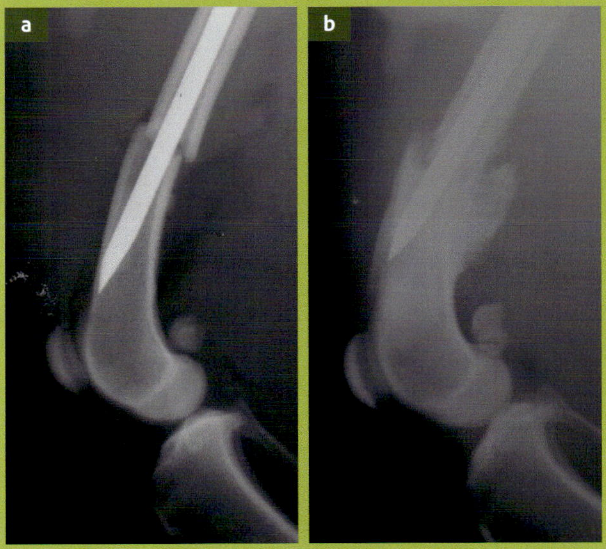

FIGURE 38. Loss of reduction of a fracture as a consequence of the use of a straight implant to fix a diaphyseal femoral fracture in a canine, whose femur presented distal curvature (a). Same fracture one month after surgery. The pin has been partially pushed out (b).

To prevent movements of rotation as much as possible (those that are not neutralised by this system), the following is useful:

- Associate intramedullary fixation to cerclages or partial external fixation.
- Insert more than one pin (Fig. 40).
- Associate the intramedullary fixation with supporting plates. This combination is more and more frequent and allows for easier alignment of the primary fragments as well as increasing resistance against forces of flexion (Fig. 41).

External fixation

Due to the anatomical particularities of the femur, external fixation of this bone is limited to the application of single-plane, unilateral fixators or, in very specific cases, of hybrid systems, tie-in systems that allow for the use of clamps in the medial portion at the stifle joint level. Normally, this type of external fixation is applied in fractures that are difficult to treat as a system associated with minimal osteosynthesis, which allows for the neutralisation of movements of rotation and collapsing of the primary fragments (Fig. 42). In some cases, they can be applied temporarily to give greater stability to other implants, or as a solution to specific problems (Fig. 43).

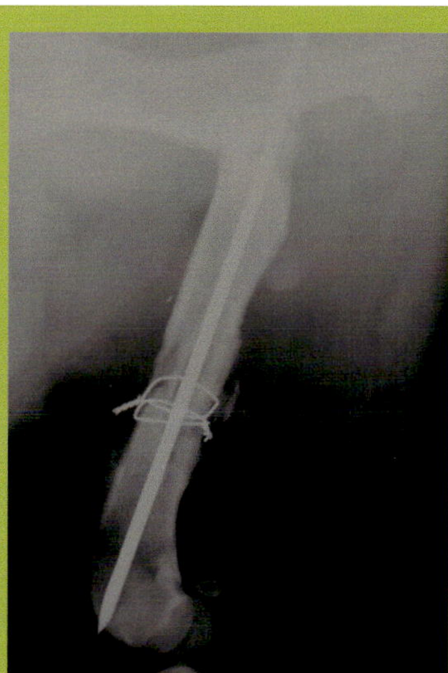

FIGURE 39. Pin invading the stifle joint.

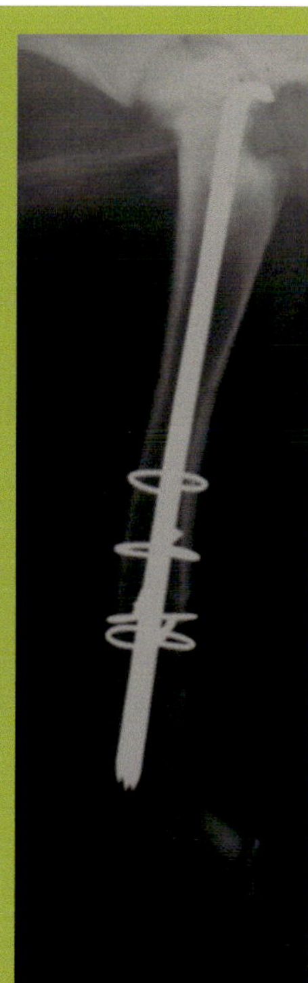

FIGURE 40. Association of pins and cerclages in a spiral fracture in a growing animal.

The localisation of the insertion points of the most external percutaneous pins of the fixator is very simple:

- The most proximal percutaneous pin is inserted in the greater trochanter of the femur, easily located by touch.
- The most distal percutaneous pin is inserted by palpating the most prominent part of the lateral condyle. The pin should be oriented towards the medial condyle. This way, there is no risk of introducing it into the joint cavity.

Percutaneous pins should only be inserted in the diaphyseal area in cases when it is strictly necessary as the pins may cause adhesions of the muscle to the bone due to their contact with the quadriceps muscle.

Generally, no external fixator should be left for longer than three weeks to avoid the possible limitations in the degree of flexion of the stifle joint.

In certain highly comminuted fractures, external fixators can be applied in a tie-in or hybrid configuration which provides more stability.

Osteosynthesis plates

Osteosynthesis plates are the most suitable fixation system in the treatment of femoral fractures, except in the rare cases of very proximal or distal fractures in which there is not enough space to insert a sufficient number of screws.

Osteosynthesis plates, whenever possible, should be applied to the tension-bearing surface of the bone due to the greater resistance of the metal against the forces of traction. This way, in fractures that affect the proximal third, the plate will be placed in a lateral position. In proximal fractures, the plate can be bent over the greater trochanter, enabling the insertion of the three necessary screws in a very reduced space. When perforating in these cases, the drill bit should be placed in an oblique manner and in different directions so that the tips of the screws do not come into contact with each other (Fig. 44).

In diaphyseal fractures, the plate should be placed on the lateral surface in an increasingly cranial direction, depending on how distal it needs to be inserted. Due to the curvature of the femur in its distal portion, the placement of a straight implant is, in many cases, complicated. To solve this problem, the plate should be placed in a slightly cranial direction, "twisting" the distal portion of the implant to prevent it from interfering in the displacement of the patella (Fig. 45).

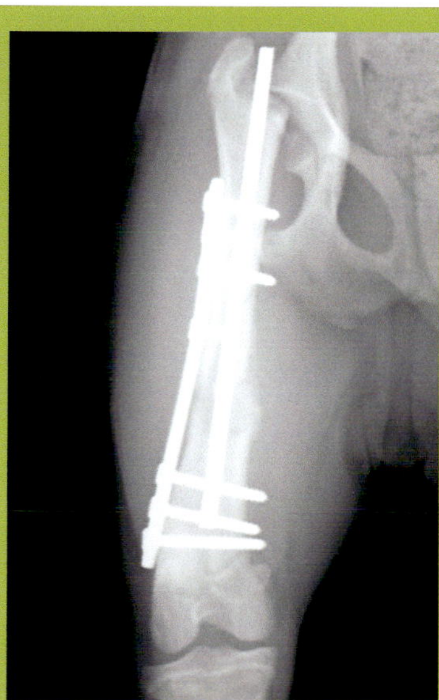

FIGURE 41. Pin associated with a supporting plate.

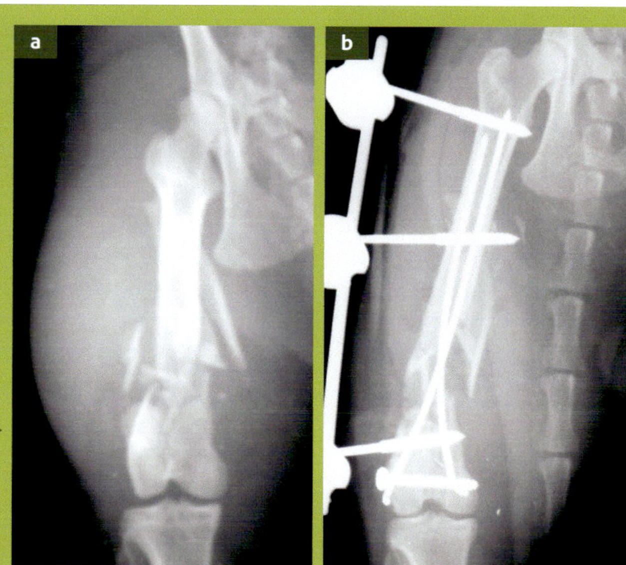

FIGURE 42. Comminuted distal fracture of the femur in a cat (a) treated with Rush pins and partial external fixation (b).

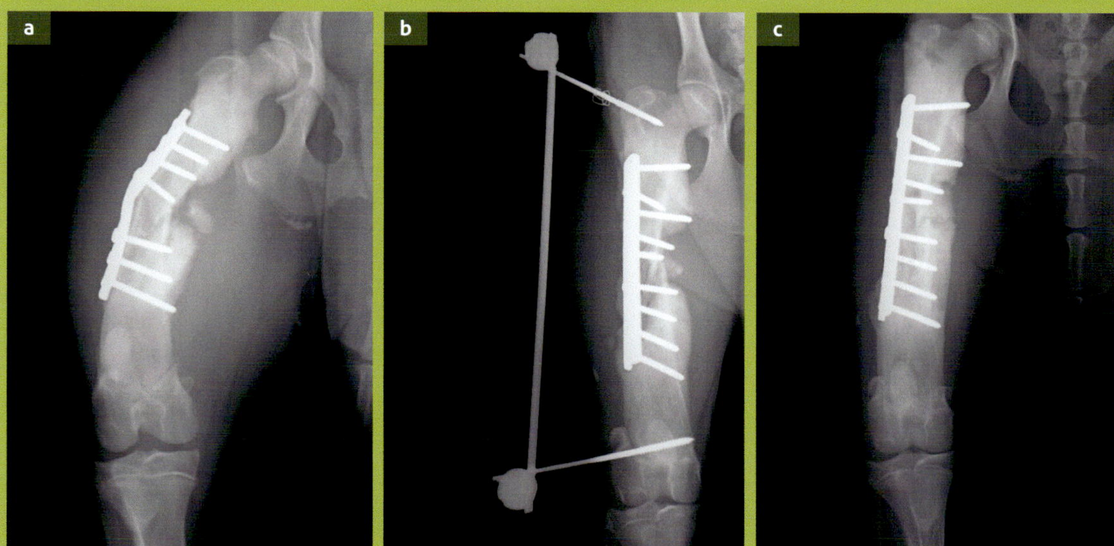

FIGURE 43. Implant failure (a) and temporary reinforcement of the new osteosynthesis by means of partial external fixation (b). The unilateral fixator is removed once the fracture callus has gained sufficient stability (c).

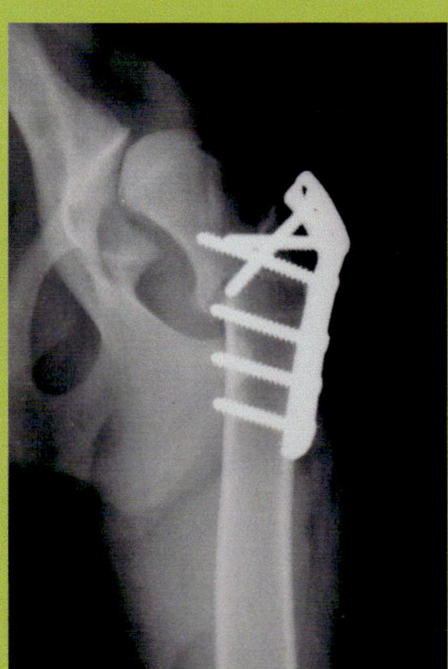

FIGURE 44. Plate moulded above the greater trochanter of the femur. The screws should be oriented so that they do not come into contact with one another.

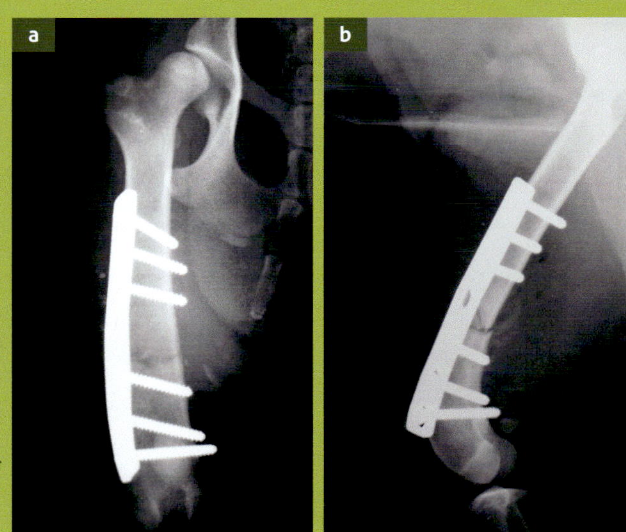

FIGURE 45. Plates moulded to adapt to the distal third of the femur (a and b).

To make this process easier, there are distal femur plates with different designs and made by different manufacturers, however, they all share certain characteristics:

- The most distal portion of the plate presents a caudal curvature to adapt it to the shape of the bone.
- Most are wider in their distal portion to hold a greater number of screws in a reduced space. This way, the implant can be properly stabilised even if the fracture is very distal.

Depending on the location of the fracture and the breed of the animal, different types of plates adapt better.

The "normal" plates can also be moulded in the direction of the wide plane using a wrench in the shape of a J. These instruments prevent the deformation of the holes given that when the plate is bent in this direction, its holes take on an oval shape which can eventually impede the introduction of the screws in said holes (Fig. 46).

The reconstruction plates are designed to be moulded in said direction, but unfortunately, they are not especially resistant, and thus, surgery could fail to achieve its purpose.

Surgical approach

The approach to femoral fractures is always performed on the lateral surface of the limb. It is a simple approach given that there are no relevant vascular or nerve structures in this area. Once the skin incision is made and the fascia lata is located, a longitudinal incision is made to demarcate the vastus lateralis and the biceps femoris muscles. After displacing the latter in a caudal direction, the entire femoral diaphysis is accessed (Fig. 47). To completely expose the most dorsal portion of the greater trochanter and be able to insert the implants in fractures very proximal to the femur, a tenotomy of the superficial gluteal muscle must be performed (Fig. 48). Once surgery is finished, the tendon is sutured in a routine manner.

In the case of very distal fractures, in which a plate cannot be placed in a cranio-lateral position because it would interfere with the displacement of the patella, it will have to be placed on the lateral surface of the condyle. In these cases, it will be easier to handle the femur as if an arthrotomy was going to be performed on the stifle, but always avoiding cutting the capsule. After exposing the distal part of the femur, the biceps and quadriceps muscles will be separated in a proximal direction for easy access to the bone.

Treatment of the most frequent fractures

In this section, the most frequent femoral fractures are described with the principal aspects to be taken into account to select the optimal stabilisation system, as well as their particularities.

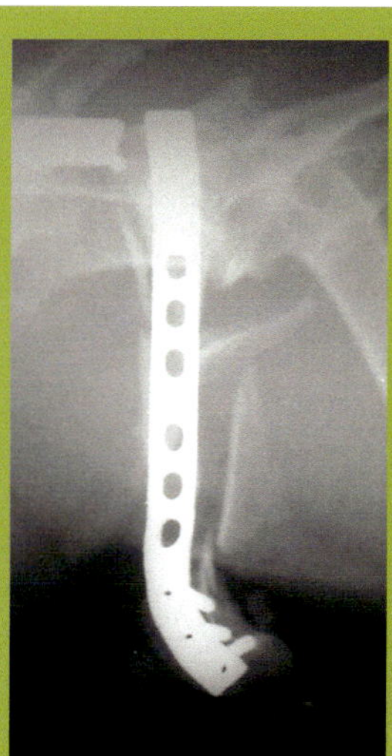

FIGURE 46. Plate moulded in the direction of the wide plane to stabilise a highly distal fracture in a Teckel breed dog.

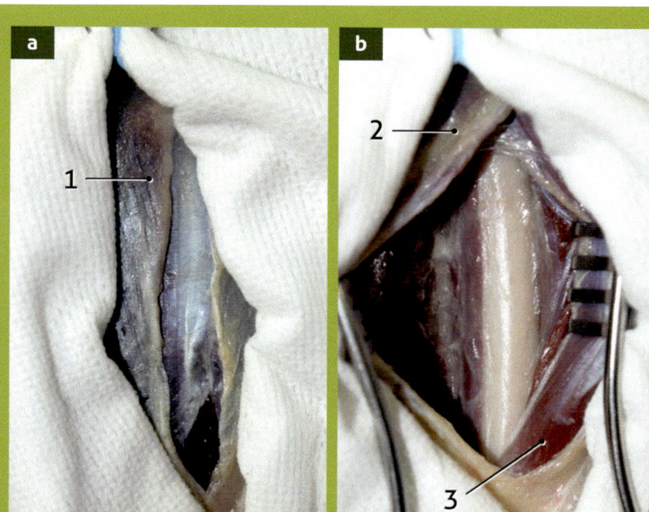

FIGURE 47. Incision of the fascia lata (a) and separation of the quadriceps femoris and biceps femoris muscles (b) to access the femoral diaphysis.
1. Fascia lata.
2. Biceps femoris muscle.
3. Quadriceps femoris muscle.

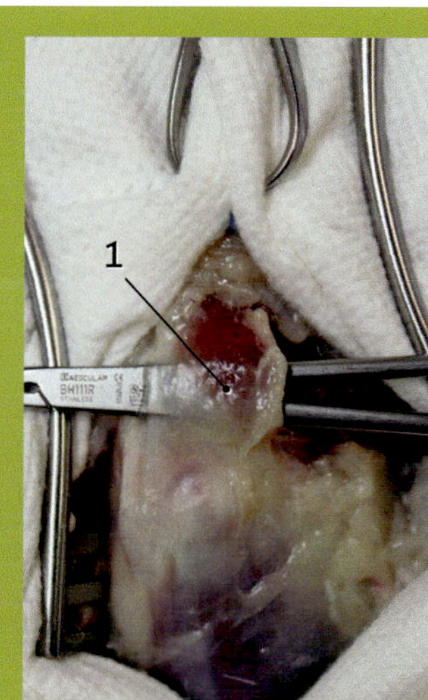

FIGURE 48. Lifting of the superficial gluteal muscle for a tenotomy using a haemostat clamp.
1. Superficial gluteal muscle.

Fractures of the proximal epiphysis

In veterinary bone surgery, fractures of the proximal epiphysis of the femur are not especially frequent. They primarily affect young patients given that the resistance of the growth plates is less than that of the tendon structures. In adult patients, if a treatment is implemented that affects said area, it is more frequent that a coxofemoral dislocation or an acetabular fracture occur than a proximal epiphyseal fracture.

Epiphysiolysis of the head of the femur

The epiphysiolysis of the head of the femur is a type I Salter-Harris fracture of the head of the femur. The growth plate separates completely, leaving the joint portion attached to the acetabulum by the round ligament (Fig. 49). In young patients, this fracture may also be accompanied by a type I Salter-Harris fracture of the greater trochanter.

The diagnosis is made by means of a ventrodorsal X-ray view of the hip. In some cases, it may be useful to take an X-ray in the "frog" position or pushing the femurs in a cranial direction for better visibility of the lesion. It must not be forgotten that, when tractioning the femurs in a ventral direction for correct placement of the patient, the fracture may become less visible or appear smaller by X-ray leading to it going unnoticed.

Due to the fact that this is a lesion to the growth plate, treatment consists of stabilisation using pins inserted in the lateral surface of the femur that cross through the plate in a perpendicular manner (Fig. 50). They should be inserted into the joint fragment as deep as possible without invading the joint.

Although the surgery is easier if an osteotomy of the greater trochanter is performed, it can also be done without it, preventing possible problems derived from the technique. To do so, the proximal portion of the femur is operated on, displacing the tensor fascia lata muscle in a ventral direction and the middle gluteal muscle in a dorsal direction. Between the tensor muscle, the deep gluteal muscle and the vastus lateralis muscle, a triangle is formed through which the head of the femur can be accessed.

Once the joint capsule is located, which is usually partially damaged, the joint is accessed and the fracture line is located. Next, the femur is rotated, placing its neck in a cranial direction. The acetabular fragment of the head will remain inside of the joint, attached to the round ligament.

The pins must be placed along the femoral neck. To insert them in the correct direction, they should be placed before reducing the fracture, confirming by palpating the fracture plane that the tips of the pins stick out in the correct position. The pins should be inserted from the lateral surface of the femur, in a slightly distal and cranial point to the insertion of the superficial gluteal muscle.

In cases of epiphysiolysis of the head of the femur, the first pin can be inserted in a retrograde manner for correct placement. This will mark the insertion point and direction of the rest of the pins.

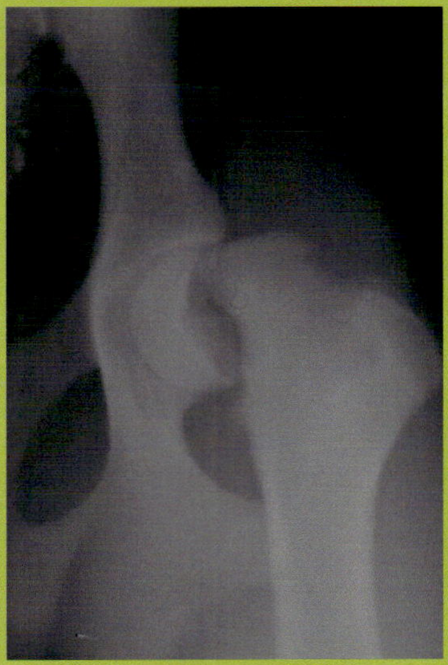

FIGURE 49. Type I Salter-Harris fracture of the head of the femur.

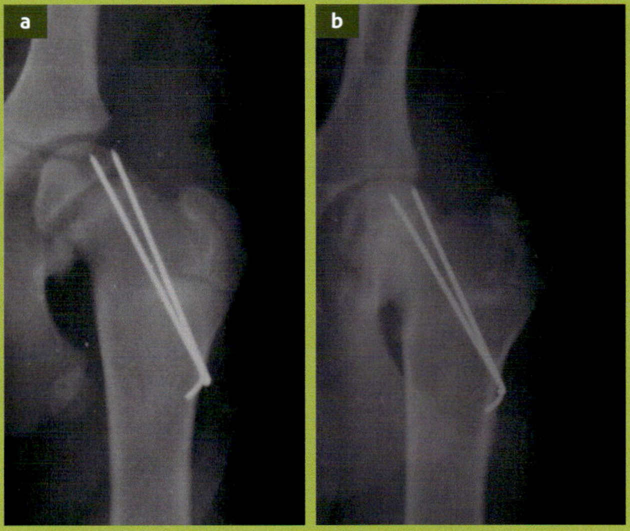

FIGURE 50. Pins inserted into the lateral surface of the femur, perpendicular to the plate. Postoperative X-ray (a) and one month after surgery (b).

The implant should impede movements of rotation and sliding of the fragment in a ventral direction as, when the patient bears weight on the limb, the fracture plane is pressured which benefits bone healing. To avoid rotation of the fragment, placing two or three pins in a slightly divergent manner is helpful. Given that the system is very stable, said pins do not have to be very thick.

> *Before reducing the fracture, the pins should be slightly removed, concealing their tips to avoid making the reduction more difficult.*

To reduce the fracture, the proximal portion of the femur must be held using fragment reduction forceps and its head should be oriented towards the joint. In this position, small movements of rotation will occur while the femur will simultaneously be tractioned in a ventral direction to finish reducing the fracture, checking that the position is correct at all times. If the fracture is properly reduced, the femur can be moved without displacing the fracture line.

To finish, the tip of the pins need to be inserted in the acetabular fragment without sticking out from the cartilaginous surface. There are two options to avoid this:

- Calculate the depth in which they should be inserted by measuring the width of the acetabular fragment in the X-ray.
- Insert, between the head and the acetabulum, a surgical instrument that is similar to a teaspoon with a slit in its central portion to be able to introduce the pins without coming into contact with the round ligament. This instrument will act as a barrier when the pin sticks out, and it will only have to be removed 1 mm to ensure that it does not damage the joint.

Lastly, the capsule and the soft tissues are sutured as usual.

Epiphysiolysis of the greater trochanter

The epiphysiolysis of the greater trochanter is infrequent and is usually associated with the epiphysiolysis of the head of the femur (Fig. 51). It is classified as a type I Salter-Harris fracture of the greater trochanter caused by the forced traction of the insertions of the middle and deep gluteal muscles. It is, therefore, an avulsion fracture and should thus be stabilised using a tension band system (Fig. 52). The surgery itself is simple and the premature closing that takes place in the growth cartilage of the trochanter should not cause any functional impediments of the affected limb. In very young patients, to interfere as little as possible in their growth, and for more aesthetic than functional reasons, the cerclage wire of said system can be substituted by a resorbable suture (Fig. 53).

Fracture of the neck of the femur

Fractures of the neck of the femur are typical in adult patients in which, due to the direction of the impact, the hip does not dislocate, and the forces are concentrated on the neck of the femur which eventually breaks.

Adequate treatment consists of the placement of a compression screw perpendicular to the fracture plane, associated with a pin placed parallel to the latter. The screw should be inserted as deep as possible in the head of the femur without reaching the joint surface. The pin, aside from providing stability to the fracture, has a primary function of preventing movements of rotation around the screw.

The surgery is performed similar to that previously described for type I Salter-Harris fractures of the head of the femur. The only difference is that the reduction of the fracture site must be as exact as possible, especially in large patients. In this case, performing an osteotomy of the greater trochanter is recommended to have better visibility of its correct reduction. The surgery will be much easier if the gliding hole of the screw is perforated from the fracture plane towards the lateral cortical bone. If the size of the patient allows for it, cancellous screws should be used. Of course, they should be completely threaded given that the tip of the screw will not be anchored to any cortical bone. Once the screw is placed, the Kirschner pin is inserted and the osteotomy of the greater trochanter is reduced and stabilised using a tension band system (Fig. 54).

In the case of non-reducible fractures or implant failure, performing an excision of the head and neck of the femur may be necessary (Fig. 55). This is also applicable to epiphysiolysis of the head of the femur.

Diaphyseal fractures

Diaphyseal fractures are the fractures that affect the femur with greater frequency. In this type of fractures, as previously commented, the plate should be placed on the cranio-lateral

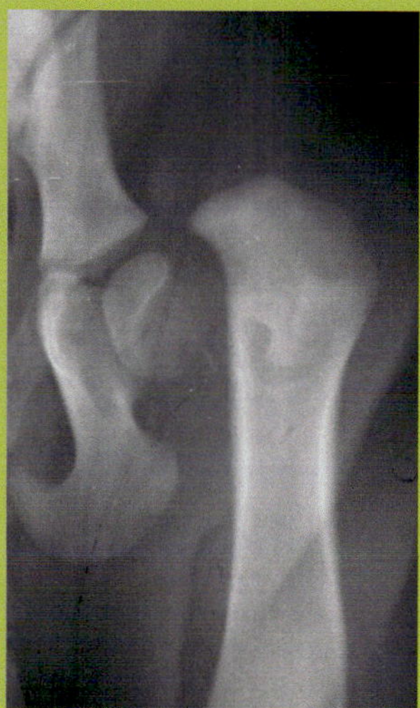
FIGURE 51. Type I Salter-Harris fracture of the head and greater trochanter of the femur.

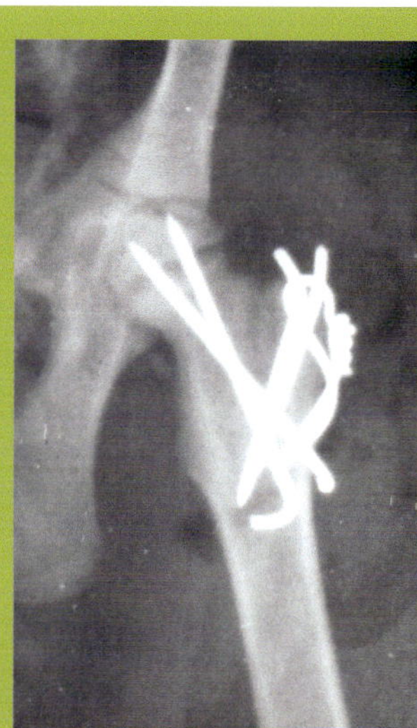
FIGURE 52. Tension band system in a type I Salter-Harris fracture of the head and greater trochanter of the femur.

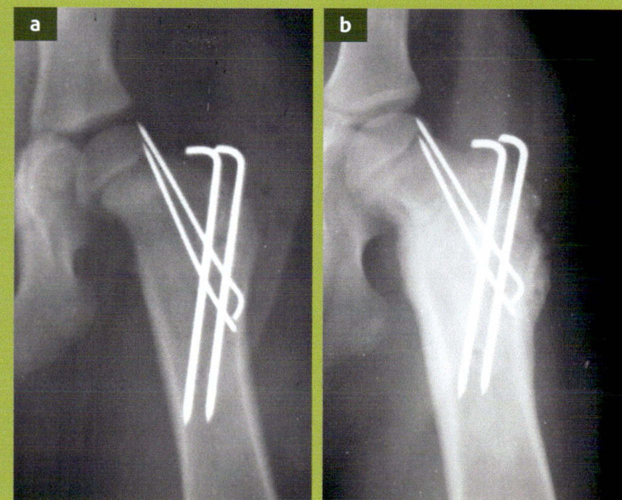

FIGURE 53. Postoperative X-ray (a) and progress of pins with a tension band, implemented with resorbable material in a very young patient (b).

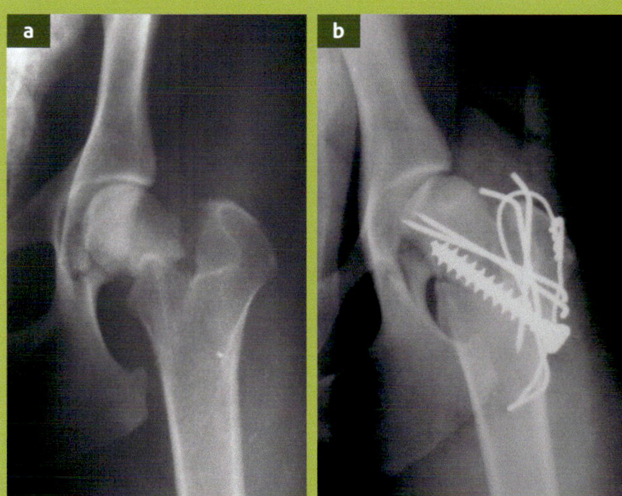

FIGURE 54. Fracture of the femur neck (a) and postoperative X-ray (b).

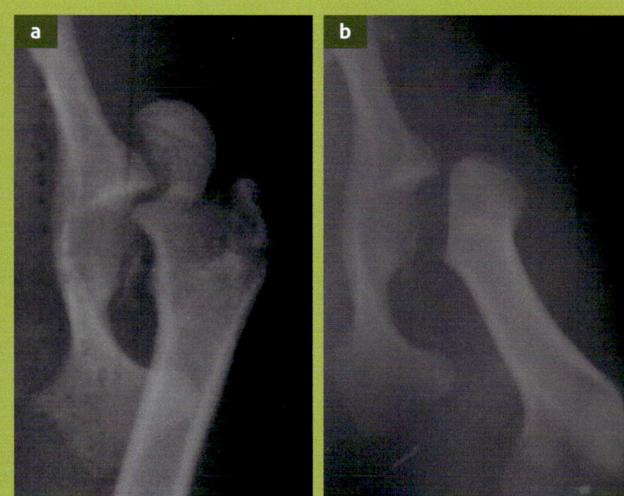

FIGURE 55. Non-reducible fracture of the head and neck of the femur (a), treated by means of resection of the head and neck of the femur (b).

surface, which is the tension-bearing surface of the bone. The choice of which stabilisation system should be used depends on the type of fracture, obviously, as well as the age of the patient and the surgeon's preferences.

The ideal system to treat diaphyseal femoral fractures are osteosynthesis plates. Generally, compression plates are used in transversal fractures (Fig. 56), neutralisation plates are used in multiple (Fig. 57) or oblique fractures, and supporting plates are used in those in which reconstruction is impossible, or biological osteosynthesis is chosen (Fig. 58).

Subtrochanteric fractures

Subtrochanteric fractures are not especially frequent. When they occur, their principal problem resides in the small size of the proximal fragment.

As previously commented in this chapter, the plate can be placed on top of the trochanter, curving it so that no great space is required to place an adequate number of screws. For its placement, a tenotomy of the superficial gluteal muscle is necessary as the plate is inserted in a slight caudal direction, just above the insertion point and anatomical trajectory of said muscle (Fig. 59).

Fractures of the middle third

Taking into account the characteristics of the femur, relatively few fractures can be adequately stabilised by the application of intramedullary pins alone. Only long oblique fractures in young patients can be treated using this kind of implant, in combination with cerclages to impede sliding movements.

Similarly, the fractures located in the distal portion of the femur should not be stabilised by means of intramedullary fixation given that the implant should not stick out through the distal epiphysis of the bone. As the distal fragment is only attached by a small portion of the pin, the stability achieved is scarce. If the natural curvature of the femur at this level is added to the previous characteristic, it is easy to understand why this type of fixation is not recommended for distal fractures.

Similar to that which occurs in fractures of the humerus, external fixation should not be the first choice for treatment of femoral fractures. The impossibility of attaching connecting rods to both sides of the bone due to anatomical reasons impedes the use of sufficiently stable structures. Unilateral, single-plane configurations or hybrid forms of said configurations are the only choice, taking advantage of the possibility to place clamps on the medial surface of the stifle in certain breeds.

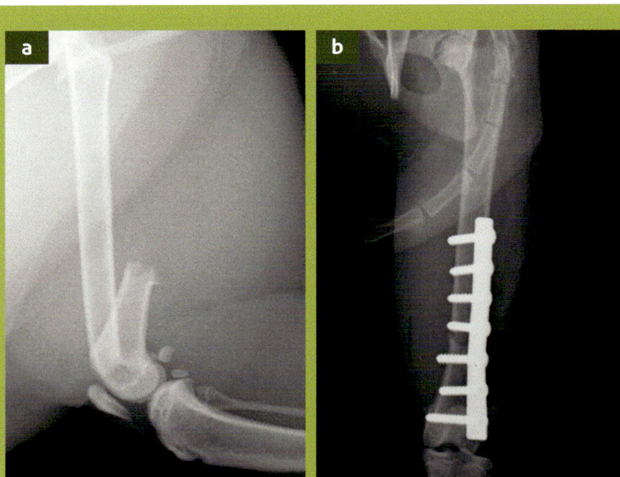

FIGURE 56. Transversal femoral fracture (a) treated with a compression plate. Due to the fact that the patient is a cat, the plate must be placed in a distal position (b).

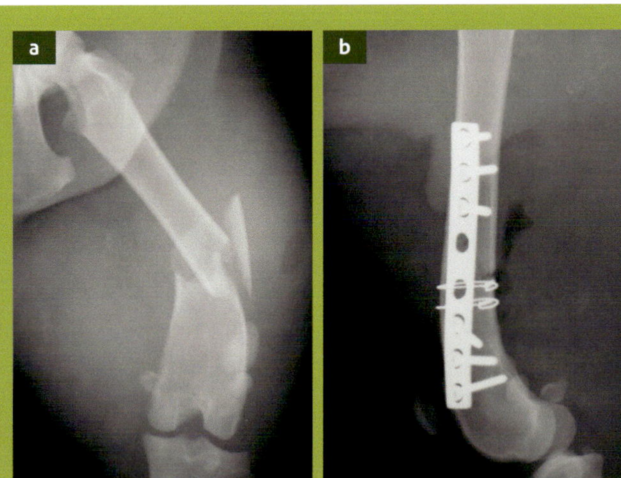

FIGURE 57. Multiple fracture of the femur (a) stabilised with a neutralisation plate and cerclages (b).

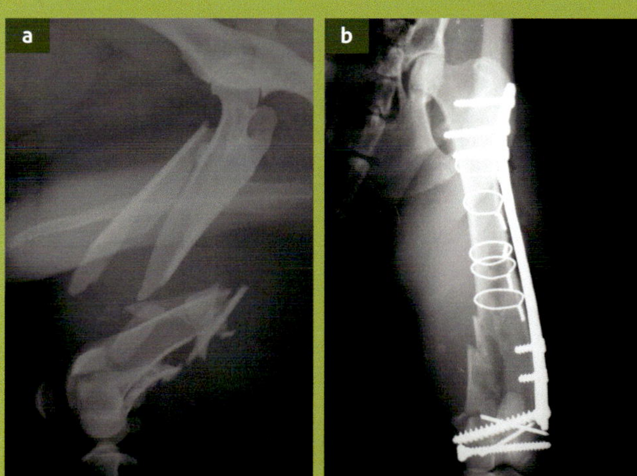

FIGURE 58. Comminuted femoral fracture (a) treated with a supporting plate (b).

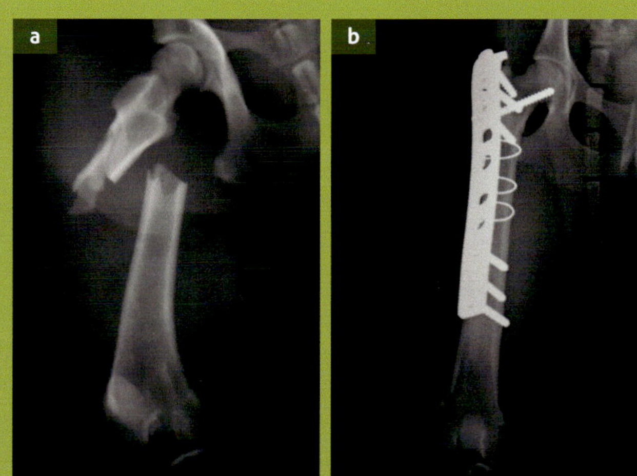

FIGURE 59. Subtrochanteric multiple fracture of the femur (a) treated with cerclages, a neutralisation plate and a compression screw for a fracture of the neck of the femur (b).

Another option is to place two connecting rods to achieve more resistance to flexion (Fig. 60). The most external rod can be removed after a few weeks to make the fixator more dynamic. However, the most stable option if external fixators must be used, is that using a tie-in type structure. The association of an intramedullary pin that neutralises the forces of flexion requires the use of only two percutaneous pins, which in turn avoids the need to place screws in muscular areas.

Another possible application of external fixation is to provide temporary stability in the case of minimal osteosynthesis or when there are doubts about the resistance of the implant. In these cases, the external fixator is removed once it is considered that the healing processes have achieved a sufficiently stable callus for the primary implant to be successful.

Without doubt, osteosynthesis plates are the ideal system for femoral fractures. The type of implant selected and its function will depend on the type of fracture.

The most frequent fractures are multiple or comminuted fractures of the middle and distal thirds. The application of neutralisation plates associated with other compressive or supporting systems will not only depend on the possibility of the reduction of the fragments, but also on the surgeon's preferences (Figs. 61 and 62). The plate must always be placed on the tension-bearing surface. If it must be placed on a very distal area, interference with the movement of the patella must be avoided.

In fractures in which stabilisation by means of biological techniques is chosen, the association of intramedullary stabilisation to the plates may be helpful. The insertion of a pin facilitates the alignment of the longitudinal axis of the bone and the separation of the primary fragments to achieve the adequate length. Later, it will only be necessary to adjust its correct position regarding the longitudinal axis formed by the "trochanter-femur head" complex. In this manner, rotational maladjustments will be avoided (Fig. 63). In reducible fractures, alignment is achieved automatically as the fragments fit together correctly.

In the case of fractures of the distal third, the possibility of anchoring the plates using an adequate number of screws should be assessed. There are special plates to compensate this lack of space (Fig. 64).

In growing patients, these implants cannot be used as the development of a rigid bridge between the metaphyseal and epiphyseal areas would impede bone growth of the femur. In these cases, if the fracture is not sufficiently stable after its reduction, stabilisation using Rush pins associated with a temporary external fixation system can be used. Of course, the fixator should never be anchored to both sides of the growth plate.

When dealing with large patients or when the fracture is not stable after reduction, one option is to use two plates

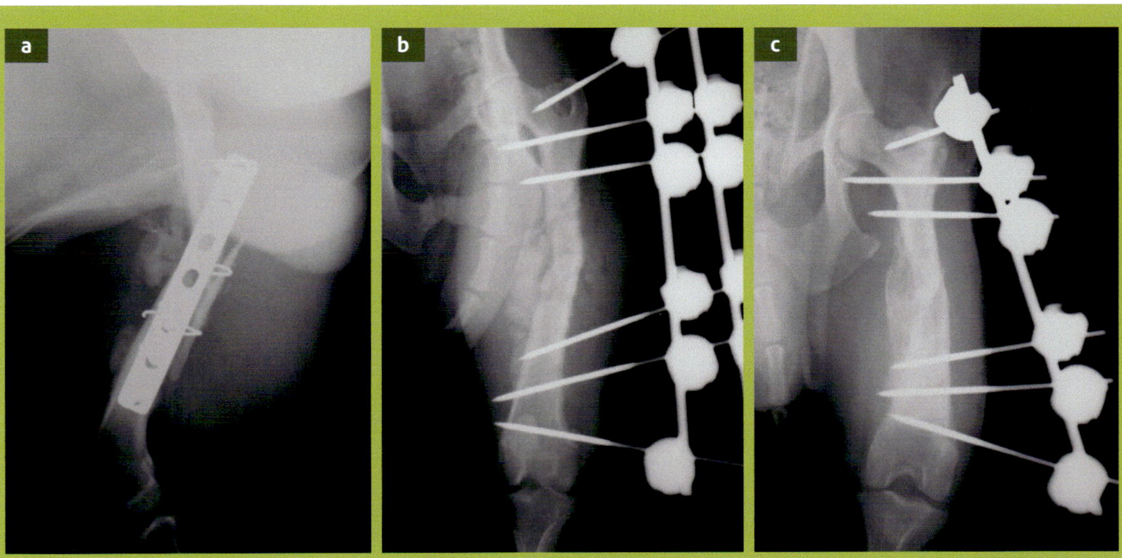

FIGURE 60. Poorly stabilised fracture (a) treated with partial external fixation with a dynamic double connecting rod (b and c).

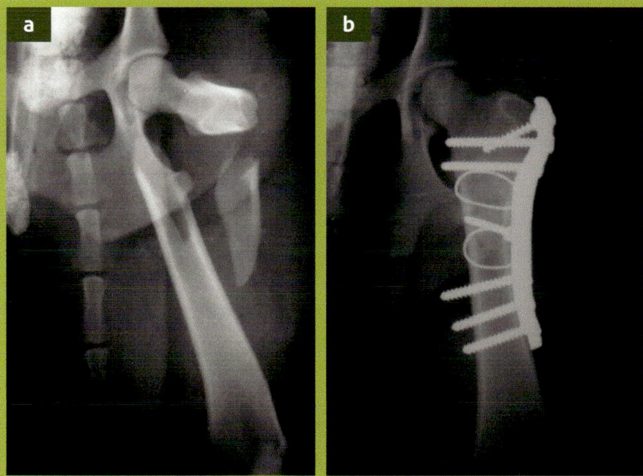

FIGURE 61. Multiple fracture (a) treated with a neutralisation plate, compression screws and cerclages (b).

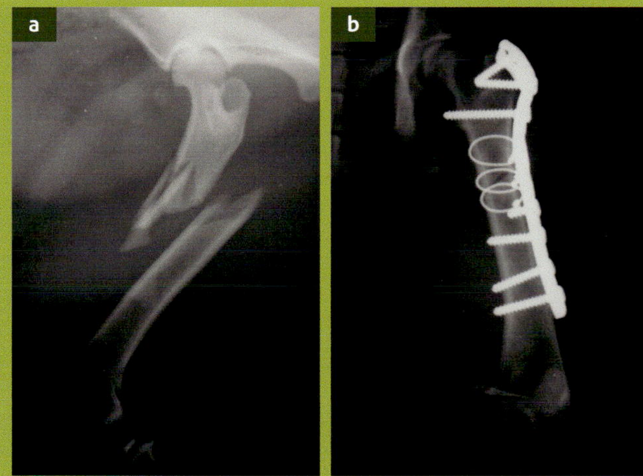

FIGURE 62. Multiple fracture (a) treated with a neutralisation plate and cerclages (without compression screws) (b).

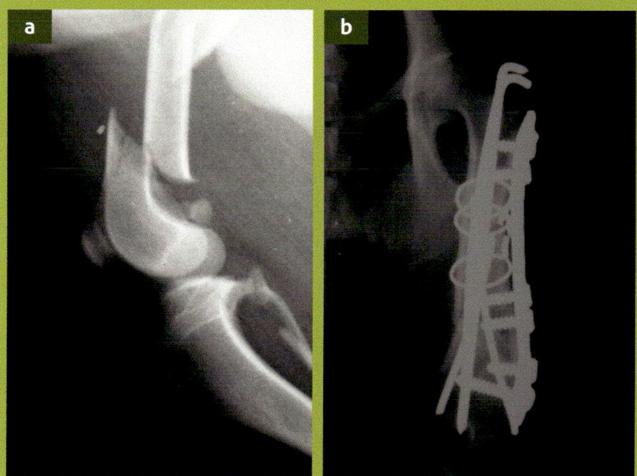

FIGURE 63. Segmental fracture (a) treated with intramedullary pins and a plate with unicortical screws (b).

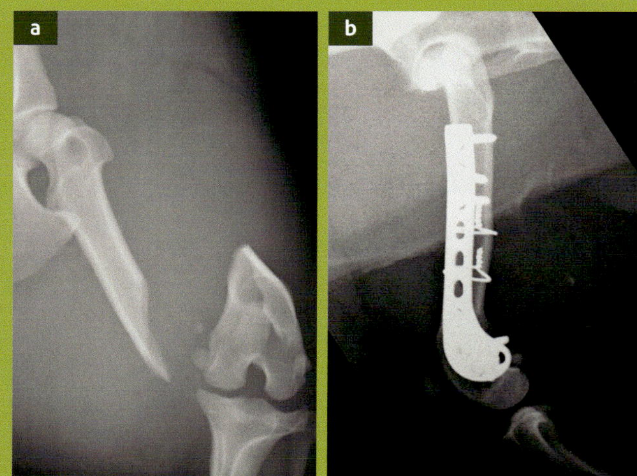

FIGURE 64. Distal fracture of the femur (a) stabilised with a "golf club" plate (b).

instead of one. This way, an adequate number of screws can be inserted between the two implants. Another option is to use locking plates which need fewer screws per fragment (Fig. 65).

Fractures of the distal epiphysis

Distal fractures of the femur are more frequent in cats than dogs. They are usually type II Salter-Harris fractures of the distal epiphysis. As is the case in most fractures that affect growth plates, the ideal treatment is the application of Rush pins to avoid interfering with the growth of the bone.

This type of fracture is not considered as a surgical emergency; however, surgery should be performed as soon as possible. Once two or three days have passed, adequate reduction becomes complicated as the bone healing processes start rapidly in young patients, especially in the periostium of the caudal portion of the metaphysis.

The surgical approach is performed by means of a cranio-lateral incision of the stifle. Once the patellar tendon is located, an incision is made in the fascia lata that is parallel to the tendon, taking care to not get too close to the tendon to minimise post-surgery pain (Fig. 66). Next, the incision is extended along the fascia lata in a proximal direction, going around the patella to the point deemed necessary. Later, the joint capsule is opened and the patella is dislocated medially. The intervention should be done with great care and sufficient tissue in the patellar area should be left

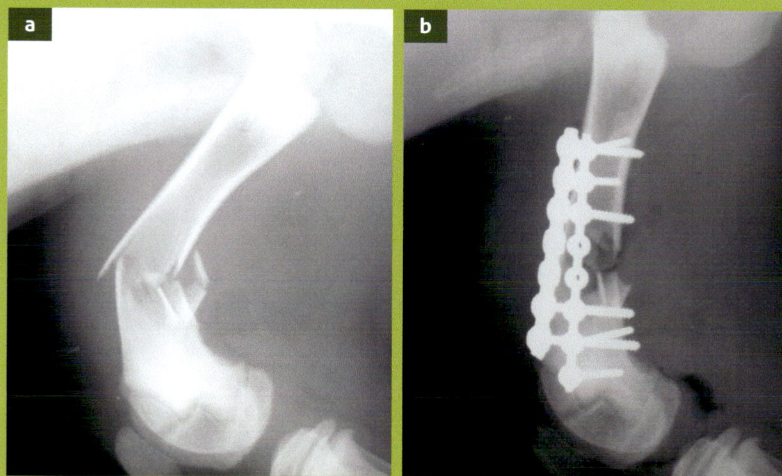

FIGURE 65. Very unstable distal fracture of the femur (a) in a young, large patient, treated with two locking plates at 90º (b).

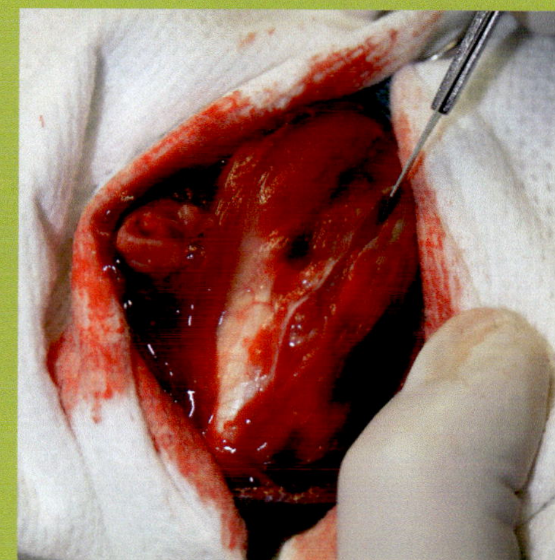

FIGURE 66. Para-patellar incision of the fascia lata, maintaining a safety margin in relation with the patellar tendon.

for proper suturing when completing the surgery. If a dehiscence occurs, the patella may dislocate.

Once the fracture is located, it is reduced, holding the tibia from its proximal portion and tractioning it in a cranial direction with the stifle in flexion (Fig. 67). In fractures that are not recent, the retraction of the periostium makes this procedure notably more difficult and said tissue may even have to be dissected completely in fractures that are several days old.

To temporarily stabilise the fracture, twin point reduction forceps are used: on of them is inserted between the condyles, and the other rests of the cranial surface of the metaphysis (Fig. 68). This will provide sufficient stability until the Kirschner pins can be inserted. These should be inserted from both sides of the ridges of the femoral trochlea, oriented towards the medullary cavity (Fig. 69). To finish, the ends are bent and cut to avoid interfering in joint movement (Fig. 70).

There are different possibilities regarding the stability to be achieved:

- Insertion of Rush pins through the medullary cavity (Fig. 71). This system hardly interferes in growth of the plate and it allows for certain movements of rotation and separation of the fragments where the pins cross. This implant should not be used in old or unstable fractures.
- Anchoring of the tip of the pins in the metaphyseal area (Fig. 72). This system is much more stable given that it hardly allows for any movement at the level of the fracture site, but it interferes in growth processes. It should not be used in patients with a high growth potential.
- Insertion of pins from the cranial metaphyseal area in a parallel manner towards the condyles. This is very stable and allows for normal bone growth. The only problem is that it requires a more extensive intervention and great care must be taken to avoid damaging the joint surface. This is the best system, especially if the potential growth of the animal is very high (Fig. 73).

In some cases, metaphyseal fractures are accompanied by joint fractures, which worsens the prognosis. They are much more frequent in cats as a result of falls from great heights. Treatment is implemented following the stabilisation principles for joint fractures, attempting to reconstruct the joint surface as anatomically as possible. To do so, compression screws will always be used if the fragment is large enough (Fig. 74). If not, pins can be used, although the stability achieved will be much less (Fig. 75).

In some fractures of the distal epiphysis of the femur, it may be helpful to perform an osteotomy of the tibial crest which provides complete visibility of the joint area for correct insertion of the implants. With this approach, as the quadriceps muscle can be lifted, all areas of the femoral condyles can be easily accessed (Fig. 76). Once the surgery is completed, the osteotomy must be stabilised using a tension band system to counteract the traction of the quadriceps femoris muscle (Fig. 77).

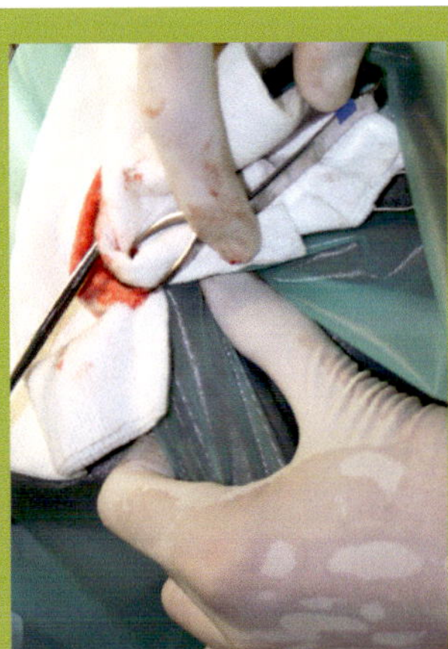

FIGURE 67. Reduction of the fracture by means of displacement of the tibia in a cranial direction.

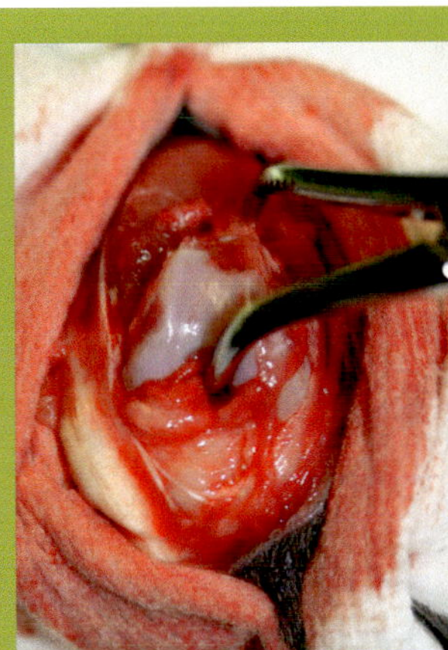

FIGURE 68. Temporary stabilisation of the fracture by means of twin point reduction forceps.

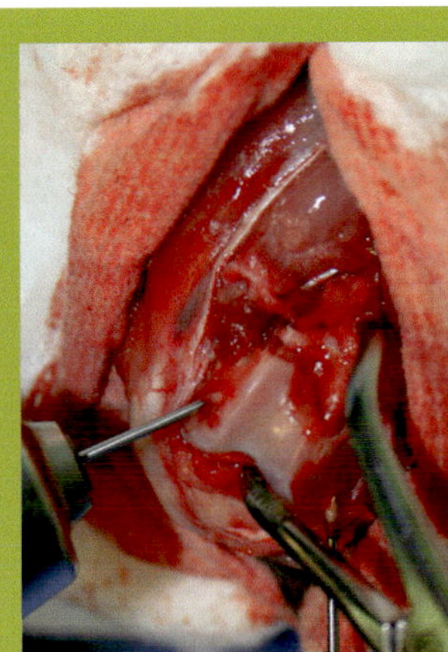

FIGURE 69. Insertion of the pins.

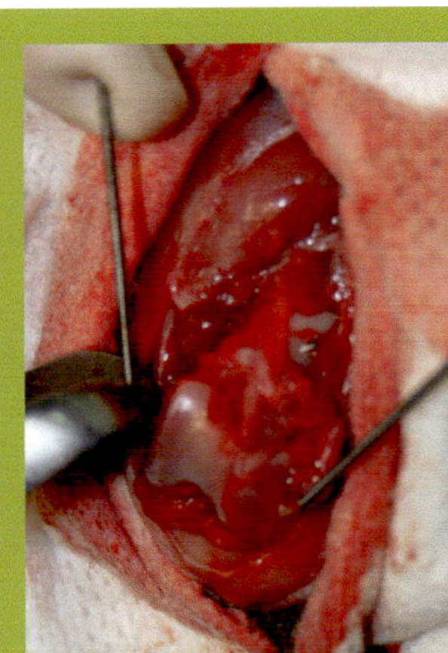

FIGURE 70. Bending and cutting of the pins.

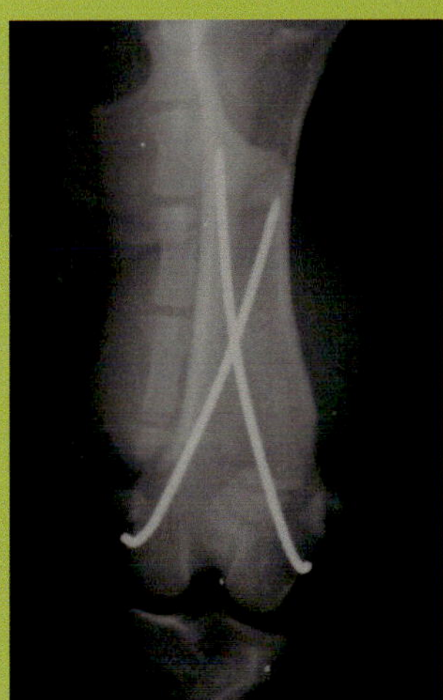

FIGURE 71. Rush pins.

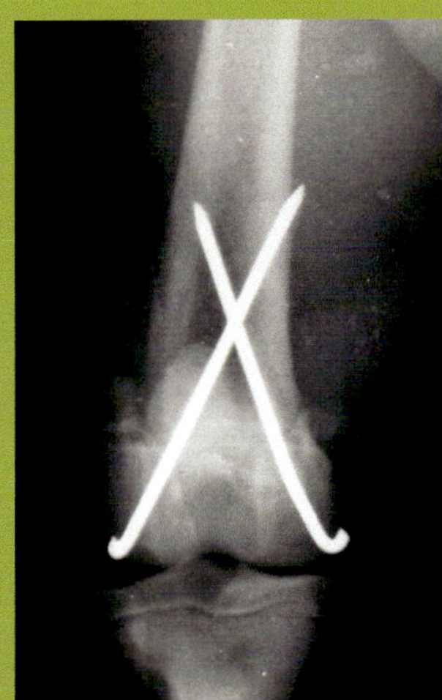

FIGURE 72. Rush pins anchored in the metaphyseal area.

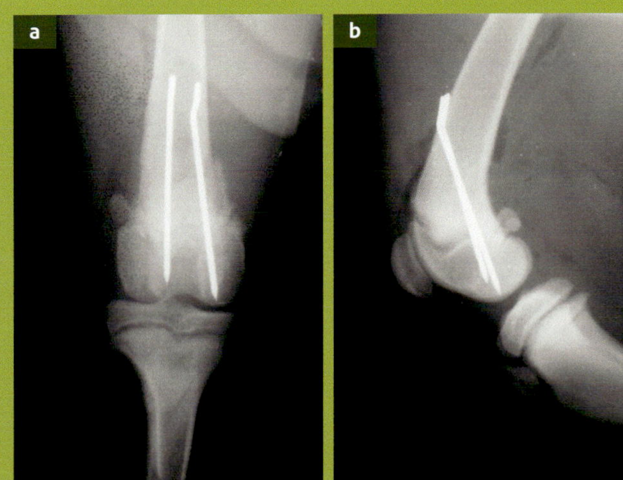

FIGURE 73. Parallel pins inserted from the metaphysis. Cranio-caudal view (a) and latero-medial view (b).

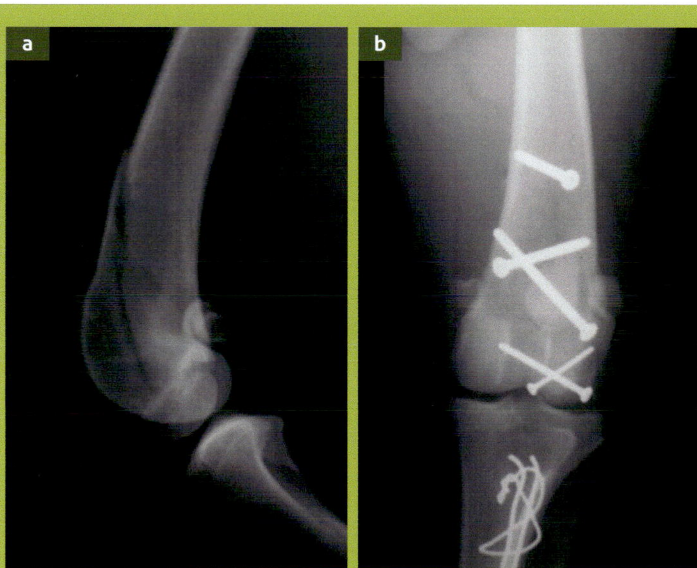

FIGURE 74. Distal spiral fracture (a) treated with compression screws (b).

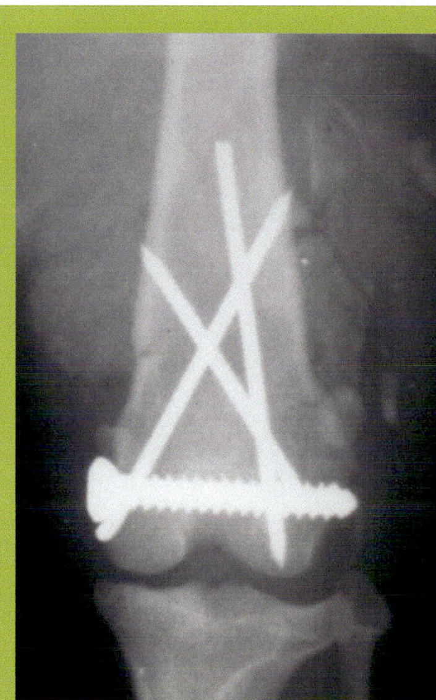

FIGURE 75. Fragments stabilised with pins and an intercondylar screw.

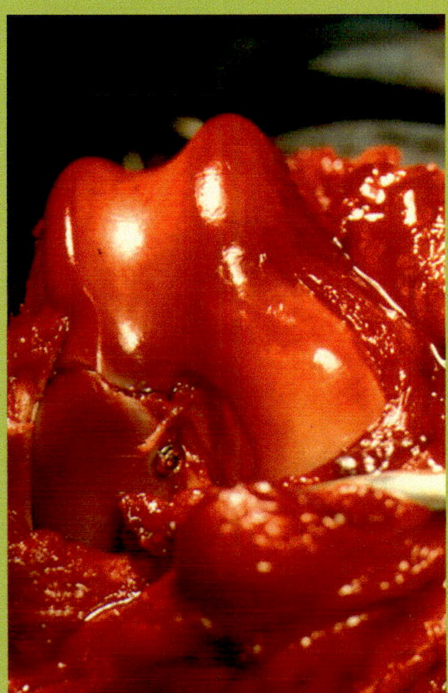

FIGURE 76. Osteotomy of the tibial crest to insert a compression screw from the internal surface of a condyle.

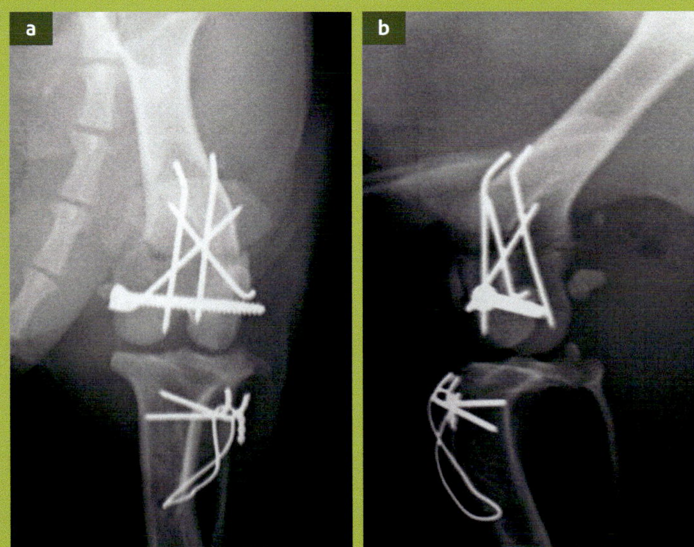

FIGURE 77. Pins with a tension band to stabilise an osteotomy. Cranio-caudal view (a) and latero-medial view (b).

FRACTURES OF THE TIBIA AND FIBULA

Statistically, the tibia is the long bone that is most infrequently fractured, with the exception of the humerus. It is usually associated with fractures of the fibula, except in certain cases (oblique fractures of the middle third in growing patients).

It is a nearly straight bone with a slight curvature in its middle diaphyseal area (Fig. 78). Its proximal epiphysis widens creating a marked concavity of the lateral and medial cortical surfaces.

The tension-bearing surface is located on the medial surface. For biomechanical reasons, it is important to highlight its section, as it is the only long bone in which it changes from a triangular shape in its proximal portion, to a circular shape in its distal third (Fig. 79). This anatomical configuration is the cause of it suffering frequent multiple or comminuted fractures with very large fragments and fracture lines that extend towards the distal epiphysis of the bone. Transversal fractures of this bone are infrequent and, when they occur, are located in the distal third, an area that acts like a typical long bone.

When a trauma has taken place that affects the tibia, the distal third should be carefully studied in the X-rays to discard any fissures that may make the correct selection of an implant to be used more difficult, primarily if a closed fixation system is going to be used (Fig. 80).

Regarding its anatomical position, its epiphyses are blocked: proximally by the joint surface of the femur, and distally by the epiphysis of the talus bone. This peculiarity makes stabilisation by means of intramedullary fixation inadequate. On certain occasions, the pin can be forced to stick out through the proximal epiphysis of the tibia, always inserting it in a normograde manner, slightly displaced towards the medial cortical surface to avoid posterior damage to the patellar tendon.

The blood supply of this bone in its most distal portion is reduced due to the fact that there is little muscle mass in this area.

Regarding the fibula, its greater anatomical importance in cats should be highlighted, given that the distal epiphysis in cats forms part of the joint surface of the tarsus, as opposed to how in dogs the distal portion is positioned laterally, in contact with the ridge of the talus, but without bearing weight.

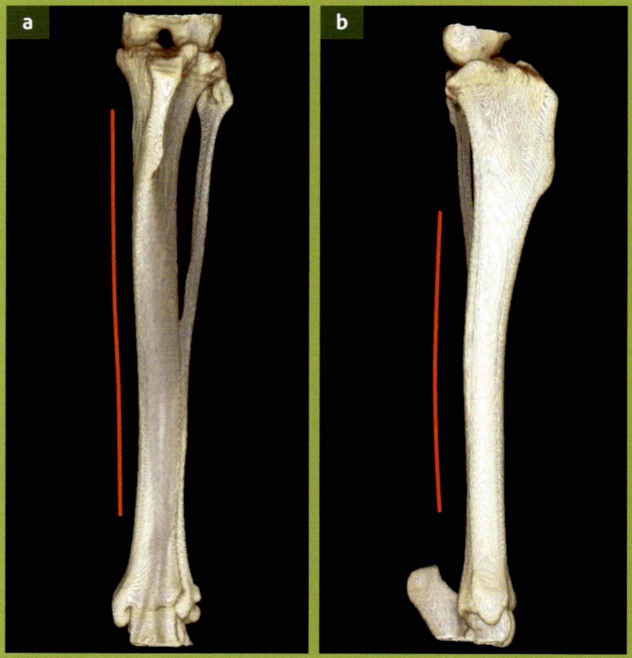

FIGURE 78. Reconstruction of the tibia using CT. The red lines represent the tension-bearing faces.

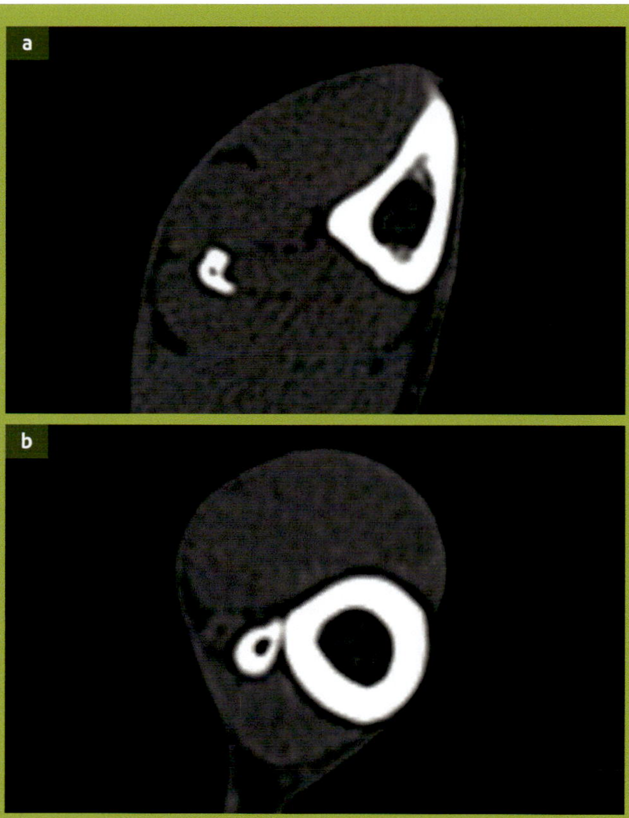

FIGURE 79. Transversal slices of the tibia. Proximal (a) and distal (b) slices. Images taken using CT.

Generally, in tibia and fibula fractures, only the tibia must be stabilised except for in cases of fractures of the distal portion of the fibula, in which it too must be stabilised. This is due to the fact that the distal epiphysis is where the collateral lateral ligaments insert and, therefore, it would affect the stability of the tarsus.

Stabilisation techniques

The tibia can be stabilised by any fixation system, including intramedullary fixation although this is not recommended.

External coaptation

Few fractures should be treated with conservative techniques. They must be highly stable fractures in young patients in which the healing processes compensate for the lack of stability. In accordance with that previously mentioned, stable fractures that affect the tibia are scarce, and thus conservative treatment is rarely used, almost exclusively in short oblique fractures without displacement in growing animals.

One detail to keep in mind when considering conservative treatment of the tibia is the integrity of the fibula (Fig. 81). Although this bone is thin and of little resistance, it acts as an internal brace, significantly decreasing the movements of the fracture site, especially against collapse during axial weight bearing.

There are many types of rigid bandages for the conservative treatment of fractures, but all are based on the application of a light Robert-Jones bandage that covers from the toes to a few centimetres above the stifle (Fig. 82). Too much padding should not be used given that it permits certain movements of the fracture site. Afterwards, a rigid component that provides stability is added. There are many types of commercial splints, but the best systems are made of fibreglass casting tapes. One detail of great importance is the need to perfectly pad the point of weight bearing of the ends of the rigid material to prevent lesions (Fig. 83). In the specific case of the tibia, the application of a splint on the cranial surface that surrounds the front portion of the toes reaching the proximal part of the metatarsus is usually sufficient.

Bivalve bandages, due to their complexity and the fact that they may cause problems due to chaffing over the calcaneus, are usually reserved for use with minimal osteosynthesis systems of the tarsus.

Intramedullary pinning

Taking into account that the tibial plateau, where the femoral condyles actually bear weight, is found to be displaced in a caudal direction, it is anatomically impossible to insert intramedullary pins. The portion of the implant that sticks out of

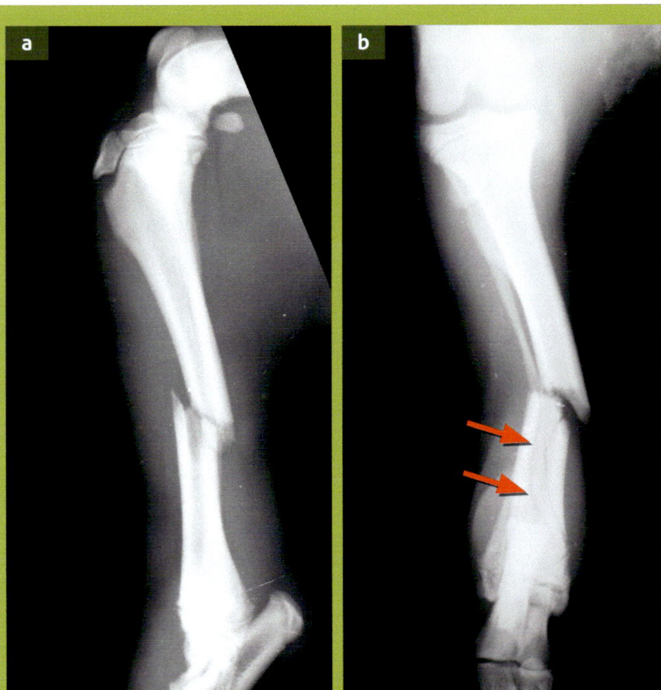

FIGURE 80. Short oblique fracture of the tibia. Note the fissures of the distal fragment in the cranio-caudal view (b).

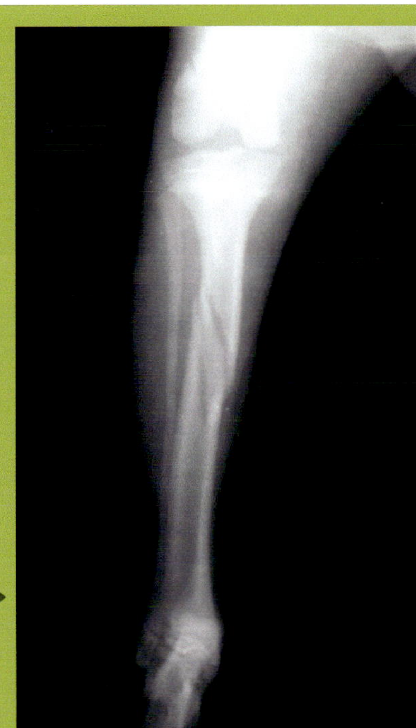

FIGURE 81. Oblique fracture of the tibia without damage to the fibula.

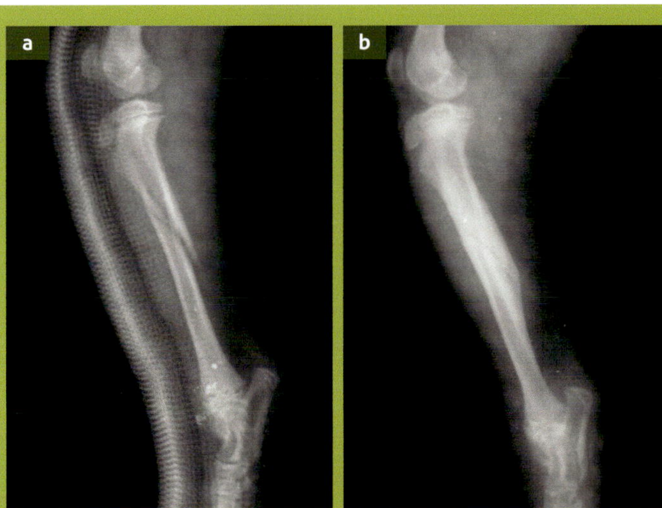

FIGURE 82. Conservative treatment by means of a splint. X-ray taken immediately after its reduction (a) and progress (b).

FIGURE 83. Proximal padding of a splint to immobilise the tibia, placed on the stifle.

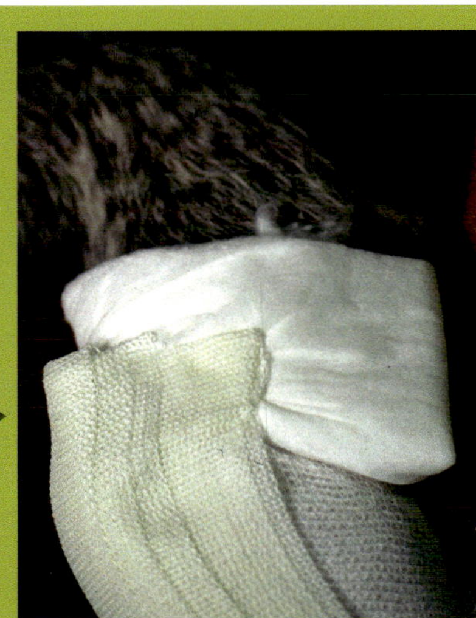

the proximal part of the tibia should be placed in a medial direction from the insertion point of the patellar tendon. Bending its end in a cranial direction is very important to avoid contact with the femur during hyperextension of the stifle. However, the high incidence of multiple and comminuted fractures, together with the possibility to apply other implants, rules out the selection of this fixation system as a system to be used alone.

Due to the boom in MIPO techniques over the last few years, the placement of an intramedullary pin before stabilisation by means of a locking plate in almost all cases has become popular.

The pin, inserted in a normograde manner, serves as an alignment system, making the surgical intervention easier. Also, it notably increases resistance against forces of flexion and, therefore, prevents premature unloosening of the screws.

External fixation

The possibility to apply all external fixation configurations and the low probability of damaging important structures when inserting the percutaneous screws in their safe corridors makes this bone the best candidate for the application of external fixation as an osteosynthesis system. On the other hand, the insertion of implants in the desired point is very simple, thanks to the fact that the medial cortical bone in its proximal third is flat with little musculature. The insertion of the pins in the distal third is also quite simple given that both the medial as well as the lateral surfaces of the tibia at this level are not covered by any musculature, which facilitates the palpation of the bone structures that guide the surgeon during surgery.

Almost all fractures of this bone can be treated by means of external fixation as long as the adequate configuration is selected.

One of the advantages of this system compared to stabilisation with others is the possibility of using external fixators in closed fractures. This way, by not damaging the soft tissues, the healing processes are much faster. The decision, as usual, depends on the type of fracture as well as the surgeon's preferences.

For better orientation and easier and safer insertion of the pins, the patient should be placed in a dorsal decubitus position with the affected limb sticking out from the edge of the operating table (Fig. 84). Movements of flexion and extension of the limb can be carried out in this position, and the anatomical references can be compared with the other limb. Primarily, this may be of great use if the fixator is to be applied in a closed fracture.

First of all, the pins should be inserted in the ends of the fixator. The most proximal percutaneous pin should be located on the caudal part of the tibia, an important aspect due to the triangular profile of this bone in this area (Fig. 85). If the pin is inserted in the normal place, that is, centred, the pin would be attached to the tibial crest. A threaded implant in this position tends to loosen easily. However, if the proximal percutaneous pin is placed closer to the caudal cortical surface, the loosening of the implant is much more difficult due to the separation between the medial and lateral cortical surfaces and the better quality of the bone.

The placement of the most distal percutaneous pin should also be in a medial to lateral direction. For correct orientation, it should be done in this direction. One of the problems to be kept in mind is that the malleolus overlaps the astragalus, for which the implant may be inserted in an intra-articular manner by mistake. The most distal limit that should never be surpassed is the beginning of the concavity immediately proximal to the medial malleolus (Fig. 86).

Once both the proximal and distal percutaneous screws are placed, they are connected to the connecting rod (or rods), depending on whether a unilateral or bilateral fixator is being used, respectively.

The structure created is sufficiently stable to confirm the correct alignment of the bone. If deemed necessary, the movements of flexion and extension of the joints can be compared along with the correct position of the bone prominences with the healthy limb.

To conclude, the rest of the external components of the chosen fixator are placed, using the connecting rods for support.

Osteosynthesis plates

The placement of the plates is determined by the position of the tension-bearing surface of the bone (in this case, the medial surface), and the simpler alternative approach (also the medial surface). For these reasons, in the tibia, almost all plates are applied to said area.

Similar to the external fixators, this implant should be placed parallel to the caudal cortical surface to anchor the proximal screws in a bone area with adequate quality.

To perform osteosynthesis by means of a plate, the patient should be placed in a lateral decubitus position with the limb resting completely on the table to facilitate the reduction and manipulation of the bone. Regarding the other limb, displacing it in a cranio-dorsal direction is recommended. In this position, the femoral condyles rest overlapping on the table and can serve as a reference if the fracture cannot be reduced.

The morphology of the tibia, practically flat, requires very little moulding of the plate, except for in certain chondrodystrophic breeds in which the curvature is more accentuated. More notable moulding is needed only in patients in which the plate must be placed very proximally to one of the epiphyses.

As most fractures that affect this bone affect a considerable portion of the diaphysis, the use of long plates that cover the entire bone is of utmost importance (Fig. 87).

It is especially important to keep in mind the anatomical concavity of the medial surface of the proximal epiphysis. When perforating to insert the screw closest to the joint, the

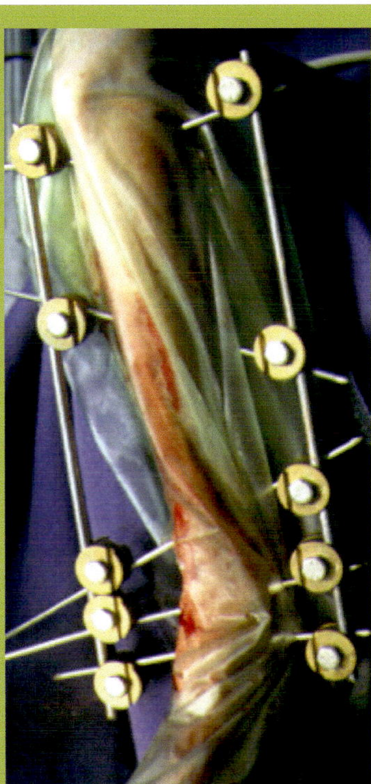

FIGURE 84. Patient in supine decubitus position with the limb positioned for easy orientation.

FIGURE 85. Medio-lateral view of a limb in which type II external fixation has been used. Note how the proximal part is displaced towards the caudal cortical surface.

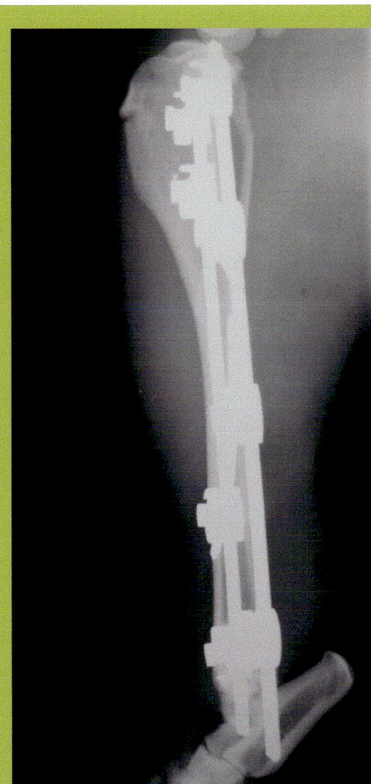

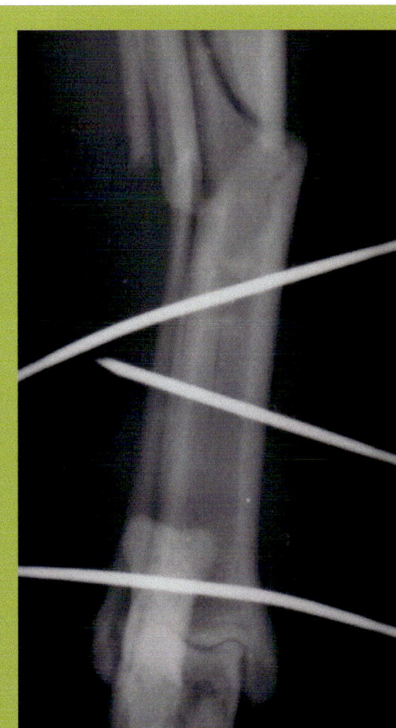

FIGURE 86. Detailed image of the distal limit for the insertion of a percutaneous pin.

drill bit should not be oriented in a direction perpendicular to the implant as it could penetrate into the joint. For this reason, to achieve the proper direction, the drill bit should be oriented towards the head of the fibula. This way, the screw will be placed parallel to the tibial plateau.

In the case of placing a plate in the distal area, the disadvantage of the scarcity of soft tissues should be highlighted as the cause of excessive tension of the skin. Therefore, it is recommended that it be slightly reduced using a light Robert Jones bandage for a few days.

Surgical approach

Except for fractures that affect the tibial crest and the lateral malleolus, the approach is always medial.

Access to the diaphysis presents no difficulties given that the only structure with which care should be taken is the saphenous neurovascular bundle that crosses the middle third of the tibia diagonally (proximo-caudal to disto-cranial). Frequently, it is located immediately on top of the fracture as its trajectory coincides with the transition zone between the triangular and cylindrical portions of the bone.

If the proximal metaphyseal area must be accessed, an incision must be made of the tendon of the semitendinosus muscle and the fascia of the sartorius muscle. Maintaining the insertion along the tibial crest is useful for suturing afterwards (Fig. 88).

Regarding the fractures that affect the tibial crest, a lateral approach is preferable. In the case of show animals or those with short hair, the incision can be made on the medial surface to avoid the scar from being visible.

Once the tibial crest is located, an incision is made to expose it along the lateral side to lift the cranial tibial muscle. If visibility of the tibial plateau is necessary, the approach is broadened towards both sides, reaching the collateral ligaments if needed. Care should be taken to avoid damaging the tendon of the common digital extensor muscle, which courses above the tibia, attached by a retinaculum, and inserts into the lateral condyle of the femur.

Most frequent tibial fractures

Fractures of the proximal epiphysis

In order to understand the characteristics of the fractures of this bone, it is important to know that the proximal epiphysis of the tibia has two secondary ossification nuclei, the first forming the tibial plateau, and the second forming the tibial crest (Fig. 89).

The fractures that affect this area usually occur in young patients and they affect the growth plates. The tendon

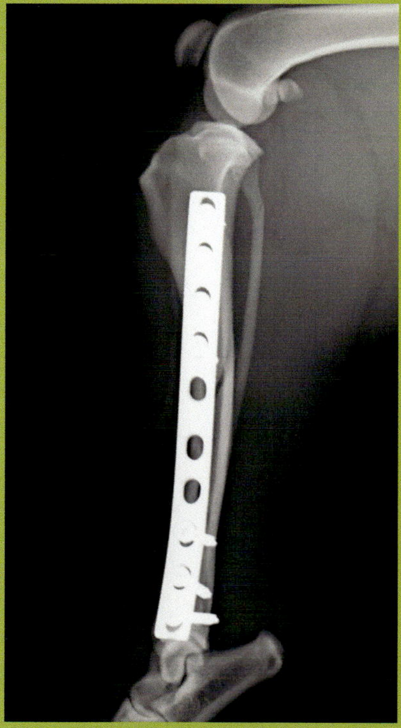

FIGURE 87. Long neutralisation plate. Note how the implant is placed close to the caudal cortical surface in the proximal metaphysis.

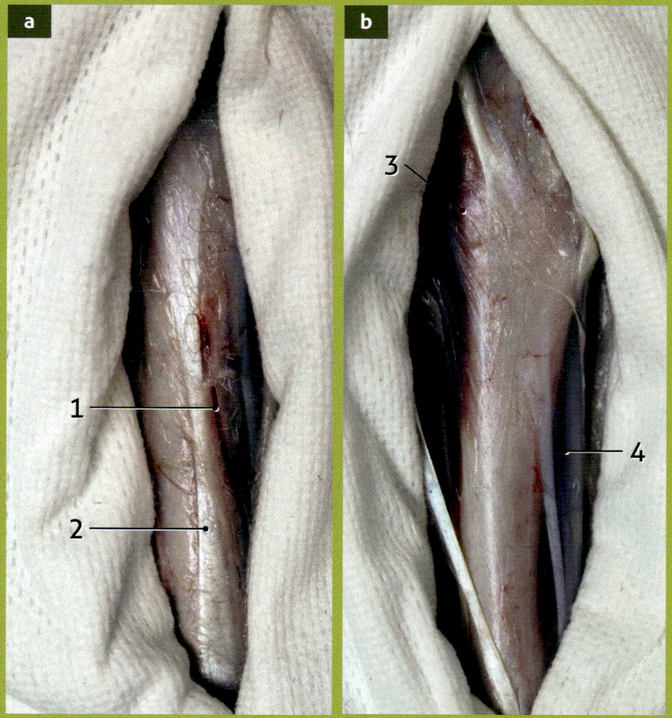

FIGURE 88. Medial approach of the tibia.
1. Medial saphenous artery and vein.
2. Medial digital flexor muscle.
3. Popliteus muscle.
4. Cranial tibial muscle.

structures, such as the collateral ligaments or the patellar tendon, are more resistant than the cartilage found in said zones during development.

This type of fractures are not excessively frequent. The most frequent, without a doubt, are type I Salter-Harris fractures of the tibial crest (Fig. 90). In some cases, this fracture may be accompanied by a detachment of the tibial plateau in a caudal direction, keeping both ossification nuclei together (Fig. 91). In special cases, the two nuclei may separate from each other, which results in three fracture lines.

In avulsions of the tibial crest, the surgeon has to work with a fragment that tends to separate itself due to the effect of the patellar tendon. The limp that the patient presents may be anywhere from slight to complete and may even go unnoticed at times. A mild case does not lead to suspicions of a fracture. In these cases, the limping persists and worsens progressively.

A proximal displacement of the patella is observed in X-rays along with a more accentuated separation of the growth line that should not be confused with the normal radiological aspect corresponding with the patient's age. When in doubt, an X-ray of the other limb should be taken with the same degree of joint flexion for comparison.

Treatment of this type of fractures consists of stabilising the tibial crests using Kirschner pins, sometimes accompanied by a tension band.

After making an incision in the skin, avoiding the cranial area of maximum cutaneous tension, the patellar tendon is located and an incision is made along the tibial crest to lift the cranial tibial muscle (Fig. 92). Once the fracture is reduced, a few pins are introduced over the insertion point of the patellar tendon, and they are oriented in a slight oblique manner towards the medullary cavity (Fig. 93). Next, a hole distal to the fracture line in the tibial crest is perforated (Fig. 94). The cerclage is passed through the perforation, crossed in front of the crest, and passed again above the pins. To conclude, it is tightened by twisting one end over the other while tractioning and the pins are bent with their tips facing in a caudal direction (Fig. 95). Adding the cerclage provides more stability against the forces of traction and is recommended in large or very active patients (Fig. 96). However, this type of cerclage causes the premature closing of the growth line which leads to a deformity in the tibial crest. The lack of normal development of this part of the bone is compensated without clinical consequences with an increase in the length of the patellar tendon (Fig. 97).

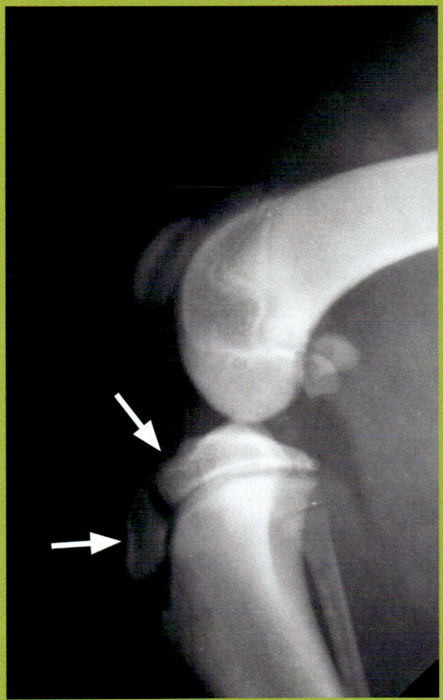

FIGURE 89. Physiological growth plates of a dog. Note the two different ossification nuclei (arrows).

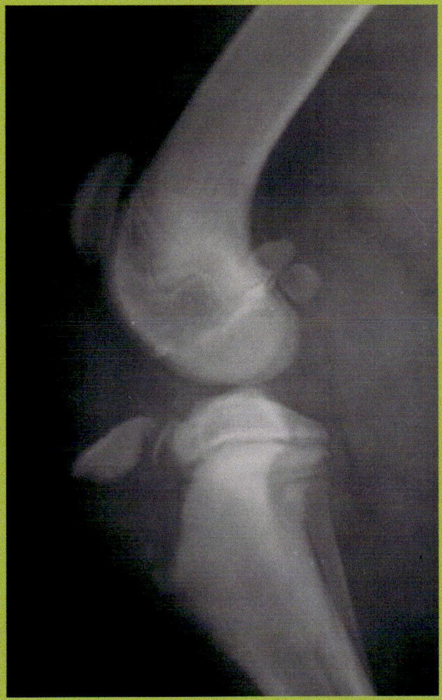

FIGURE 90. Detailed image of an avulsion of the tibial crest.

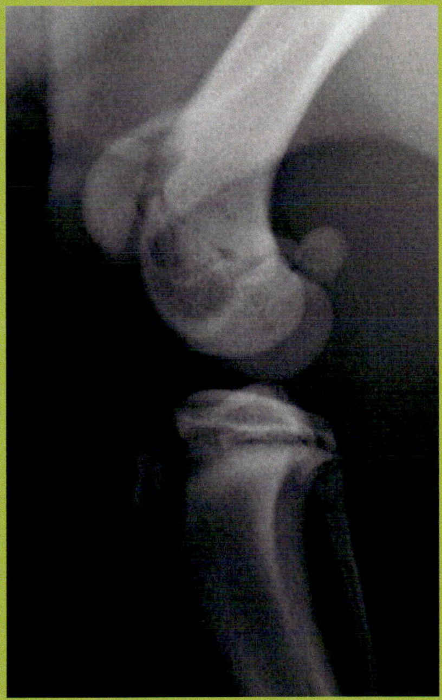

FIGURE 91. Caudal detachment with little displacement of the plateau and the crest.

The fracture can be stabilised using pins without a tension band in small patients. In this case, the pins should be inserted parallel to the tibial plateau to prevent them from being ripped out by the traction exerted by the patellar tendon (Fig. 98).

The fractures that affect the tibial plateau are usually type I or II Salter Harris fractures (Fig. 99). This lesion should always be treated surgically. Implementing conservative treatment is an error based on the reduced displacement of the fracture. The reason resides in that the physiological position of the stifle when bearing weight and the forces that it is subjected to cause progressive displacement of the proximal fragment in a caudal direction. By affecting young patients and the fact that it is a relatively stable fracture, it eventually heals, but the plateau will remain excessively inclined in a caudal direction. This inclination is likely to cause problems in the anterior cruciate ligament over time.

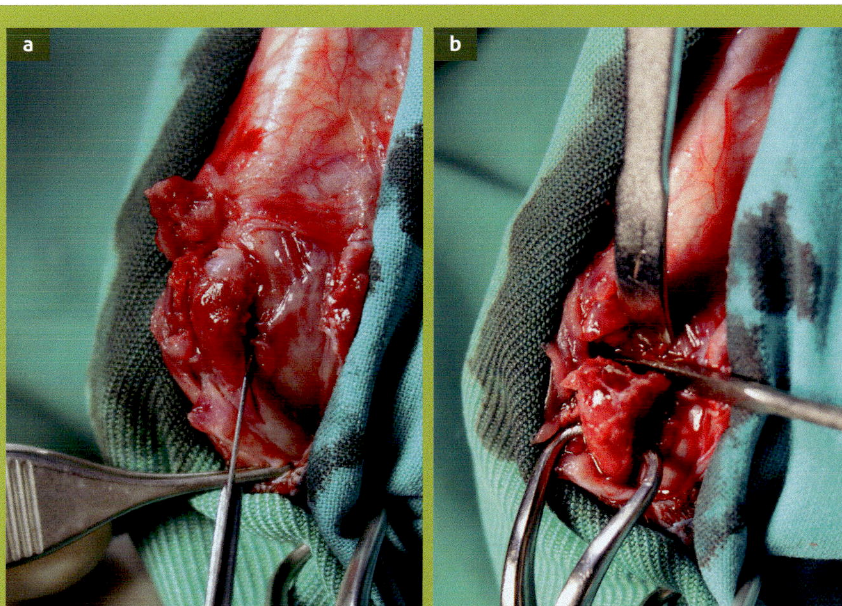

FIGURE 92. Approach of the tibial crest.

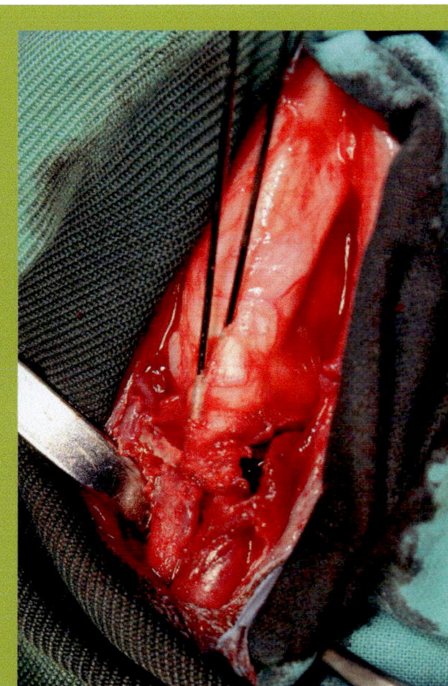
FIGURE 93. Insertion of the pins.

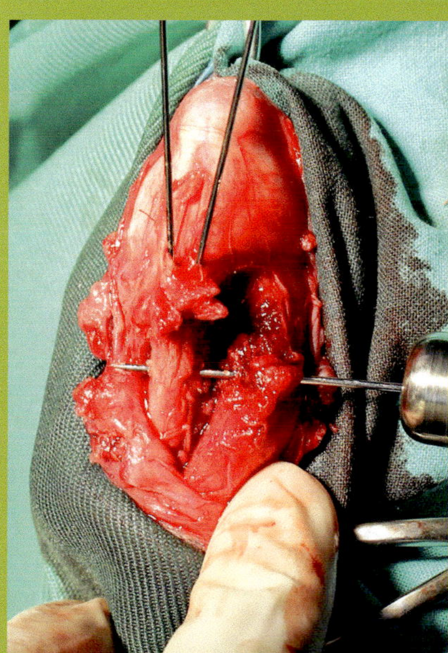
FIGURE 94. Perforation of the tibial crest.

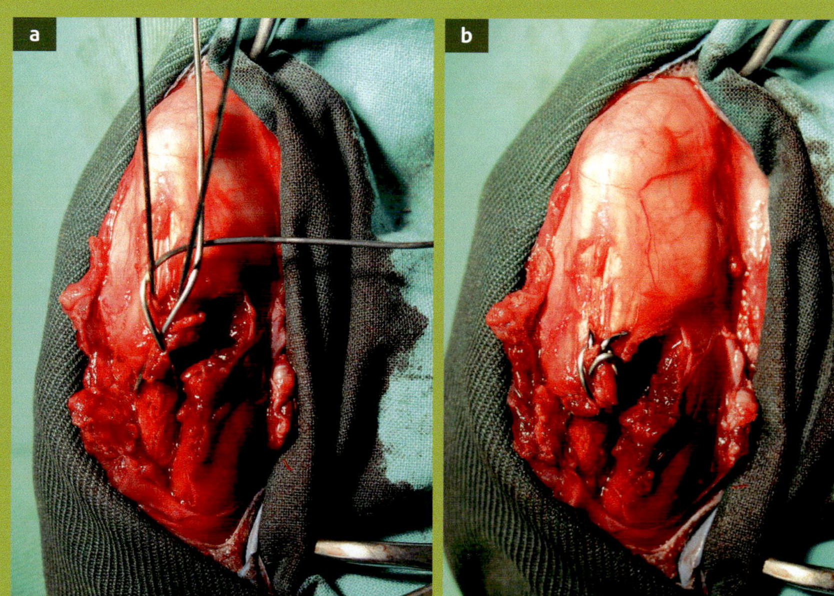

FIGURE 95. Placement of the cerclage. The cerclage crosses through the tibial crest, crossing it in a cranial direction and then passes over the pins (a). Completed tension band (b).

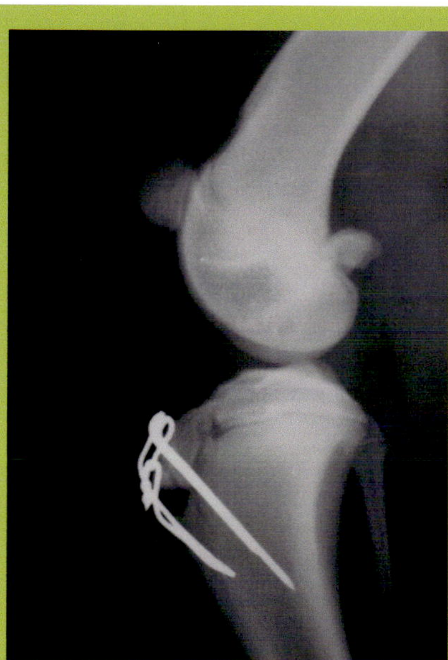

FIGURE 96. Post-surgery X-ray after resolution of the avulsion of the tibia.

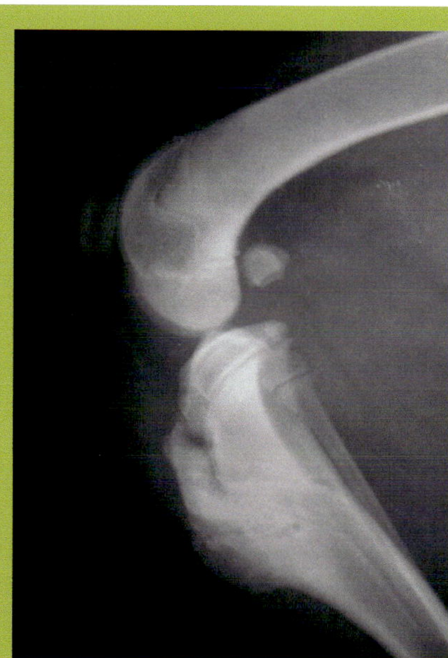

FIGURE 97. Effect of the implants on the growth plate. Note how, although the tibial crest has affected its growth, the patella is located in its normal anatomical position.

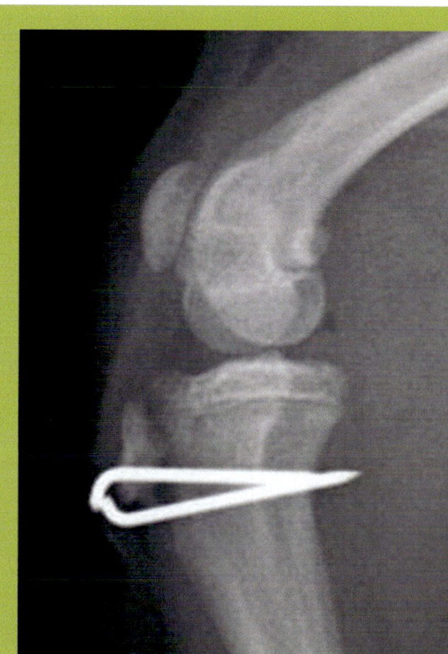

FIGURE 98. Treatment with pins without a tension band. The pins are inserted parallel to the tibial plateau.

Treatment of this fracture consists of stabilisation using pins that are inserted from the sides of the tibial plateau. These pins can be inserted into the joint, however, logically, they should never interfere with the movements of the stifle.

Normally, pins with tension bands are necessary to stabilise the tibial crest although it depends on the type of fracture (Fig. 100).

Metaphyseal fractures are infrequent in veterinary medicine. Fractures in the form of an inverted U occur occasionally only in small breeds with strong muscle masses (Fig. 101). Due to the small size of the proximal fragment, they are treated in the same manner as the previously described tibial plateau fractures.

Diaphyseal fractures

All fractures that affect the diaphysis can be treated by means of external fixation or with plates. The decision depends on the type of fracture as well as the surgeon's preferences.

Generally, stabilisation using osteosynthesis plates is preferable as postoperative care is much simpler and with less incidents. However, given that this bone frequently suffers from highly comminuted fractures with large and splintered fragments, which easily tear the skin leading to open fractures, and taking into account that this bone tolerates external fixation perfectly, this system is frequently chosen.

It has been mentioned several times in different chapters that one of the greatest advantages of external fixation is that it can be applied to closed fractures. On the other hand, the tibia is a long bone in which it is easy to locate the reference points. Nonetheless, assessing the existence of

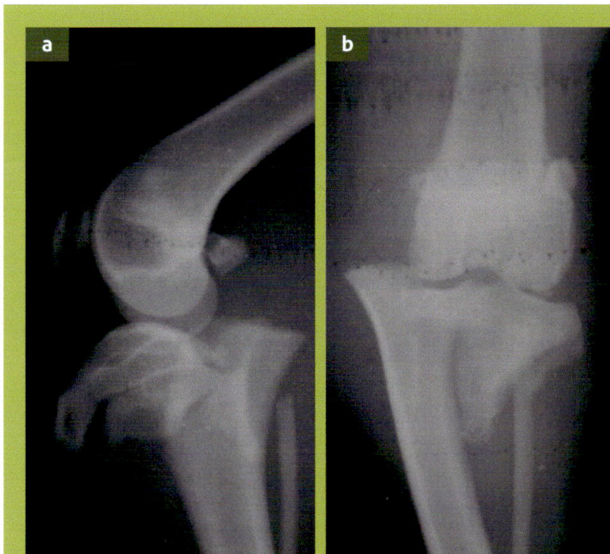

FIGURE 99. Salter II fracture of the proximal epiphysis. Latero-lateral view (a) and cranio-caudal view (b).

fissures in the distal fragment that are frequent in this bone is very important as, if they exist, and depending on their location, when inserting percutaneous pins in a closed fracture there is a risk of further fracturing the bone.

When in doubt, the intervention should be done opening the fracture, protecting the fissures with compressive systems and applying an osteosynthesis plate. Another possibility, if the fissures allow for it, is to compress them using compression screws (Fig. 102).

The tibia tolerates all types of external fixation structures and thus the ideal system should be selected depending on the patient's age, and the location and type of fracture.

As a general rule, the greater the age, weight and activity, the more rigid the structures need to be (type II and III). On the contrary, if the patient is young, simpler (type I) structures can be chosen. One fundamental detail of which the stability of a fracture depends greatly, especially regarding the collapsing of the fracture site, is if the fibula is affected or not (Fig. 103).

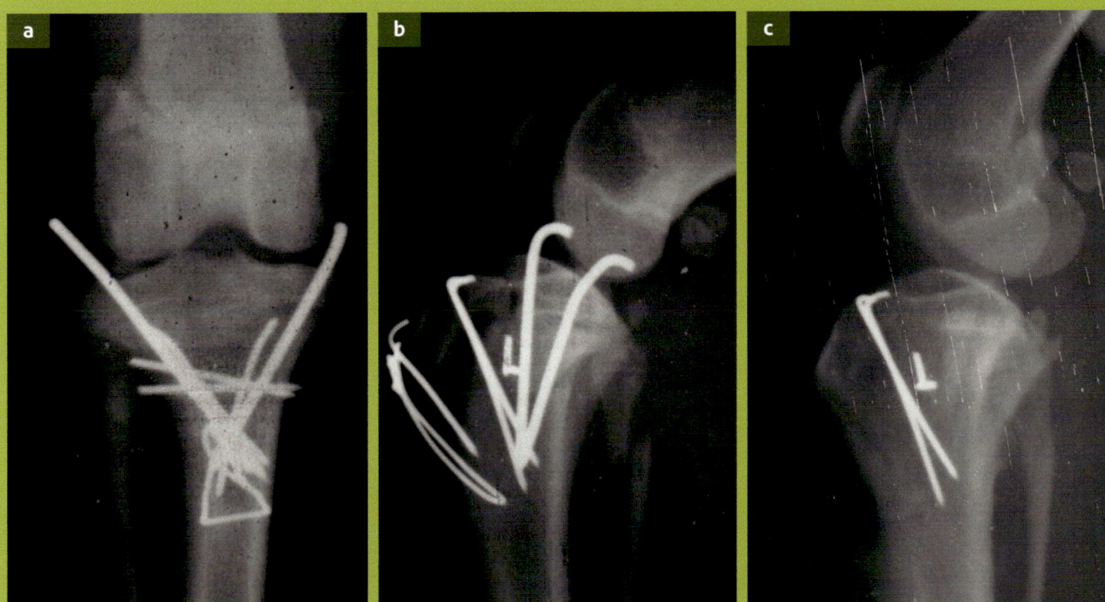

FIGURE 100. X-ray of the previous case after resolution of the fracture. Cranio-caudal view (a), latero-lateral view (b) and after partial removal of the implants (c).

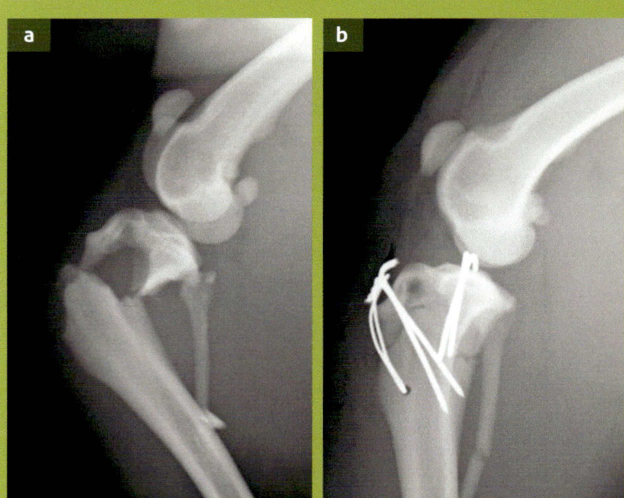

FIGURE 101. Metaphyseal fracture of the tibia. X-ray before resolution (a) and once treatment with pins with a tension band was implemented associated with Rush pins to increase the stability of the tibial plateau (b).

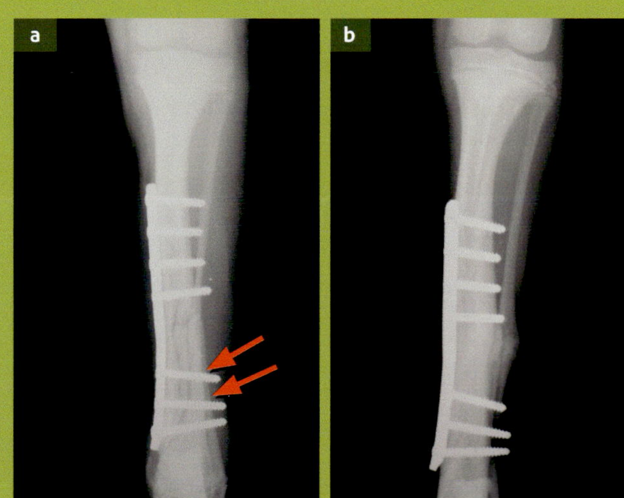

FIGURE 102. Fissures treated using a neutralisation plate and two compression screws (arrows) through the plate. X-ray after the intervention (a) and once the fracture healed (b).

The technique of fixation using plates is well tolerated in this bone. Due to the infrequency of short fractures of the tibia, compression plates are rarely applied. On the contrary, the elevated frequency of comminuted fractures together with the tendency in the last few years of implementing biological osteosynthesis are why supporting plates are the most frequently used plates (Fig. 104).

The tibia is the bone where MIPO can be performed more easily than in other bones.

Due to the cylindrical form of the distal third of the tibia, the bone in this area behaves in a more classic manner, with a greater incidence of oblique fractures that can be stabilised using compressive systems (Fig. 105). Preferably, compression screws are used for this purpose instead of cerclage. The application of cerclages becomes more difficult with the presence of the fibula on the lateral surface as its most distal third is completely attached to the tibia (Figs. 106 and 107).

When plates or external fixation are applied to very distal fractures, it must be kept in mind that the medial malleolus overlaps the astragalus and therefore there is a risk of introducing the implant into the joint. The reference point that marks the distal limit is the point of maximum concavity of the transition zone between the malleolus and the tibia (Fig. 108).

Fractures of the distal epiphysis

These fractures are infrequent and usually affect the growth plate. The distal part of the tibia usually suffers from type I or sometimes type II Salter-Harris fractures (Fig. 109).

Treatment is implemented with pins that are inserted from both malleolus perpendicular to the plate to interfere as little as possible in their growth (Fig. 110).

The insertion of the pin from the medial malleolus is simple. Insertion from the lateral malleolus, however, must be more inclined as it is part of the fibula, taking care to not penetrate the joint.

Fractures of the medial malleolus can also occur. This lesion produces great instability in the tarsus joint given that it is the insertion point of the medial collateral ligament.

This fracture should be considered as an avulsion fracture as the malleolus is subjected to forces of traction when the limb bears weight. In some cases, stress X-rays should be taken to make the fracture more visible (Fig. 111).

Treatment consists of the insertion of a few pins with a tension band (Fig. 112). Due to the small size of the fragment, temporary immobilisation of the joint may be useful, especially if it is associated with other fractures. In certain

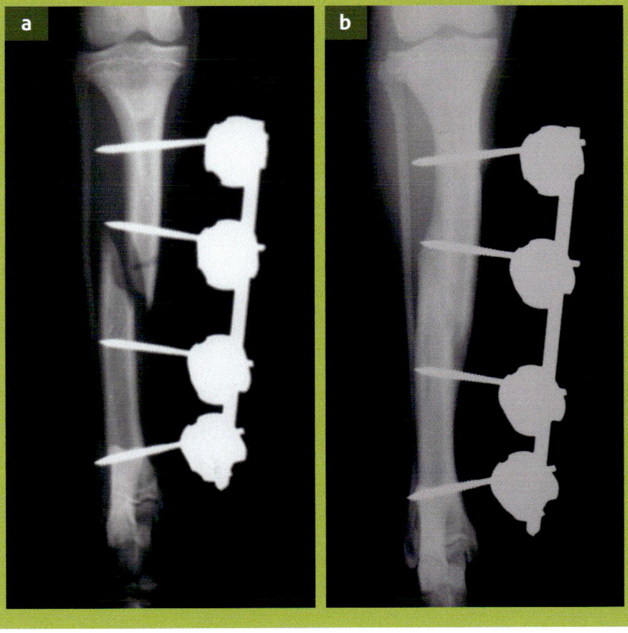

FIGURE 103. Tibia fracture without damage to the fibula treated by means of partial external fixation. X-ray image after the intervention. Note the integrity of the fibula (a) and the correct progress of the fracture in spite of the separation of the fragments (b).

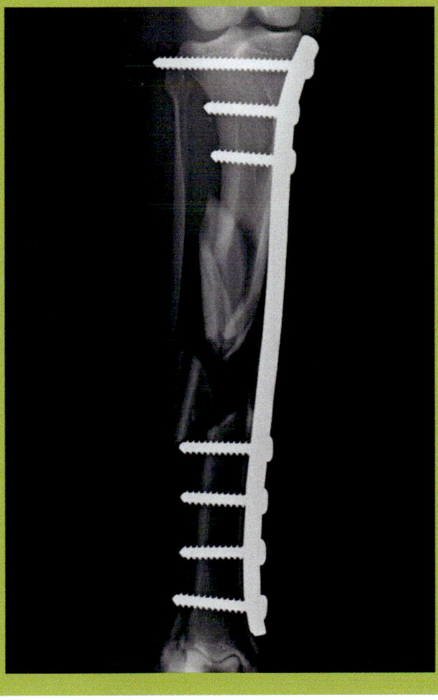

FIGURE 104. Comminuted fracture treated with a supporting plate.

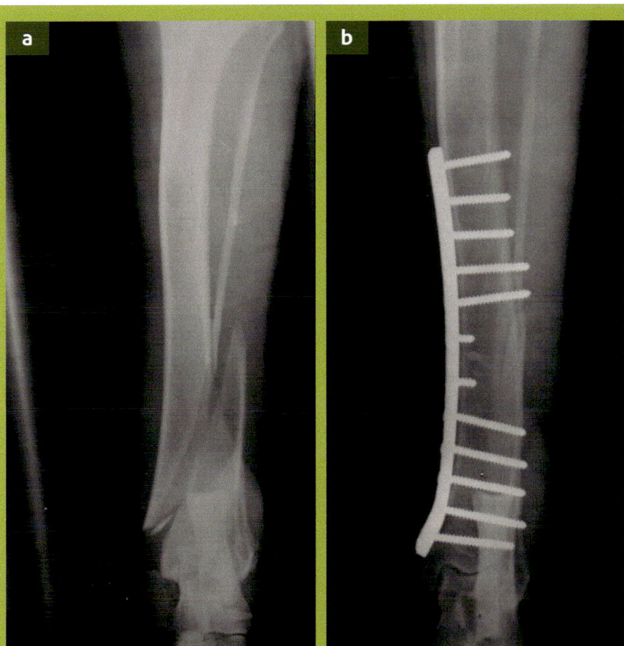

FIGURE 105. Long oblique distal fracture (a) treated with a neutralisation plate with compression screws (b).

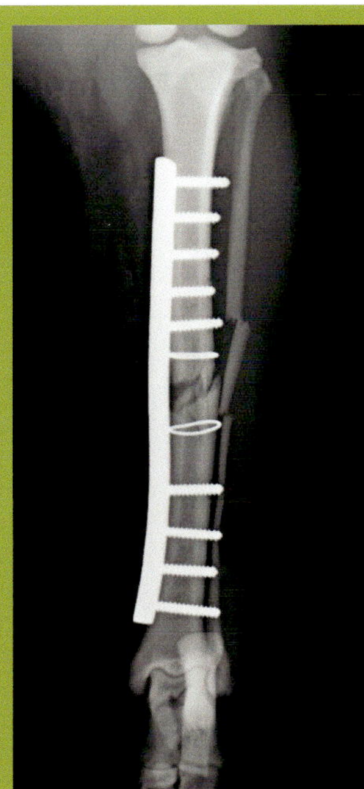

FIGURE 106. Cerclage placed between the tibia and the fibula.

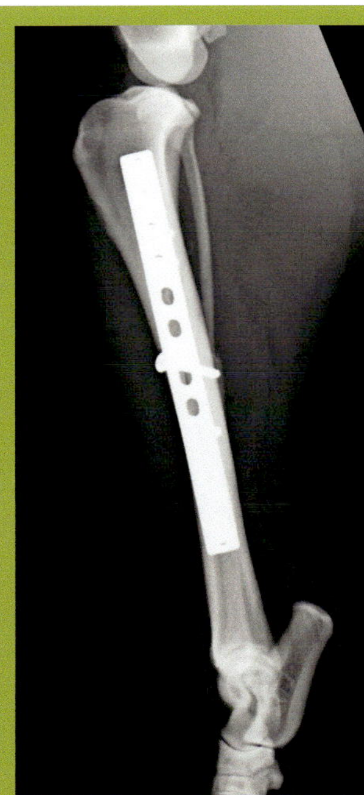

FIGURE 107. Compression screw with a neutralisation plate.

circumstances, the placement of a temporary trans-articular external fixator may be recommended.

Most frequent fractures of the fibula

Given the small amount of weight that this bone bears, fibula fractures do not need to be stabilised, with the exception of fractures of the distal malleolus that requires surgical treatment.

The diagnosis is made through a standard X-ray exam. However, in cranio-caudal X-rays, as the calcaneus overlaps the distal part of the fibula, it may be difficult to correctly examine its integrity. When in doubt, sky line X-rays should be taken, placing the metatarsi perpendicular to the X-ray table. This allows for its examination with greater precision (Fig. 113). In other cases, a CT scan may be necessary to assess the extension of the lesion (Fig. 114). Treatment is necessary as it serves as an insertion point for the long and short collateral lateral ligaments which intervene in the stabilisation of the tarsal joint.

Treatment basically consists of that described for the stabilisation of the lateral malleolus (Fig. 115), although the stability achieved through surgery is less than that achieved for the medial malleolus, and thus, temporary external immobilisation of the joint is recommended (Fig. 116).

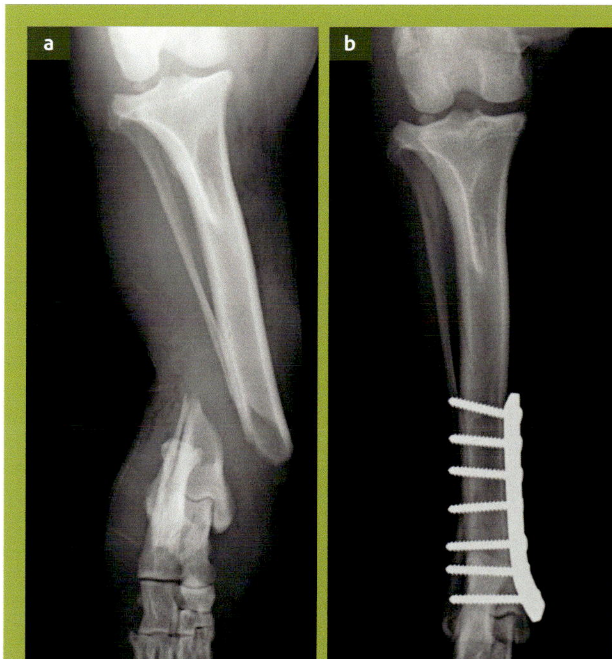

FIGURE 108. Very distal oblique fracture (a). Note where the limit to place the most distal screw is located (b).

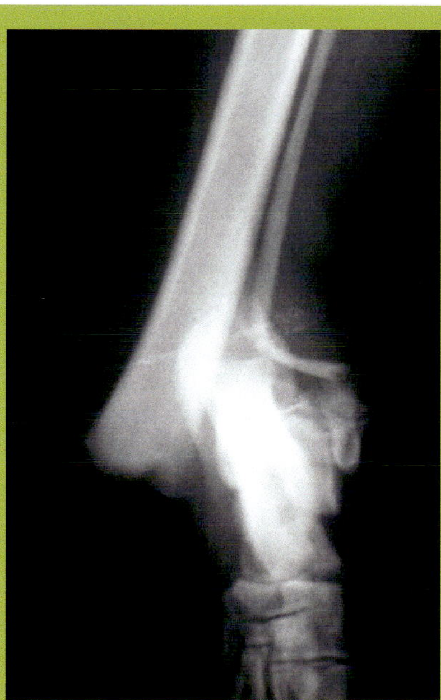

FIGURE 109. Type I Salter-Harris fracture of the distal epiphysis of the tibia.

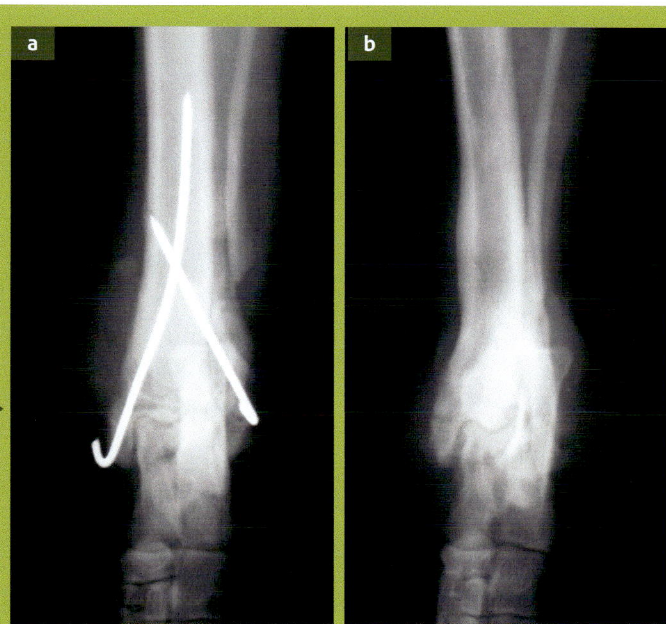

FIGURE 110. X-ray of the previous case after inserting the pins (a) and once the implants have been removed (b).

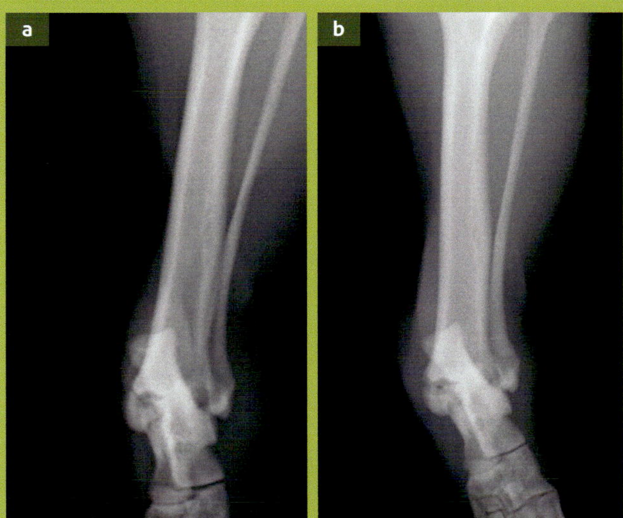

FIGURE 111. Fracture of the medial malleolus in a normal position (a) and in a stress position to make the fracture visible (b).

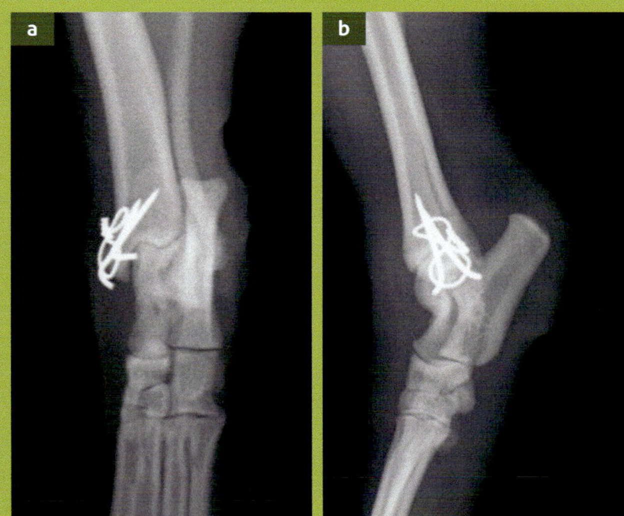

FIGURE 112. Stabilisation of a medial malleolar fracture using pins and a tension band. Oblique (a) and medio-lateral (b) views.

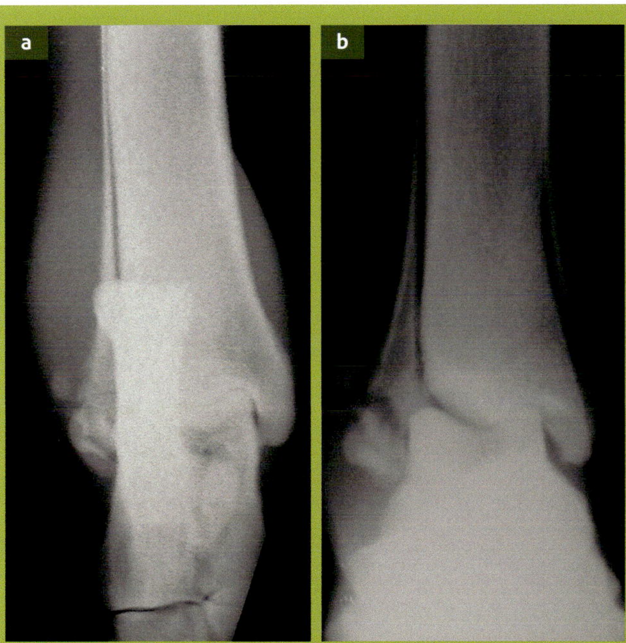

FIGURE 113. X-ray in a normal position (a) and in a sky line position (b) of a fibula fracture. Note how more detail of the fracture can be observed in the second X-ray.

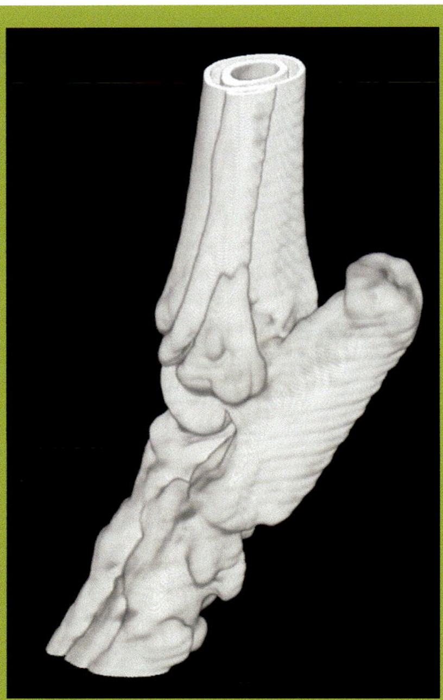

FIGURE 114. Longitudinal fracture of the distal malleolus of the fibula. Reconstruction using CT.

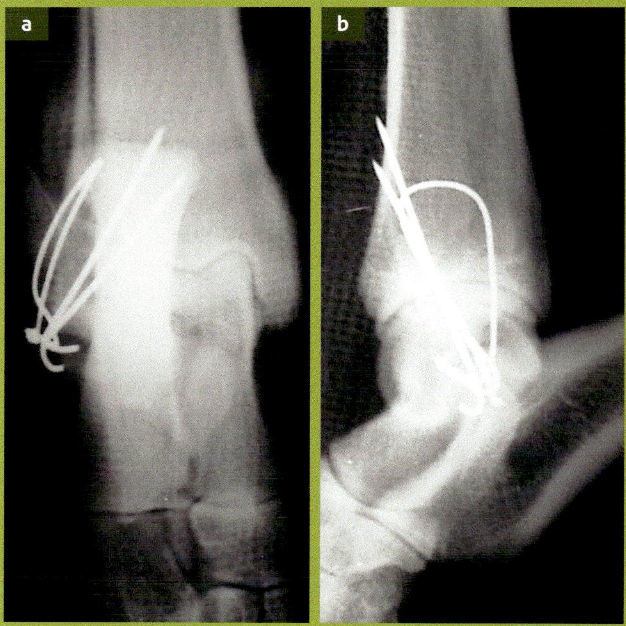

FIGURE 115. Malleolar fracture treated with pins with a tension band. Cranio-caudal view (a) and medio-lateral (b) views.

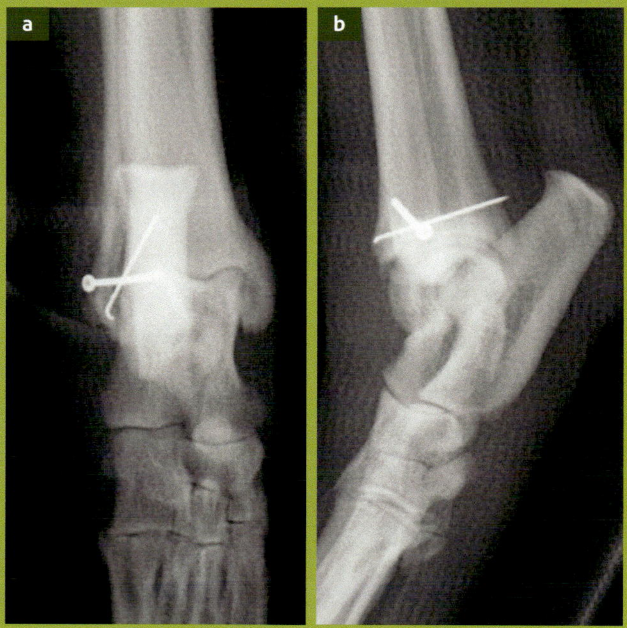

FIGURE 116. Treatment of a longitudinal fracture of the fibula by means of a compression screw and a pin. Temporary stabilisation with a bi-valve cast. Cranio-caudal view (a) and medio-lateral (b) views.

TARSAL FRACTURES

The lesions that affect the tarsal bones are not frequently seen in veterinary practice. Secondary joint degeneration processes, such as arthritis, produce evident clinical symptoms in this joint due to the complete anatomical adaptation that exists between the bones involved. This is why a pantarsal or tarsometatarsal arthrodesis frequently must be performed depending on the location of the lesion. The arthrodesis option is a first option or a secondary resource in the patient's secondary joint degeneration cannot be compensated. That said, there is a great difference regarding the aesthetic and functional results of both surgeries.

Two joints are involved in the tarsus, the tibiotarsal joint, involved in almost all of the joint movement of the tarsus, and the tarsometatarsal joint that, together with the intertarsal joint, hardly intervenes in any movement. The latter basically act as a shock absorber and to adapt to the irregularities of the terrain.

Permanent immobilisation of the tarsometatarsal joint is an excellent first option for lesions produced at this level as it produces practically no impediments in the animal's gaits, and is simple to implement. There are different techniques for its application, however, the most recommended is stabilisation by means of a plate, covering from the calcaneus to the fifth metatarsus (Fig. 117). The second option, in the case of distal lesions of the calcaneus, consists of applying plates and screws with a tension band between the tarsal and metatarsal bones (Fig. 118).

However, the tibiotarsal joint is very different. Its permanent immobilisation, although it solves the clinical problem, leads to a mechanical limitation of the limb and the owner of the patient should be informed regarding said limitation before surgery. The patient will not be able to flex its tarsus and will thus walk with a certain amount of abduction of the limb and will take on anomalous postures when sitting. This surgical technique which is considerably more complex that the previous one, should be reserved for situations in which other types of treatment do not give good results.

The tarsometatarsal arthrodesis obtains functional results that are much better than the pantarsal arthrodesis. Also, it is much easier to perform.

The technique consists of eliminating the cartilaginous surfaces and stabilising the fracture using a plate (Fig. 119). Although the tension-bearing surface of the tarsus is located on the plantar surface, as implants cannot be placed in said area, angled plates have been designed that can be placed on the medial surface of the joint (Fig. 120). These

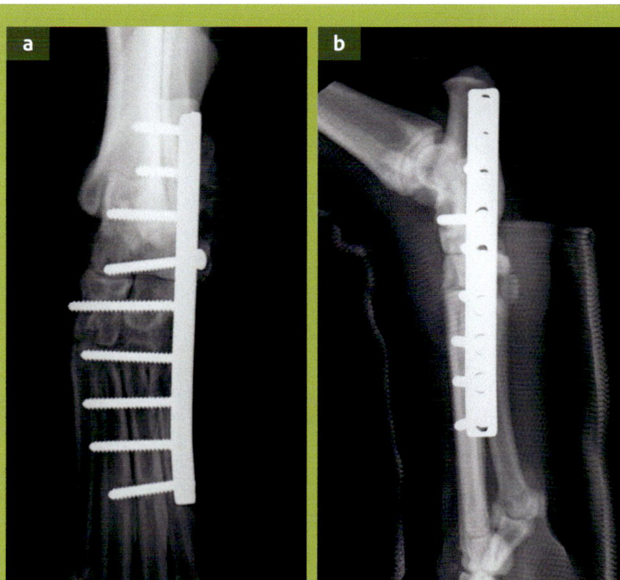

FIGURE 117. Tarsometatarsal arthrodesis.

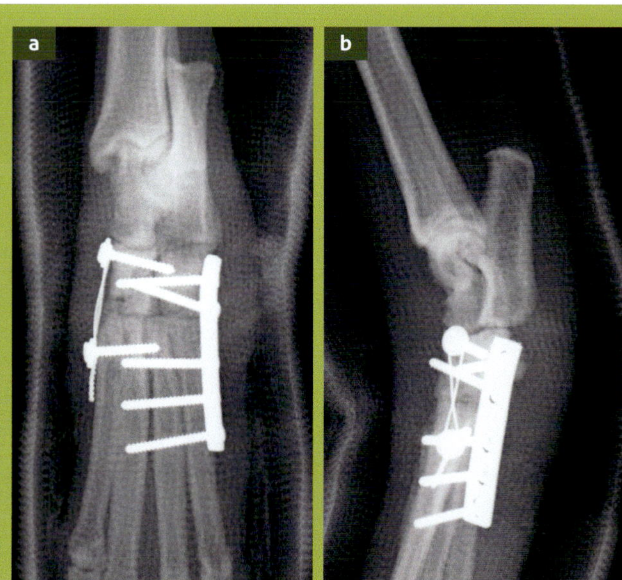

FIGURE 118. Tarsometatarsal hemiarthrodesis.

plates achieve good results although there are other surgical options such as fixation using plates on the cranial surface or external fixation.

The fractures produced in the distal epiphysis of the tibia are basically those that affect the malleoli. Their treatment has been described in the previous chapter (page 203).

Calcaneus fractures

Among the fractures that affect the tarsus, the most frequent is most likely that which affects the calcaneus (Fig. 121). This fracture occurs as a consequence of an abrupt tractioning of the tendon of the gastrocnemius muscle. The patient typically presents a limp without bearing weight on the affected limb, or, in a plantigrade manner. The extensor system of the tarsus is not functional.

Treatment consists of reducing and stabilising the calcaneus, neutralising the traction of the gastrocnemius muscle, that is, as it is an avulsion fracture that is usually resolved using pins with a tension band.

The approach is lateral. The fracture is located and then reduced. Two intramedullary pins are inserted, preferably in a normograde manner, being careful not to damage the common digital flexor tendon. This tendon is found along the groove of the calcaneus, stabilised by a retinaculum, and inserting the pins in a lateral to medial direction towards this tendon is preferable (Fig. 122).

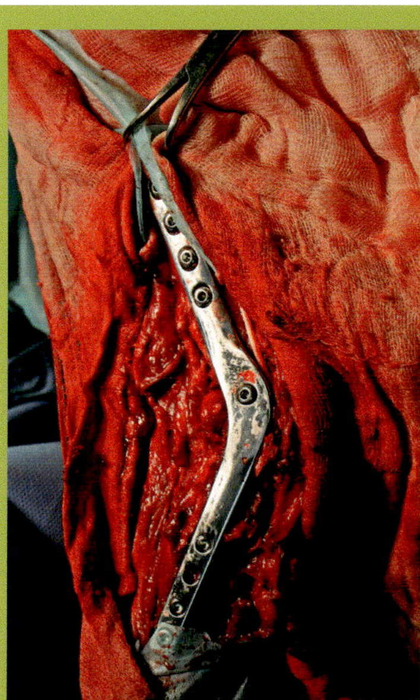

FIGURE 119. Hybrid pantarsal arthrodesis plate. It is adapted to the angle of the joint.

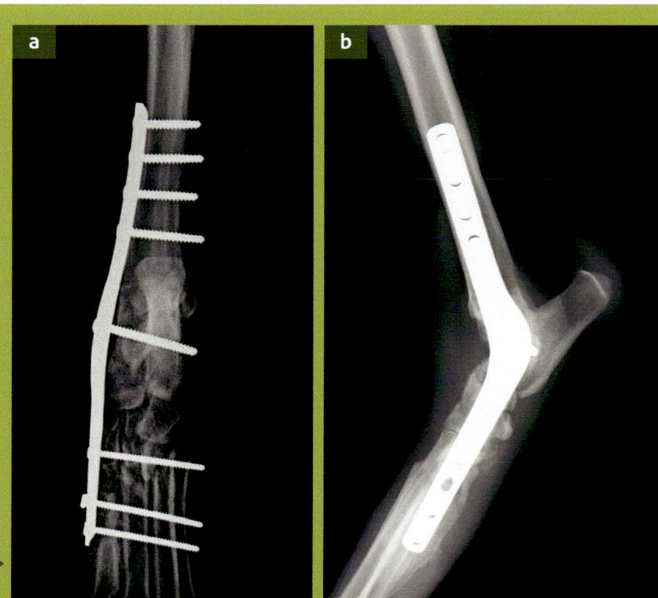

FIGURE 120. Pantarsal arthrodesis.

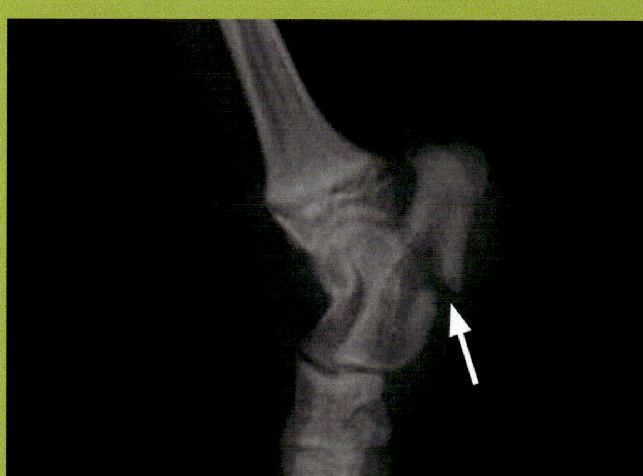

FIGURE 121. Calcaneus fracture.

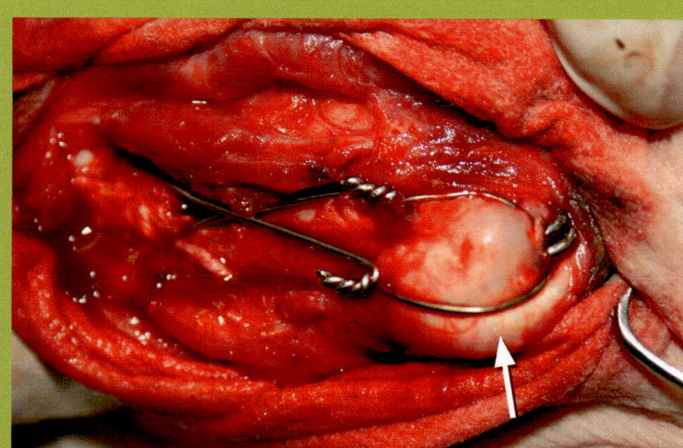

FIGURE 122. Tension band pin system. Note how the digital flexor tendon remains in a lateral position to avoid being damaged (arrow).

The depth to which the pins should be inserted depends on the level in which the fracture has occurred. In young patients, a type I Salter-Harris fracture can occur at the level of the proximal growth plate. In these cases, the pin does not need to be inserted very deeply.

When dealing with fractures in the central area of the tarsus, but in young patients, making a second perforation is preferable in the proximal fragment to pass the cerclage over the pins to avoid interfering with the animal's growth. This also prevents iatrogenic damage to the digital flexor tendon (Fig. 123).

In the case of fractures of the base, given the small distal fragment, it is recommended that the pins be partially inserted into the IV tarsal bone. The articulation of the calcaneus with this bone does not have a relevant function and it can thus be sacrificed. A noticeably better stability is achieved this way.

In some large patients, it may be useful to stabilise using a plate that covers the entire length of the bone to treat the fracture.

Lastly, in highly comminuted fractures or in those where there is not enough space in the distal fragment, a tarsometatarsal arthrodesis should be performed with the previously described technique.

Astragalus fractures

The astragalus is the bone over which the tibia rests all of its weight. The intimate anatomical relationship with the distal epiphysis of the tibia makes it more sensitive to degenerative changes.

Fractures of the astragalus are usually produced from jumping or by introducing the hindlimb in holes in the terrain when exercising. The limp presented by these patients is usually very noticeable, although after a few days, they may bear weight on the affected limb. Due to the intensity of the trauma needed to fracture the bone, there are usually other associated lesions.

Fractures of this bone usually cause the detachment of one or more fragments of the trochlear ridges or even a fracture to the central area (Fig. 124). Both fractures have a poor prognosis and the possibility of performing a permanent arthrodesis to the entire tarsus should be considered as a first option.

If surgical treatment is selected, it is preferable that the fracture be stabilised using compression screws. To access the fractured area, an osteotomy of the malleolus of the corresponding side is usually necessary (Fig. 125). This way, by lifting the collateral ligament, the entire trochlear ridge can be observed. Once the surgery is finished, the osteotomy is stabilised using pins with a tension band (Fig. 126).

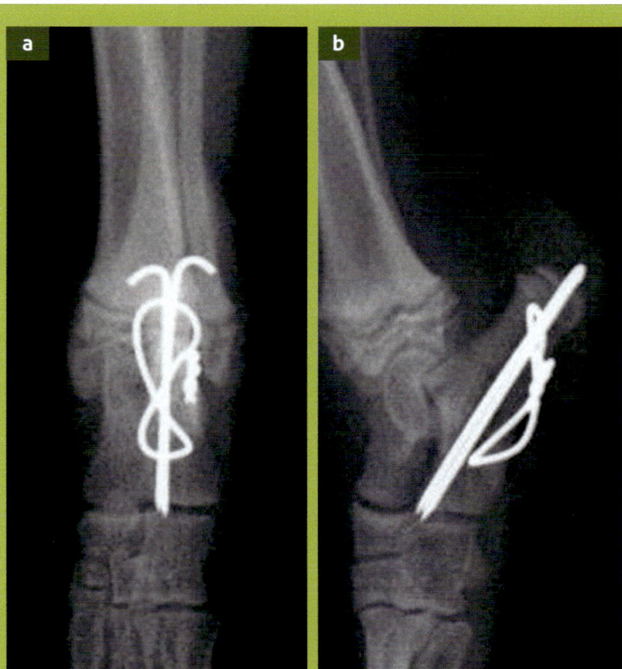

FIGURE 123. Calcaneus fracture, shown in Fig. 121, resolved with a cerclage fastened to two perforations.

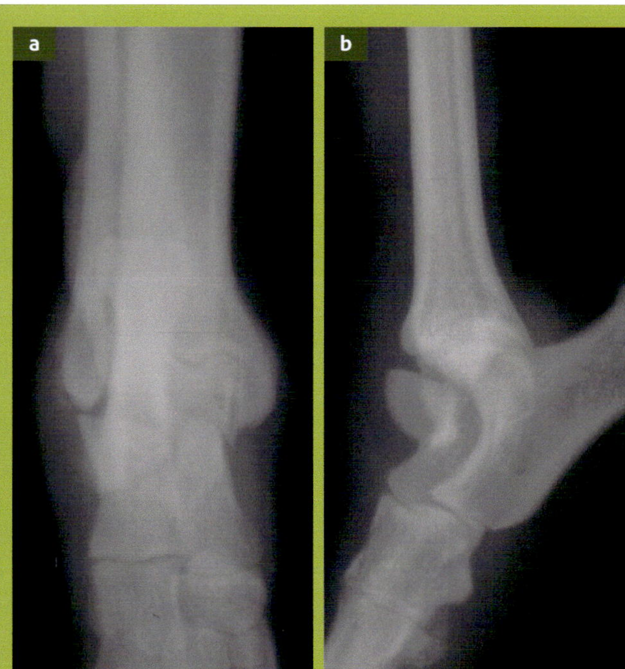

FIGURE 124. Astragalus fracture.

Due to the reduced stability of the osteosynthesis systems that are applied as a consequence of the small size of the fragments, it is best to provide additional stability using temporary systems of external coaptation (Fig. 127). If the osteosynthesis systems applied do not produce the desired results, the last option is to perform a pantarsal arthrodesis.

In the osteosynthesis systems fail, a pantarsal arthrodesis can always be performed.

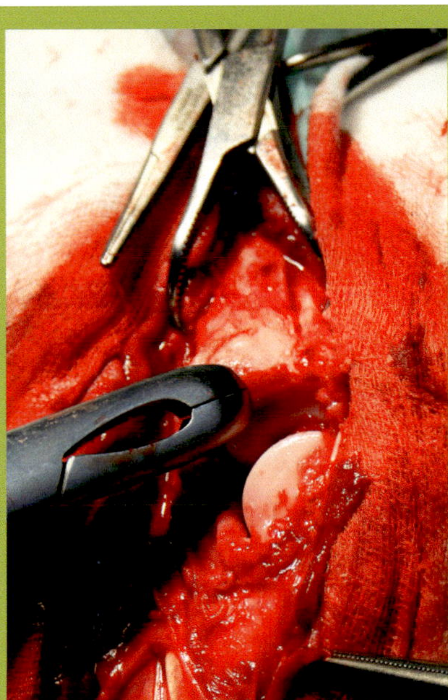

FIGURE 125. Medial approach with osteotomy of the malleolus.

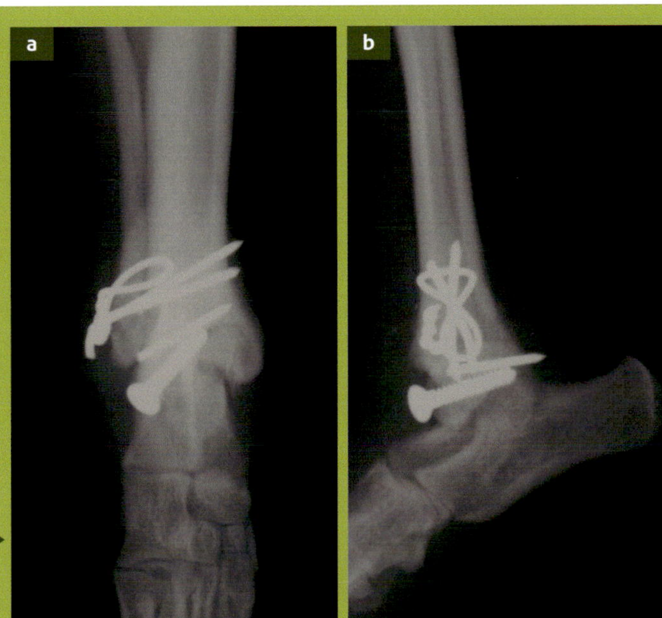

FIGURE 126. Fracture of the lateral ridge of the astragalus.

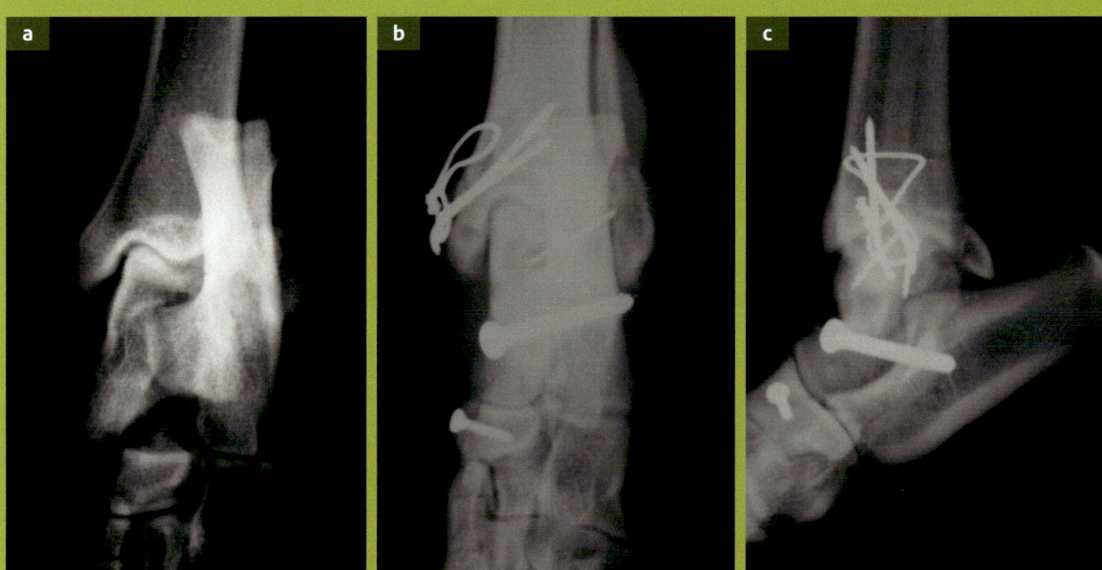

FIGURE 127. Fractures of the astragalus and central tarsus treated with minimal osteosynthesis.

Clinical cases of uncommon fractures

10

Case 1 SALTER-HARRIS III FRACTURE OF THE LATERAL COCHLEA OF THE TIBIA

Author: Andrés Somaza (Veterinary Clinic Somaza-Pérez)

Patient profile

- **Breed:** American Staffordshire Terrier.
- **Age:** 9 months old.
- **Diagnosis:** Salter Harris III fracture of the lateral cochlea of the tibia.

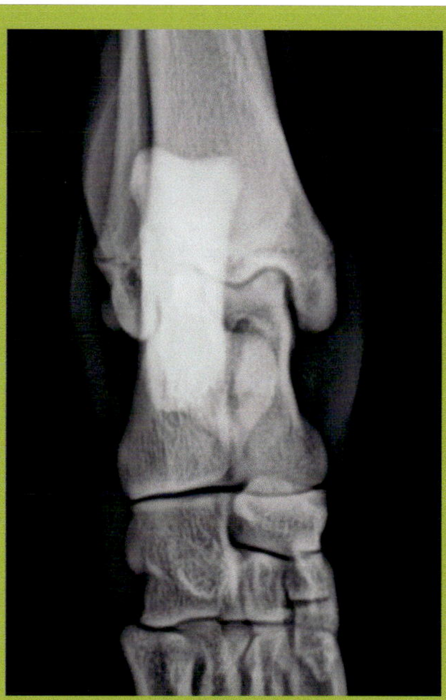

FIGURE 1. Cranio-caudal X-ray of the tarsus.

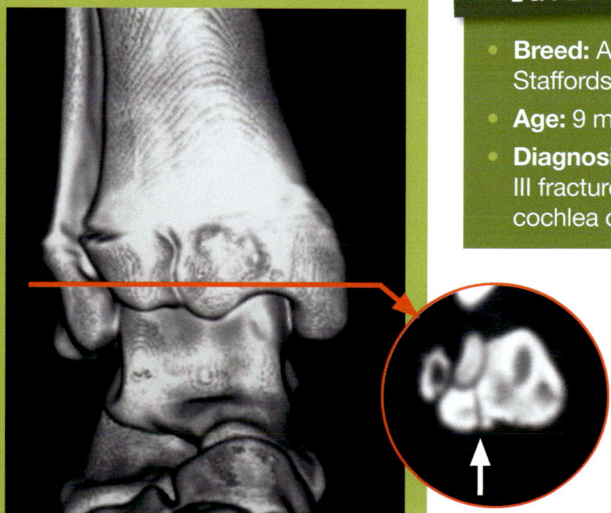

FIGURE 2. 3D computerised tomography reconstruction.

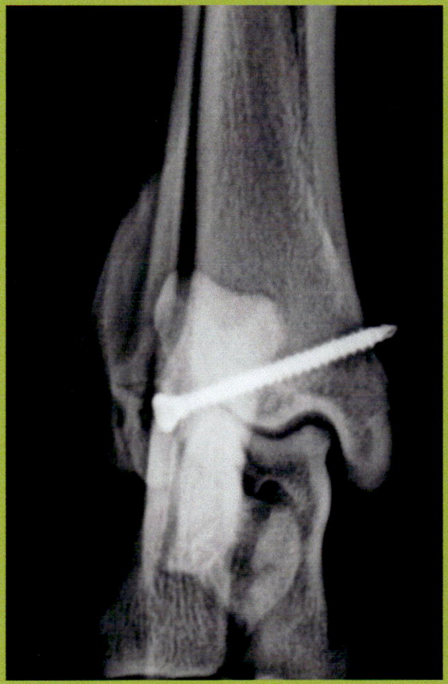

FIGURE 3. Post-surgery cranio-caudal X-ray. Note the direction of the screw.

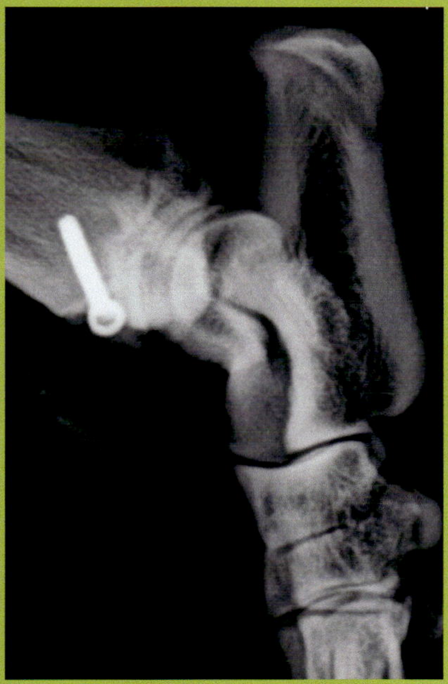

FIGURE 4. Post-surgery medio-lateral X-ray.

Treatment

2.0 compression screw. Lateral approach in front of the distal epiphysis of the fibula. The screw is inserted without excessive manipulation of the fragment, perfectly reducing the joint surface.

Justification

Intra-articular fractures should be stabilised using compression systems to ensure perfect reduction of the joint surface and recovery of joint function as soon as possible.

Case 2 SALTER-HARRIS II FRACTURE OF THE DISTAL EPIPHYSIS OF THE TIBIA

Author: Andrés Somaza (Veterinary Clinic Somaza-Pérez)

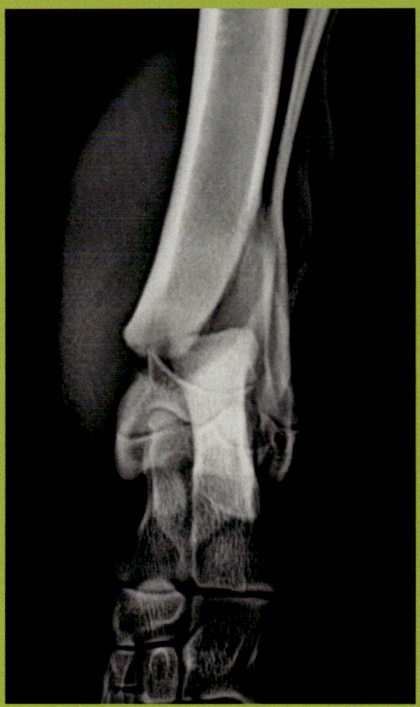

FIGURE 1. Cranio-caudal X-ray of the tarsus. Note the fracture line.

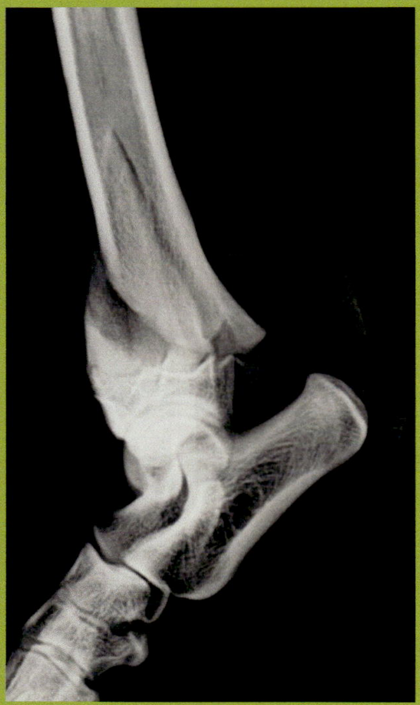

FIGURE 2. Medio-lateral X-ray.

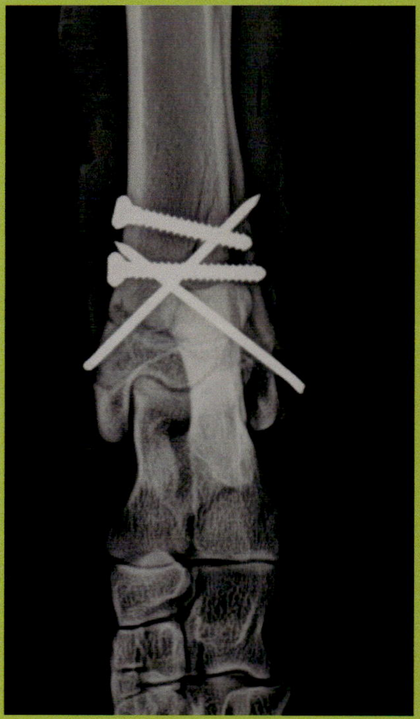

FIGURE 3. Post-surgery cranio-caudal X-ray. Note the tips of the screws anchored in the smaller fragment.

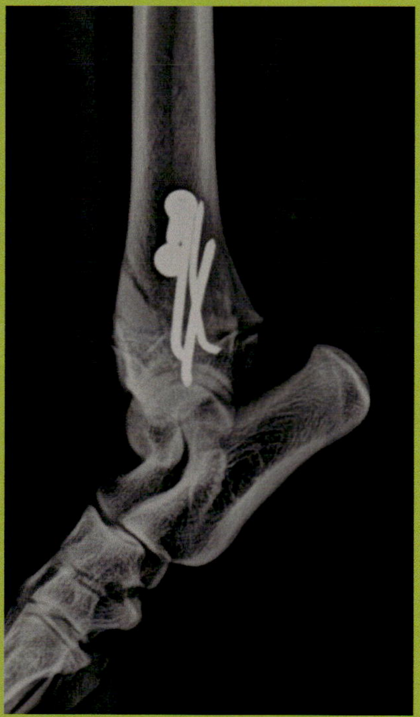

FIGURE 4. Medio-lateral X-ray.

Patient profile

- **Breed:** Griffon.
- **Age:** 7 months old.
- **Diagnosis:** Type II Salter-Harris fracture of the distal epiphysis of the tibia.

Treatment

2.7 compression screws and Rush pins anchored to the metaphysis. Medial approach for the insertion of the screws and one of the pins. The contralateral pin is inserted in a mini-approach. It is preferable the tip of the screw to be anchored in the smaller fragment.

Justification

The obliqueness of the fracture allows for the use of compression screws with two pins to reinforce their stability. Given the scarce growth potential of the patient due to its age, there is no problem in providing more stability to the fracture by anchoring the pins to the metaphysis.

Case 3 OBLIQUE FRACTURE OF THE CRANIAL PORTION OF THE OLECRANON

Author: Andrés Somaza (Veterinary Clinic Somaza-Pérez)

Patient profile

- **Breed:** Cocker Spaniel.
- **Age:** 9.5 years old.
- **Diagnosis:** Oblique fracture of the cranial portion of the olecranon.

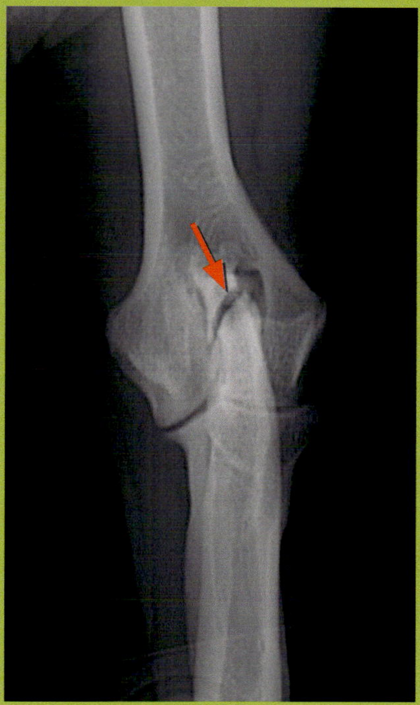

FIGURE 1. Cranio-caudal X-ray of the elbow. Note the fracture in the cranial portion of the olecranon.

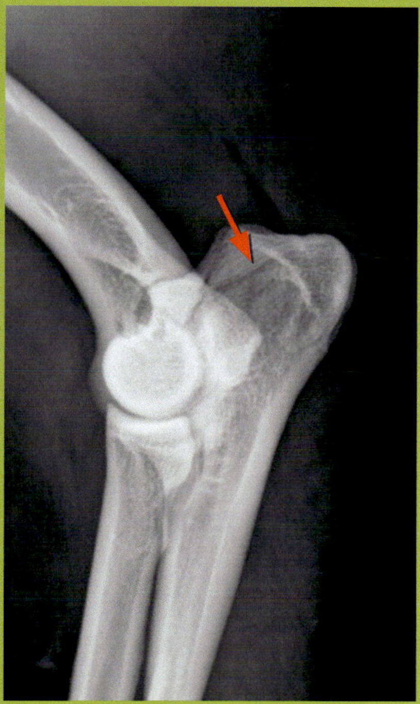

FIGURE 2. Medio-lateral X-ray of the elbow.

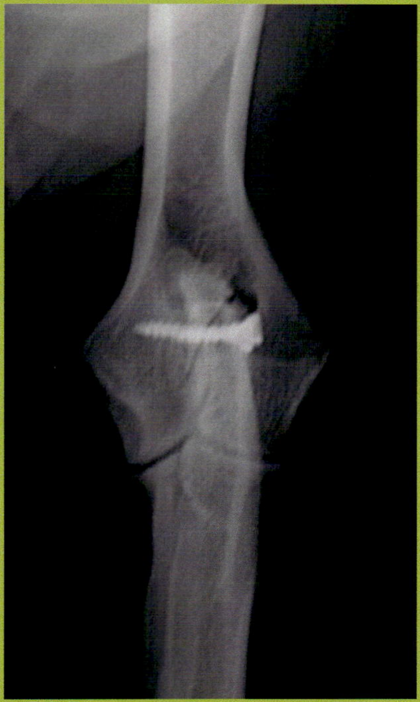

FIGURE 3. Cranio-caudal X-ray of the elbow. Note the transversal position of the screws.

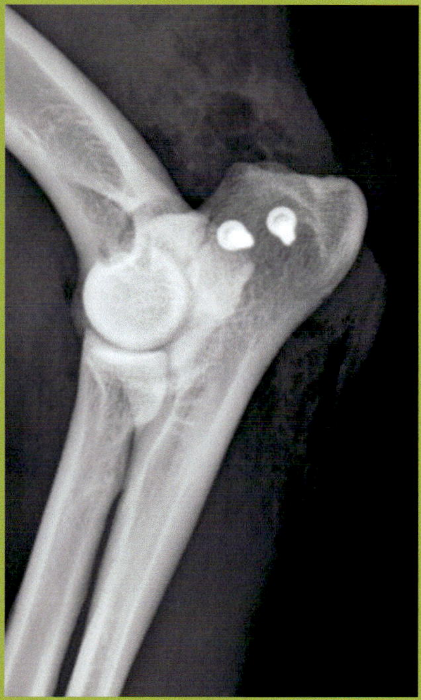

FIGURE 4. Medio-lateral X-ray of the elbow.

Treatment

A lateral approach is carried out to insert the screws, with the traction hole located in the smaller fragment.

Justification

As this is an oblique fracture, preferably, it should be compressed to accelerate healing. The application of two screws is sufficient as the fragment located in a cranial position from the insertion of the tendon of the triceps muscle is not subjected to any forces of traction.

Case 4 FRACTURE OF THE ACETABULUM AND THE BODY OF THE ILIUM

Author: Ángel Rubio (Veterinary Centre Indautxu)

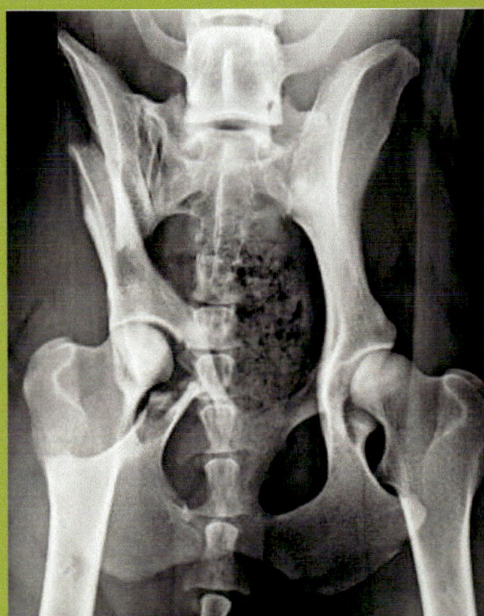

FIGURE 1. Ventrodorsal X-ray of the hip. Fracture of the body of the ilium and the acetabulum.

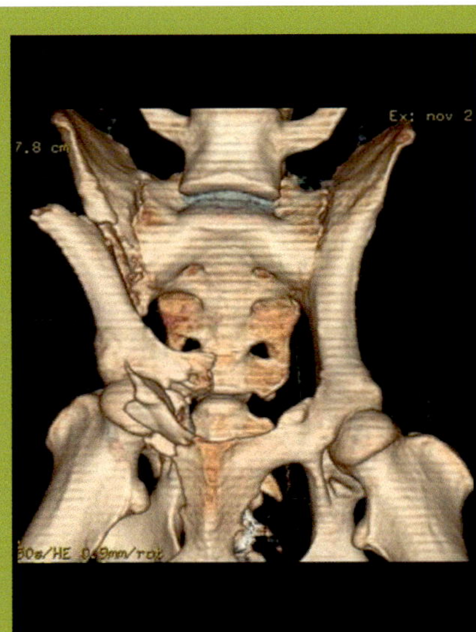

FIGURE 2. 3D CT scan reconstruction of the hip.

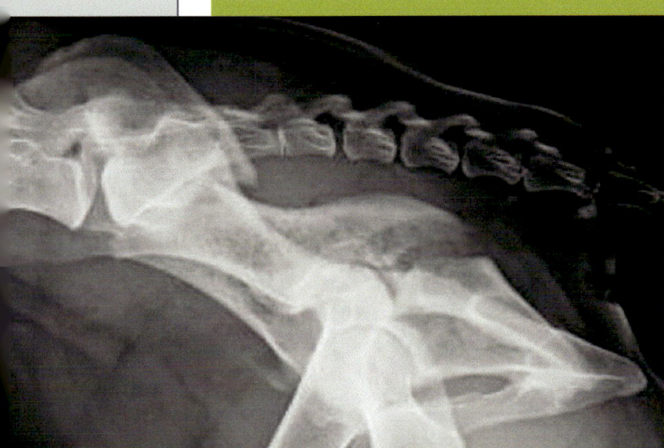

FIGURE 3. Latero-lateral X-ray.

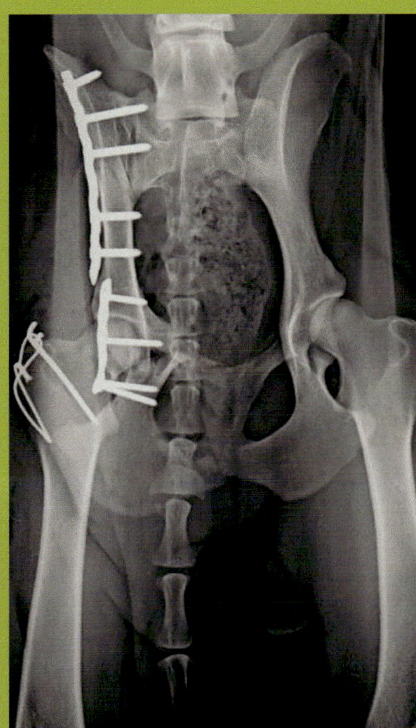

FIGURE 4. Post-surgery ventrodorsal X-ray.

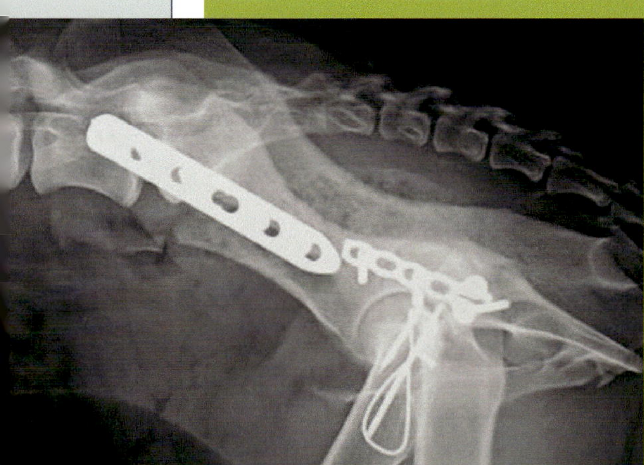

FIGURE 5. Post-surgery latero-lateral X-ray.

Patient profile

- **Breed:** German Shepherd.
- **Age:** 7 years old.
- **Diagnosis:** Fracture of the acetabulum and the body of the ilium.

Treatment

Lateral approach with osteotomy of the greater trochanter. 3.5 locking plate in the ilium and 2.7 T plate in the acetabulum. Pins with a tension band for the osteotomy of the greater trochanter.

Justification

Locking plates are ideal to treat hip fractures, especially those affecting the acetabulum in which, when the screws are tightened, the reduction is not modified even if the moulding of the plate does not completely correspond with the bone.

Case 5 JAW FRACTURE

Author: Ángel Rubio (Veterinary Centre Indautxu)

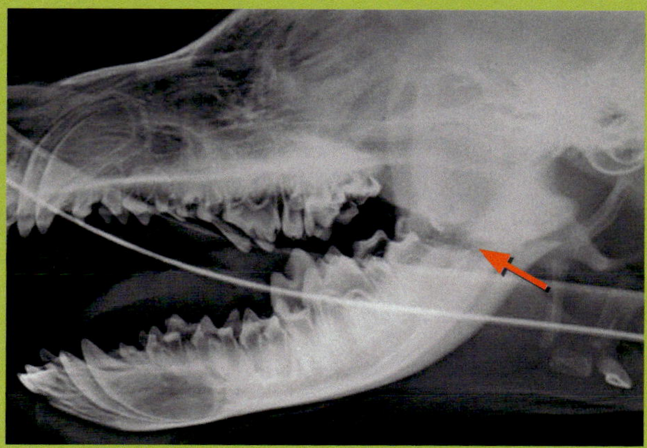

FIGURE 1. Latero-lateral X-ray of the cranium. Transversal fracture of the mandibular branch.

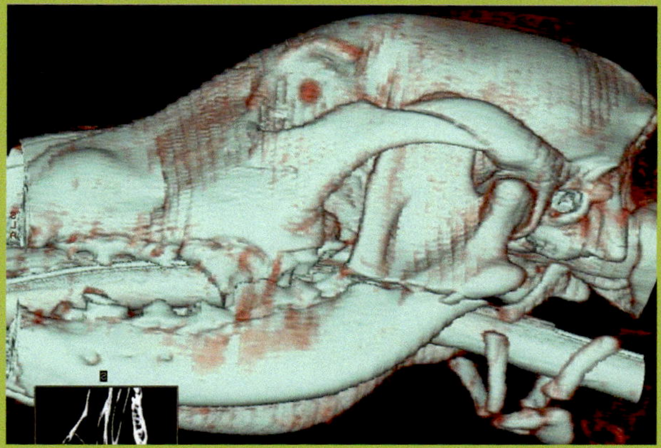

FIGURE 2. 3D CT scan reconstruction of the cranium.

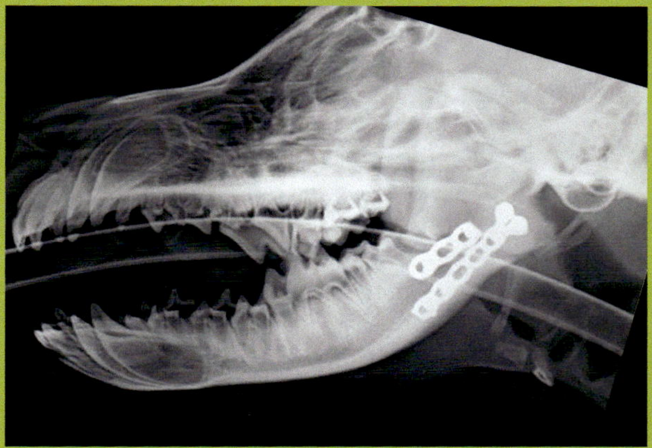

FIGURE 3. Post-surgery latero-lateral X-ray.

FIGURE 4. Post-surgery dorsoventral X-ray.

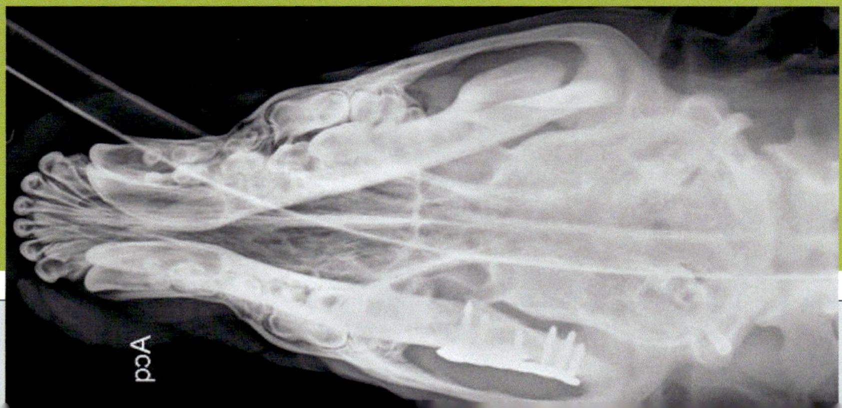

Patient profile

- **Breed:** German Shepherd.
- **Age:** 1.5 years old.
- **Diagnosis:** Jaw fracture.

Treatment

T locking plates and 2.4 LCP. A lateral approach is performed on the jaw through the skin, partially lifting the masseter muscle.

Justification

The caudal portion of the mandibular branch is formed by a thin bone in which the screws easily loosen. The use of a locking T plate makes it possible to firmly anchor the screws in a fragment of small dimensions. The LCP plate provides stability against rotation.

Case 6 FRACTURES OF THE GLENOID TUBEROSITY

Author: **Ángel Rubio** (Veterinary Centre Indautxu)

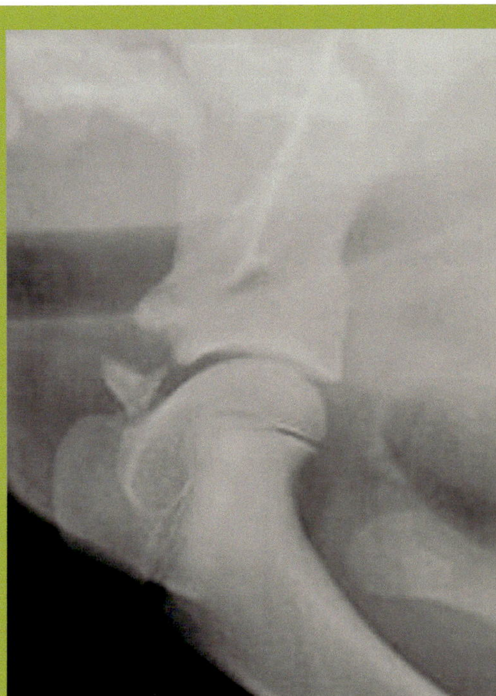

FIGURE 1. Medio-lateral X-ray of the glenohumeral joint.

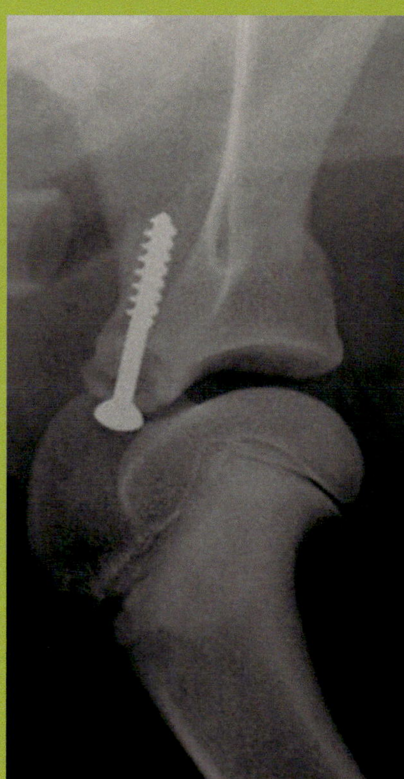

FIGURE 2. Post-surgery medio-lateral X-ray.

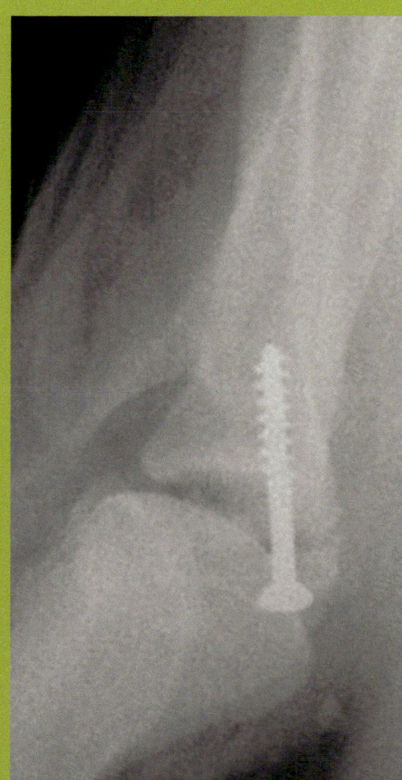

FIGURE 3. Post-surgery caudo-cranial X-ray.

Patient profile

- **Breed:** Labrador Retriever.
- **Age:** 6 months old.
- **Diagnosis:** Fractures of the glenoid tuberosity.

Treatment

Cranio-lateral approach. A 4.0, 50 % threaded cancellous compression screw is inserted instead of pins with a tension band (routine technique).

Justification

The forces of traction that the fragment is subjected to due to the insertion of the tendon of the biceps muscle is counteracted by a compression screw. The choice of a cancellous screw is made based on the weakness of the bone in this area as well as the fact that said screw does not stick through the cortical surface of the bone.

Case 7 MONTEGGIA FRACTURE

Author: Javier Tabar (Veterinary Hospital Raspeig)

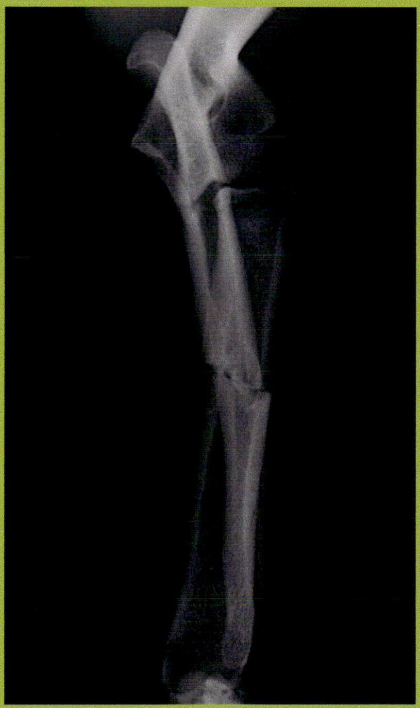

FIGURE 1. Cranio-caudal X-ray of the forearm.

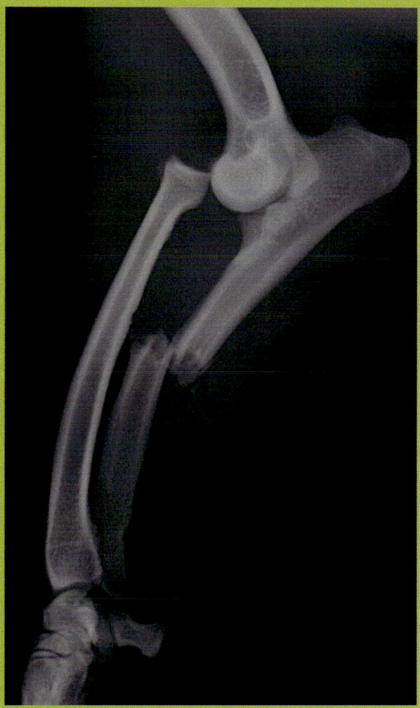

FIGURE 2. Medio-lateral X-ray. Transversal fracture of the ulna and cranial dislocation of the head of the radius.

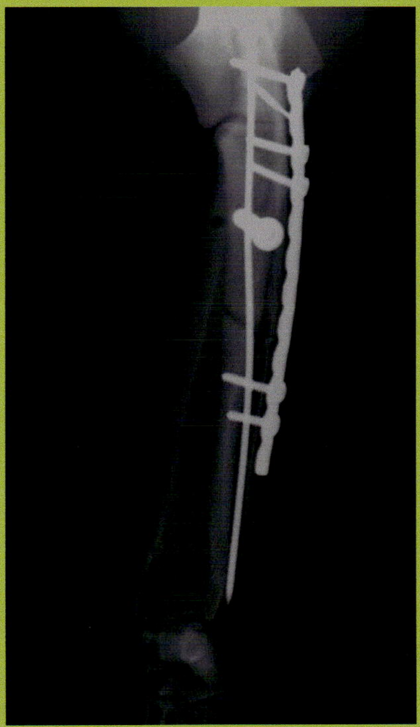

FIGURE 3. Post-surgery cranio-caudal X-ray.

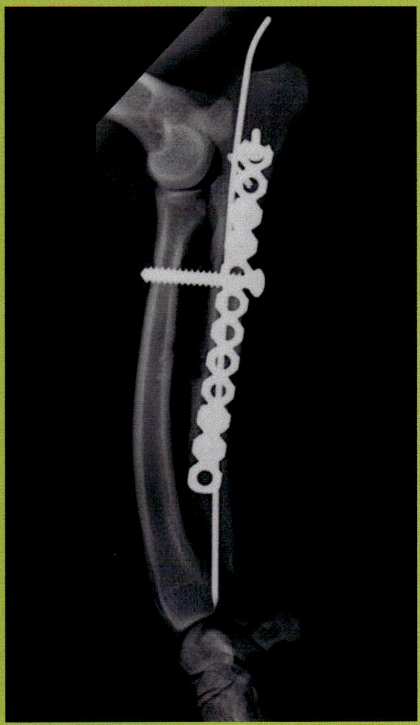

FIGURE 4. Post-surgery medio-lateral X-ray.

Patient profile

- **Breed:** Beagle.
- **Age:** 4 years old.
- **Diagnosis:** Monteggia fracture.

Treatment

3.5 ulna-radial compression screw with a supporting plate associated with marrow nailing by means of a caudal approach.

Justification

The compression screw prevents the radius from dislocating itself again in a cranial direction. The marrow nail aligns the longitudinal axis of the ulna while the reconstruction plate provides the system with stability.

Case 8 FRACTURE OF THE LATERAL CONDYLE OF THE FEMUR

Author: Javier Tabar (Veterinary Hospital Raspeig)

Patient profile

- **Breed:** German Shepherd.
- **Age:** 1.5 years old.
- **Diagnosis:** Fracture of the lateral condyle of the femur.

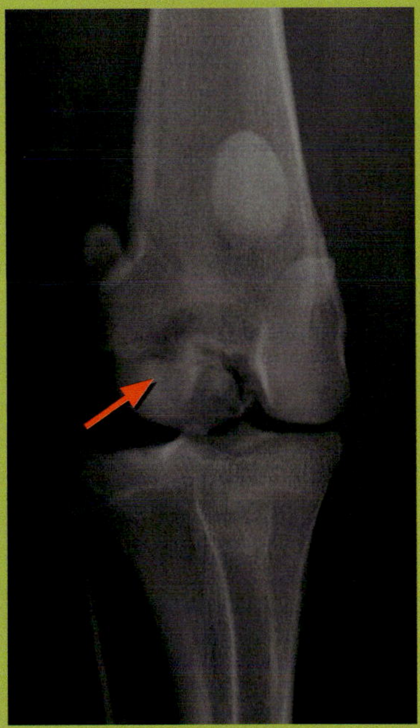

FIGURE 1. Cranio-caudal X-ray of the stifle. Note the condylar fragment (indicated with an arrow).

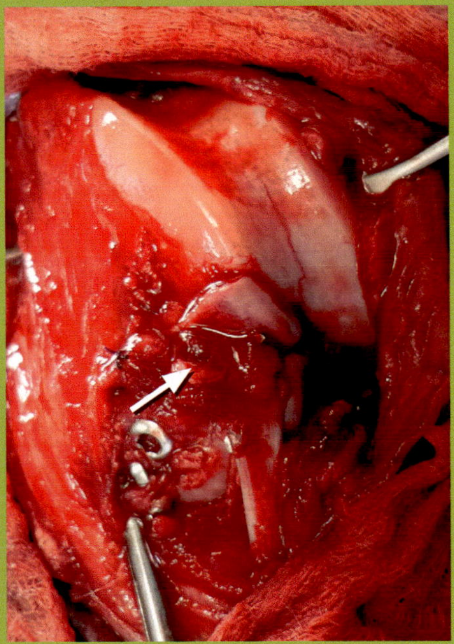

FIGURE 2. Intraoperative image that shows the placement of the screws without interfering in joint movement. Note the condylar fragment (indicated with an arrow).

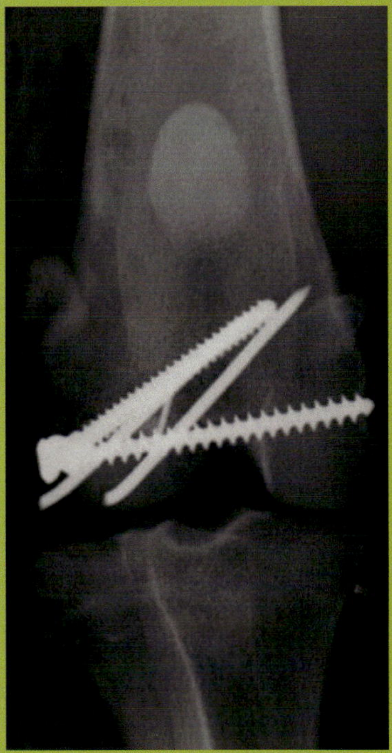

FIGURE 3. Post-surgery cranio-caudal X-ray.

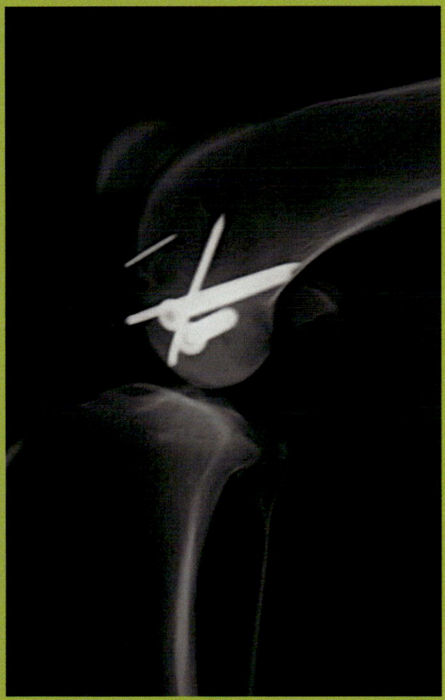

FIGURE 4. Post-surgery medio-lateral X-ray.

Treatment

Cranio-lateral approach of the stifle. 3.5 intercondylar cancellous compression screw associated with a 3.5 cortical positioning screw with an anti-rotational function with three Kirschner pins.

Justification

The compression screw keeps the fracture plane reduced while the positioning screw primarily prevents rotation of the fragment, as well as its displacement in a proximal direction. The pins work together with the positioning screw and fixate the loose bone fragments.

Case 9 COMMINUTED SUPRACONDYLAR FRACTURE OF THE HUMERUS

Author: Javier Tabar (Veterinary Hospital Raspeig)

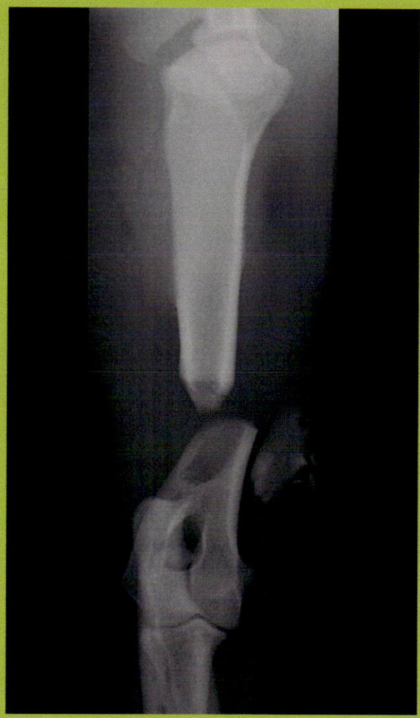

FIGURE 1. Cranio-caudal X-ray of the humerus.

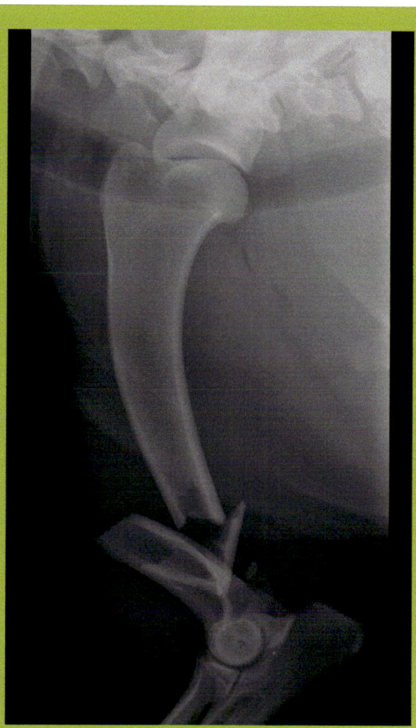

FIGURE 2. Medio-lateral X-ray of the humerus.

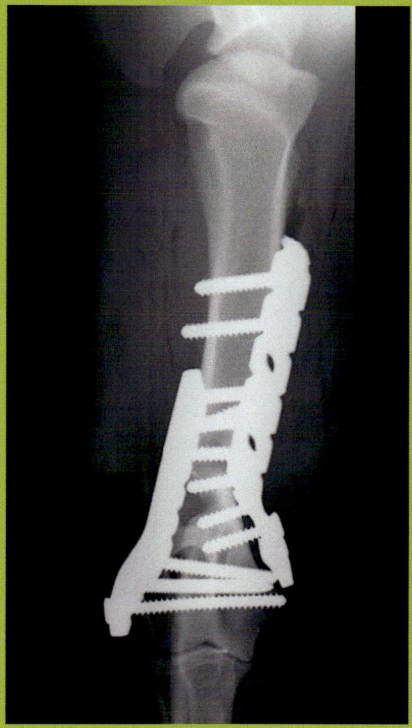

FIGURE 3. Post-surgery cranio-caudal X-ray.

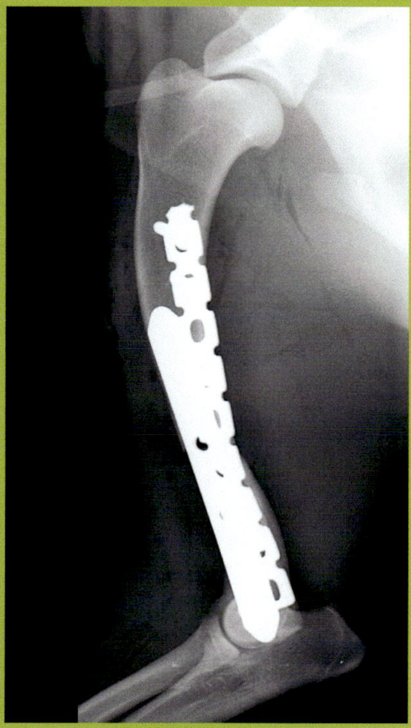

FIGURE 4. Post-surgery medio-lateral X-ray.

Patient profile

- **Breed:** Shar Pei.
- **Age:** 3 years old.
- **Diagnosis:** Comminuted supracondylar fracture of the humerus.

Treatment

Double approach: first medial, then lateral. 3.5 locking plate in the medial surface associated with a 3.5 reconstruction plate in the lateral surface.

Justification

The great instability of this fracture together with the small size of the distal fragment justify the use of one plate on each side of the bone. The locking plate allows for the correct orientation of the distal fragment while the reconstruction plate, due to being more malleable, better adapts to the lateral portion of the humerus.

Case 10 SUPRACONDYLAR FRACTURE OF THE FEMUR

Author: Juan Pablo Zaera (ULPGC-HVSM)

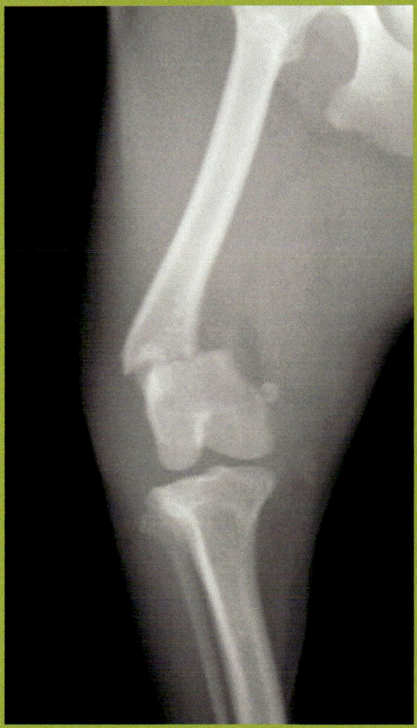

FIGURE 1. Cranio-caudal X-ray of the femur.

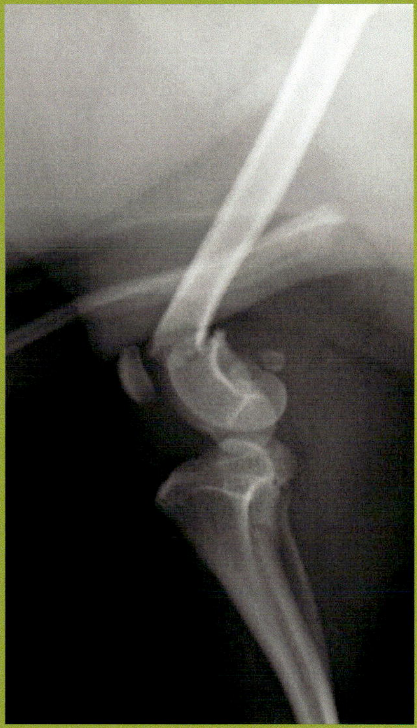

FIGURE 2. Medio-lateral X-ray of the femur.

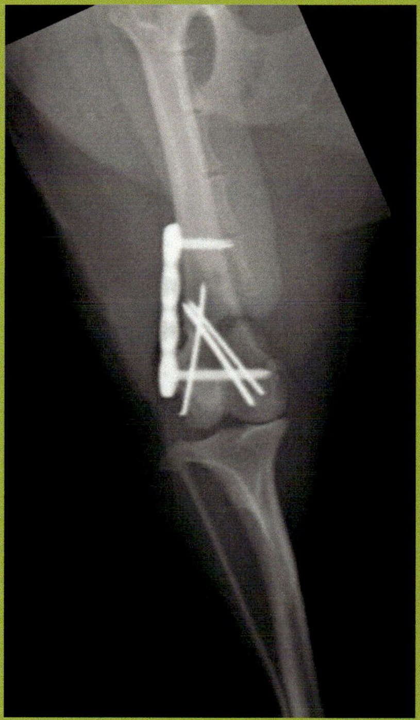

FIGURE 3. Cranio-caudal X-ray of the femur.

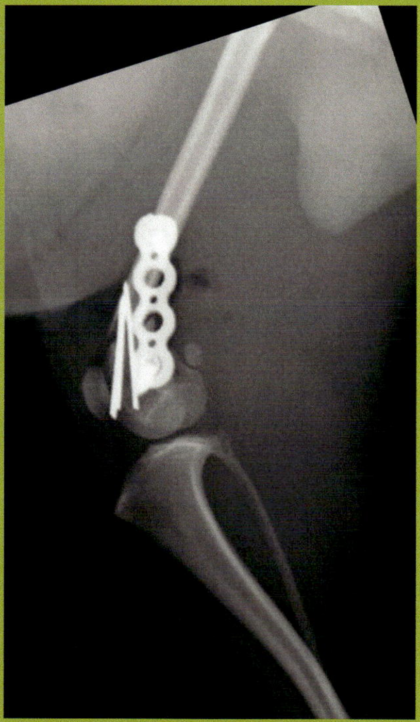

FIGURE 4. Medio-lateral X-ray of the femur.

Patient profile

- **Breed:** Yorkshire Terrier.
- **Age:** 10 years old.
- **Diagnosis:** Extremely distal supracondylar fracture of the femur.

Treatment

Medial approach of the stifle. Reduction of the fracture and stabilisation by the placement of three 0.8 mm Kirschner pins and a 2.0 locking plate fixated with two screws.

Justification

Supracondylar fractures can be treated with Rush pins or distal femur plates. In this case, this combination of implants was selected due to the small size of both the patient and the fragment, along with the significant curvature of the distal third of the femur. The pins prevent lateral displacement of the fracture site, and the plate, locked with one screw per fragment, acts like a type I fixator, impeding movements of rotation and collapse.

Case 11 FRACTURE OF THE FRONTAL AND NASAL BONES

Author: Juan Pablo Zaera (ULPGC-HVSM)

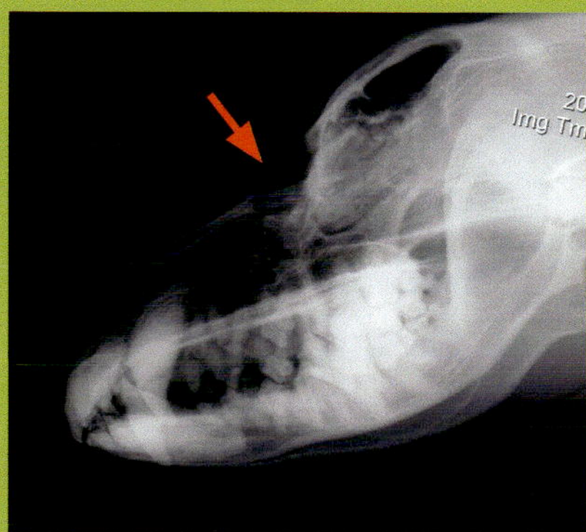

FIGURE 1. Latero-lateral X-ray of the cranium.

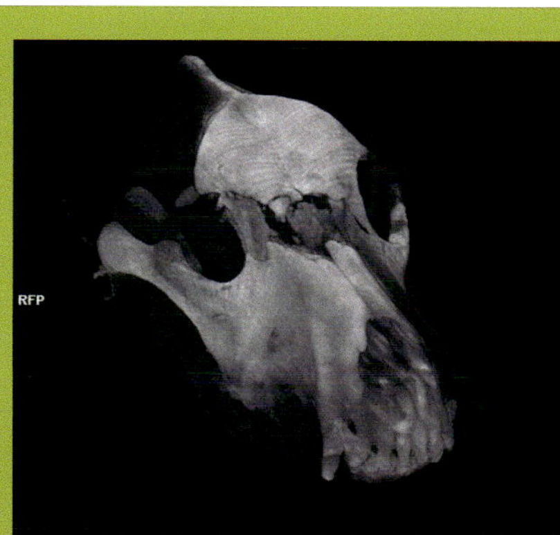

FIGURE 2. 3D reconstruction of the cranium using CT.

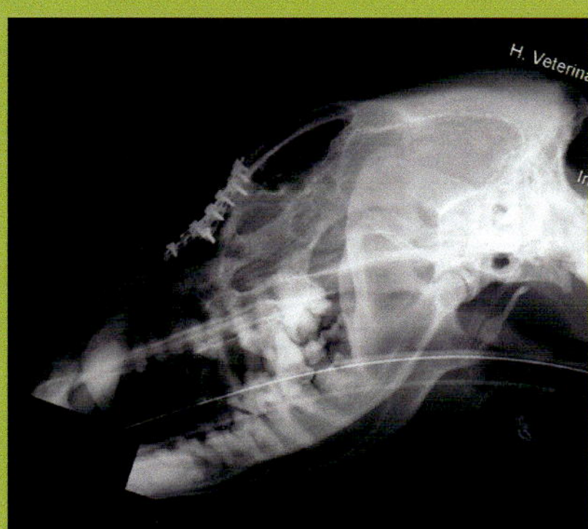

FIGURE 3. Latero-lateral X-ray of the cranium showing the position of the plate.

FIGURE 4. Dorsoventral X-ray of the cranium.

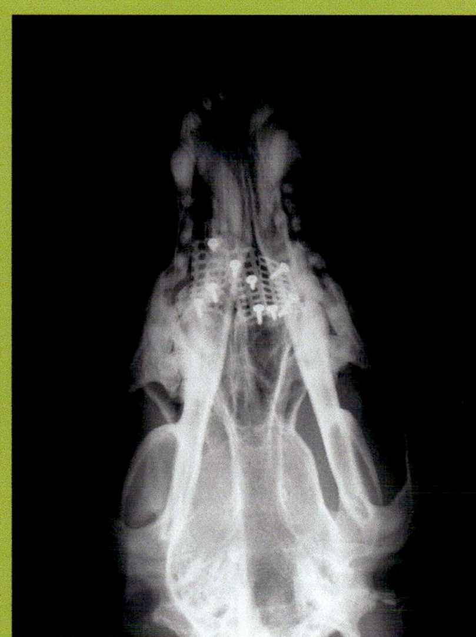

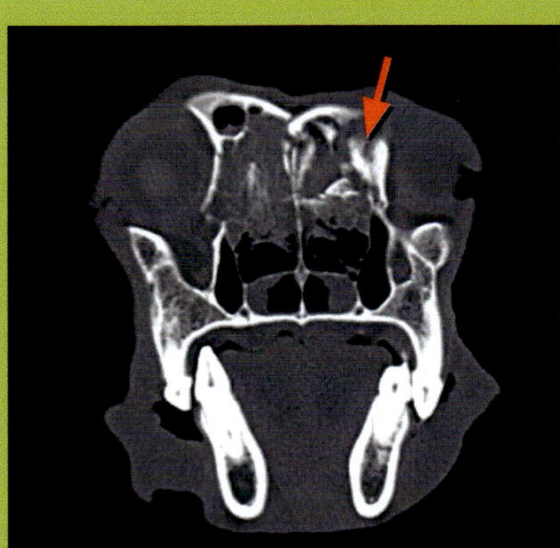

FIGURE 5. CT scan image. Sagittal slice at the level of the fracture. Note the sinking of the frontal bone (arrow).

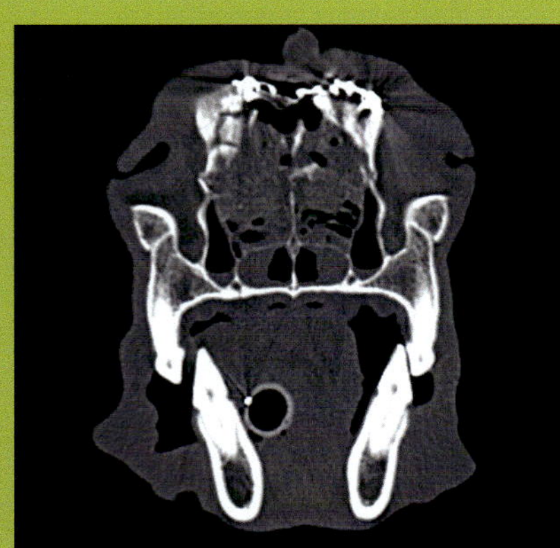

FIGURE 6. CT scan image. Sagittal slice at the level of the implants. Note how the anatomical morphology of the affected bones has been almost entirely recovered.

Patient profile

- **Breed:** German Shepherd.
- **Age:** 7 years old.
- **Diagnosis:** Fracture of the frontal and nasal bones from being kicked.

Treatment

Cranial approach. Elevation of the larger fragments and stabilisation using three pieces of adjustable plate and 2.0 screws.

Justification

The communication with the nasal cavity make treatment of this fracture mandatory. The cuttable plates are the best implant for this purpose given that, thanks to their thinness, they can be moulded in all directions, providing optimal cosmetic results.

Case 12 FRACTURE OF THE MANUBRIUM STERNI

Author: Juan Pablo Zaera (ULPGC-HVSM)

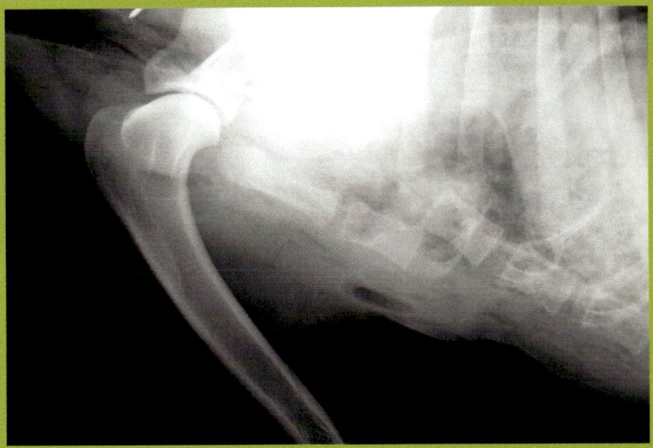

FIGURE 1. Latero-lateral X-ray of the thorax that shows the sternal fracture.

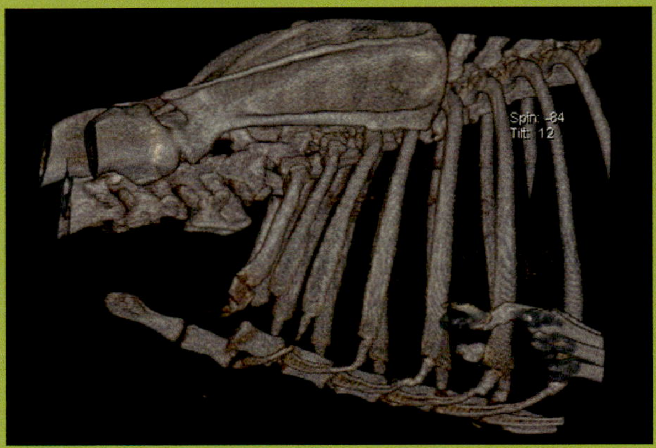

FIGURE 2. 3D reconstruction of the ribcage using CT. Note the fracture at the level of the second and third sternebrae.

Patient profile

- **Breed:** Pointer.
- **Age:** 3 years old.
- **Diagnosis:** Fracture of the manubrium sterni.

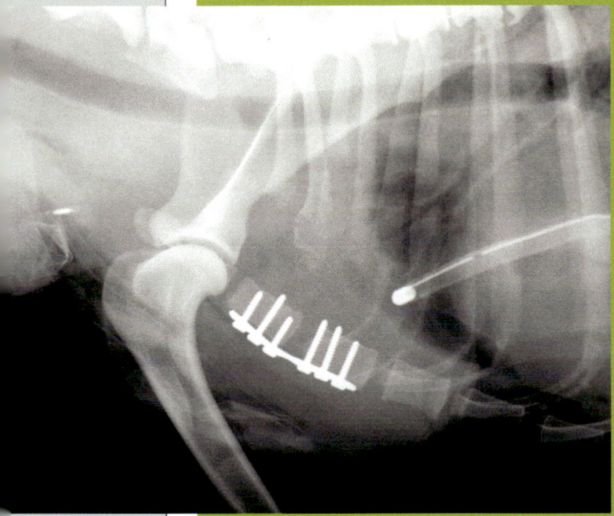

FIGURE 3. Latero-lateral X-ray of the thorax.

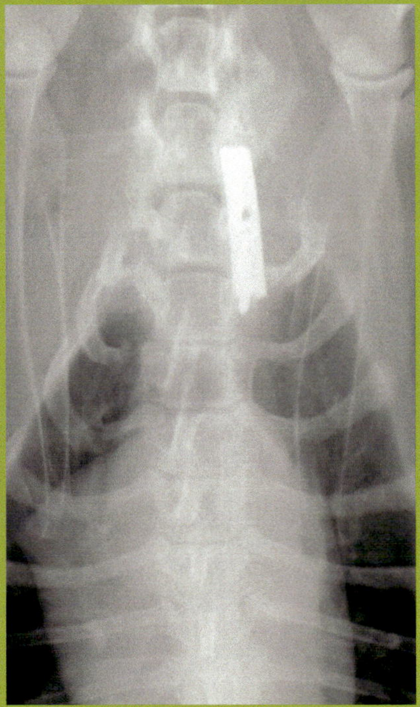

FIGURE 4. Ventrodorsal X-ray of the thorax.

Treatment

Cutaneous incision over the area of the projection of the fracture. Reduction of the fracture and stabilisation using a 2.7 adjustable plate. Placement of a chest tube.

Justification

Sternal fractures do not usually require surgical treatment. If the fragments damage the pulmonary parenchyma or affect respiratory function, they will need to be stabilised.

Case 13 COMMINUTED FRACTURE OF THE PROXIMAL THIRD OF THE ULNA

Author: Juan Pablo Zaera (ULPGC-HVSM)

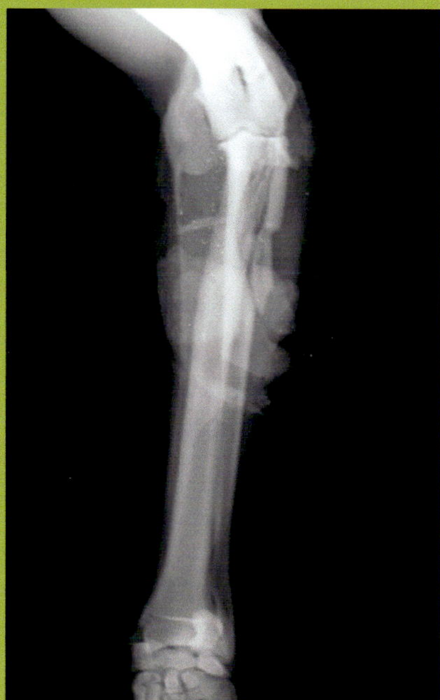

FIGURE 1. Cranio-caudal X-ray of the radius and ulna.

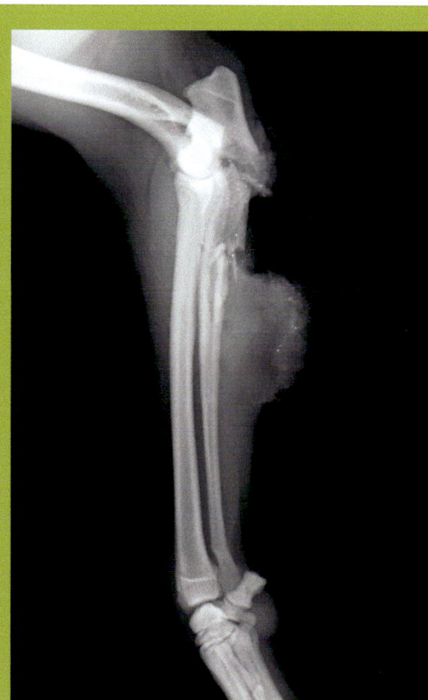

FIGURE 2. Medio-lateral X-ray of the radius and ulna. Note the laceration of the soft tissues.

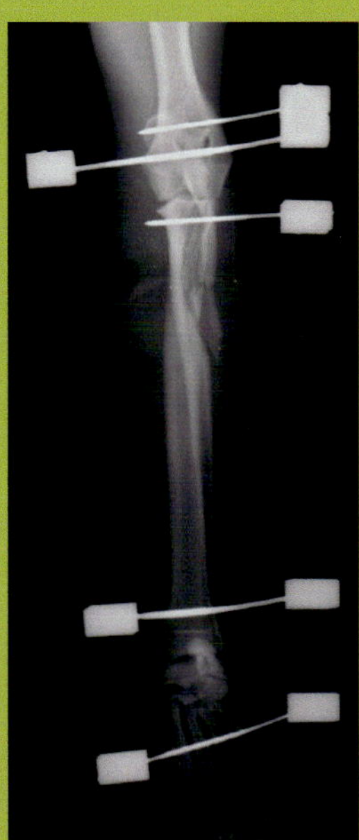

FIGURE 3. Cranio-caudal X-ray of the radius and ulna that shows the position of the external fixation system and the anchoring of its last pin to the metacarpals.

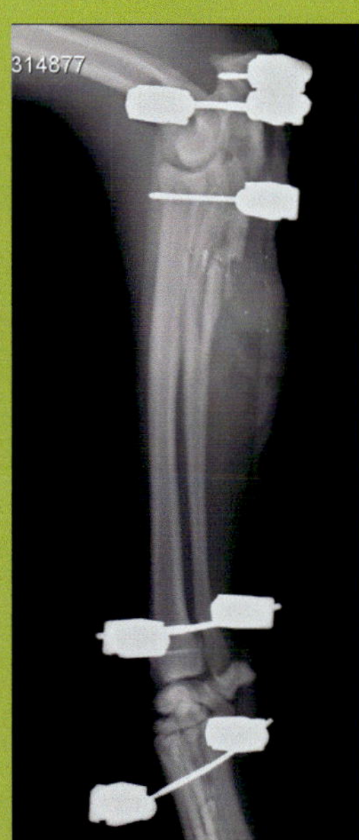

FIGURE 4. Medio-lateral X-ray of the radius and ulna.

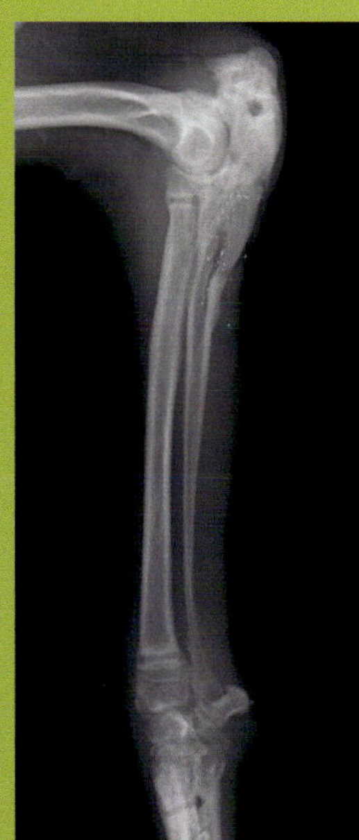

FIGURE 5. Medio-lateral X-ray of the radius and ulna after removing the implants three months after surgery.

Patient profile

- **Breed:** Podenco.
- **Age:** 2 years old.
- **Diagnosis:** Comminuted fracture from an animal bite with loss of a great amount of soft tissues in the proximal third of the ulna.

Treatment

Caudal approach. Removal of necrotic tissues from the fracture site, suturing of the rest of the flexor muscles and stabilisation of the fracture by means of single-plane, bilateral, trans-articular external fixation placed at the level of the carpus.

Justification

Fractures that affect the olecranon are subjected to forces of traction and thus they are frequently treated with pins with a tension band or plates. In this specific case, due to the great loss of soft tissues and thinness of the ulna in its distal portion, an external fixation system is chosen anchored to the radius in its distal portion. When anchoring the last percutaneous pin to the metacarpals, extension of the carpus is avoided, allowing for the proximal portion of the damaged flexor system of the forearm to heal.

Case 14 THREE-WEEK-OLD DISTAL COMMINUTED FRACTURE OF THE HUMERUS

Author: Juan Pablo Zaera (ULPGC-HVSM)

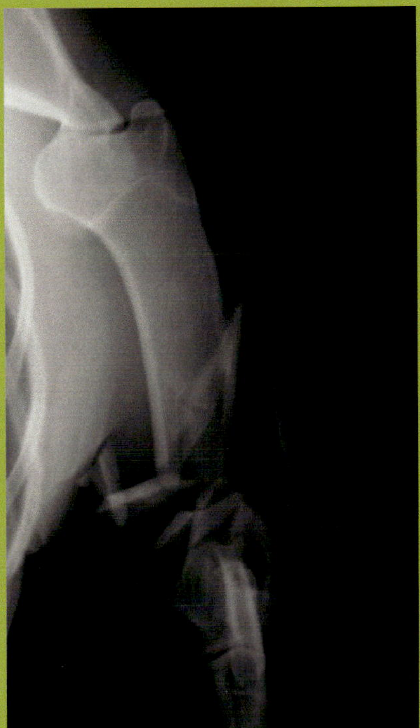

FIGURE 1. Cranio-caudal X-ray of the fractured humerus.

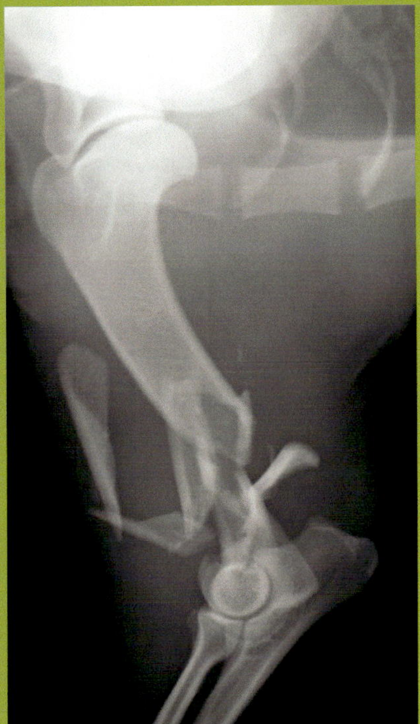

FIGURE 2. Medio-lateral X-ray.

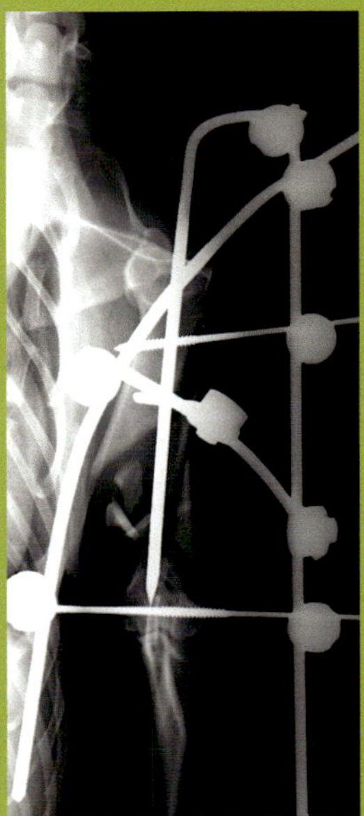

FIGURE 3. Cranio-caudal X-ray of the humerus. Note the position of the curved rod.

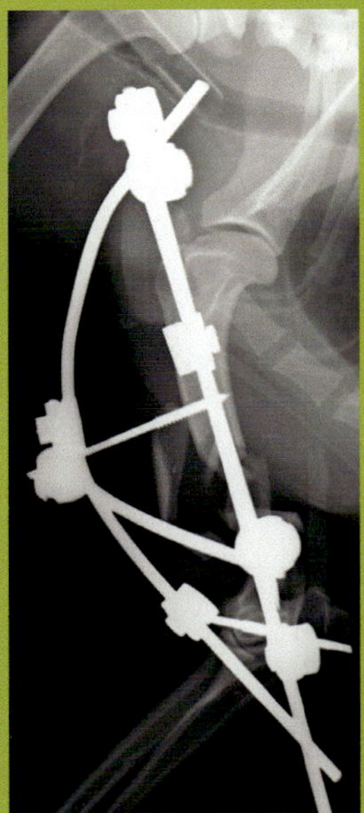

FIGURE 4. Medio-lateral X-ray.

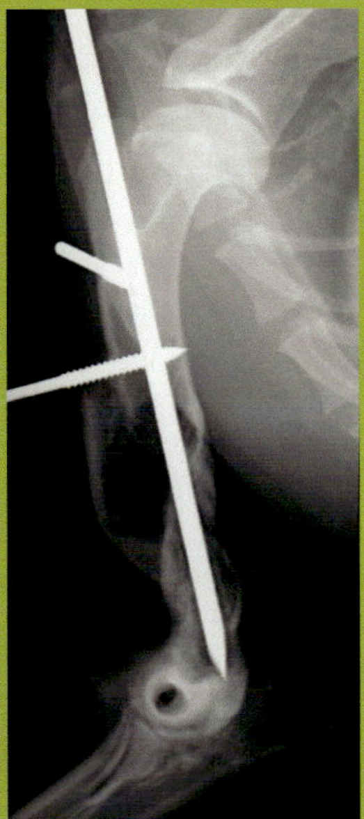

FIGURE 5. Medio-lateral X-ray of the humerus after partial removal of the implants four months after the intervention.

Patient profile

- **Breed:** Water dog.
- **Age:** 3 years old.
- **Diagnosis:** Comminuted fracture of the distal third of the humerus.

Treatment

Closed placement of a tie-in configuration of a hybrid external fixator.

Justification

The fractures that affect the humerus are usually treated using osteosynthesis plates. In this case, the high degree of comminution of the fracture site along with the time passed since the fracture occurred, makes the correct application of osteosynthesis plates much more difficult. Consequently, the application of a closed-fracture fixation system is chosen which will preserve the healing phenomena that have already began. The possibility of placing a bilateral fixation in the distal part of the humerus allows for the placement of a curved cranial rod that provides good rotational stability.

Case 15 ASTRAGALUS FRACTURE AND OPEN COMMINUTED FRACTURE OF THE TIBIA AND FIBULA

Author: Juan Pablo Zaera (ULPGC-HVSM)

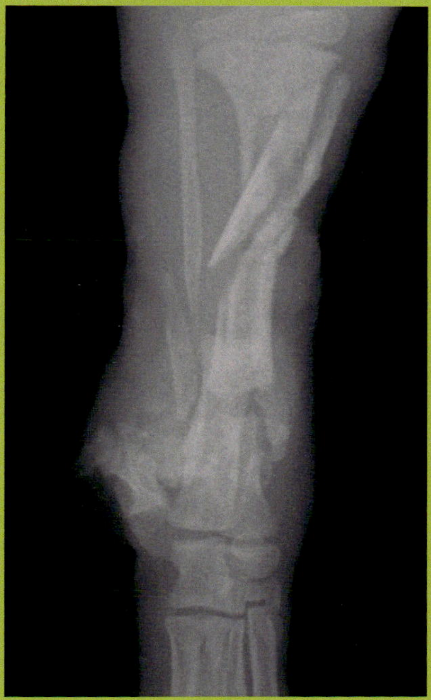

FIGURE 1. Cranio-caudal X-ray of the tibia showing multiple fragments.

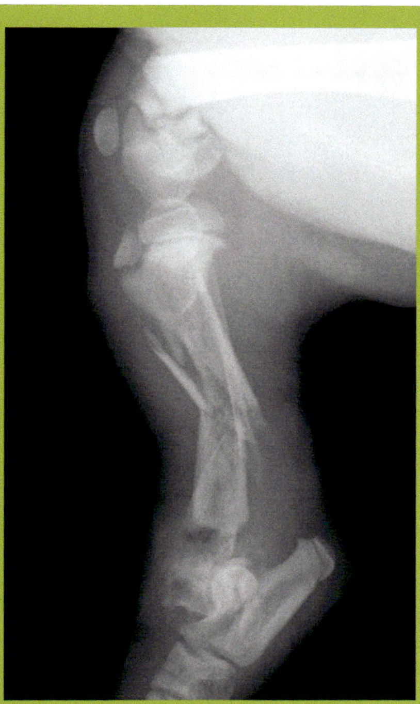

FIGURE 2. Medio-lateral X-ray.

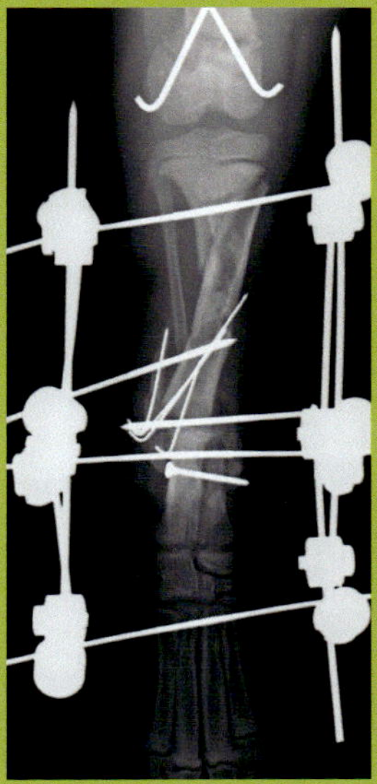

FIGURE 3. Cranio-caudal X-ray. Note the position of the Rush pins and the compression screw, as well as the different anchoring points of the external fixation system.

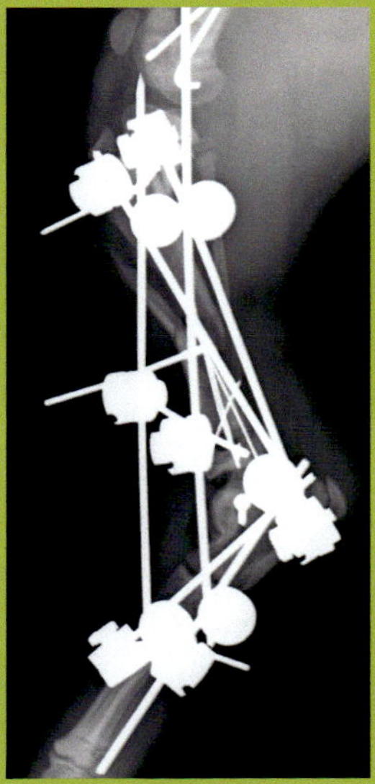

FIGURE 4. Medio-lateral X-ray.

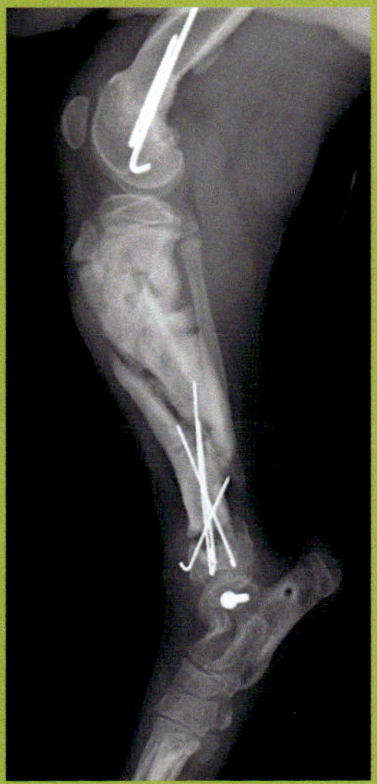

FIGURE 5. Medio-lateral X-ray four weeks after the intervention once the fixator has been removed.

Patient profile

- **Breed:** Mixed breed.
- **Age:** 3.5 months old.
- **Diagnosis:** Open comminuted fracture of the tibia and the fibula, and fracture of the astragalus.

Treatment

Medial approach of the tibia. Reduction of the fracture of the astragalus and stabilisation using a 2.7 compression screw. Reduction of the fracture of the distal epiphysis of the tibia and lateral malleolus, and stabilisation using Rush pins in the central fragment. Alignment of the tibia and stabilisation using a three-dimensional trans-articular external fixator anchored to the calcaneus and to the proximal portion of the metatarsals.

Justification

The young age of the patient is vital for the resolution of this fracture. The fracture of the astragalus is stabilised using a compression screw after extensive cleansing of the tarsal joint as the fracture is open. The Rush pins enable stabilisation of the small fragments without invading the joint. The stabilisation of all of the involved parts is done using a trans-articular fixator due to that lack of space in the distal portion of the tibia.

Published by Servet editorial - Grupo Asís Biomedia S.L.